Parkinson's Disease

Parkinson's Disease

Neurobehavioral Aspects

Edited by

STEVEN J. HUBER, Ph.D.

Director, Neuropsychology Laboratory
Assistant Professor of Neurology and Psychiatry
The University of Kansas Medical Center
Kansas City, Kansas

JEFFREY L. CUMMINGS, M.D.

Director, UCLA Alzheimer's Disease Center
Associate Professor of Neurology and Psychiatry & Behavioral Sciences
UCLA School of Medicine

Chief, Behavioral Neuroscience Section, Psychiatry Service
West Los Angeles Veterans Affairs Medical Center
Los Angeles, California

New York   Oxford
OXFORD UNIVERSITY PRESS
1992

Oxford University Press

Oxford   New York   Toronto
Delhi   Bombay   Calcutta   Madras   Karachi
Kuala Lumpur   Singapore   Hong Kong   Tokyo
Nairobi   Dar es Salaam   Cape Town
Melbourne   Auckland

and associated companies in
Berlin   Ibadan

Published by Oxford University Press, Inc.,
200 Madison Avenue, New York, New York 10016

Oxford is a registered trademark of Oxford University Press

Library of Congress Cataloging-in-Publication Data
Parkinson's disease : neurobehavioral aspects
edited by Steven J. Huber, Jeffrey L. Cummings.
p. cm.   Includes index.
ISBN 0-19-506969-2
1. Parkinsonism–Psychological aspects.
I. Huber, Steven J., 1955–
II. Cummings, Jeffrey L., 1948–
[DNLM: 1. Parkinson Disease—complications.
2. Parkinson Disease—drug therapy.
WL 359 P2513]   RC382.P265   1992   616.8′33—dc20
91-39677

9 8 7 6 5 4 3 2 1

Printed in the United States of America
on acid-free paper

Dedicated to our wives
   Edie and Inese
and children
   Joseph, Ellen, and Juliana

Preface

Compelling advances in the understanding and treatment of Parkinson's disease (PD) prompted us to organize this book. First, Parkinson's disease is one of the most common neurological illnesses, affecting approximately 100 per 100,000 population. Moreover, its frequency is age-related. The age-specific incidence rises from approximately 50 per 100,000 at age 60 to approximately 130 per 100,000 at age 75. Almost 1.5 percent of individuals age 70–79 suffer from PD. With the changing demographics of world societies and the increasing number of aged individuals, the needs of PD patients will become steadily more urgent. We hope that the information in this volume will aid clinicians and practitioners to respond to these patients more comprehensively.

Second, PD has major behavioral as well as motor dimensions. Much of the available information on the disease concerns motor aberrations—tremor, bradykinesia, and rigidity. Only in the recent past has attention been focused on the neurobehavioral manifestations. Although areas of controversy remain, enough is known to justify a comprehensive survey of the behavioral abnormalities of PD. No previous volume has provided a thorough review of the current status of the neuropsychological deficits, depression, and treatment-related behavioral abnormalities associated with this disease.

Third, the neurobiology of PD is increasingly well understood. There are sizable gaps in our knowledge, but the pathology and neurochemistry of PD have been studied carefully. When the behavioral alterations are considered in light of this emerging neurobiology, tentative hypotheses can be developed regarding the neurological basis of the cognitive and mood changes associated with PD. Thus, the disease can serve as a model for understanding the neurochemical and neuropathological alterations that may underlie a variety of behavioral syndromes, in particular the relation of subcortical structures and their neurotransmitter systems to human cognition and emotional function. Wherever possible, we have tried to provide information linking behavioral and neurobiological data.

Fourth, rapid advances have been made in the treatment of PD. Dopaminergic function can be enhanced by precursor therapy and receptor stimulation, neuronal death may be delayed or prevented by inhibition of monoamine oxidase, and transplantation of neuronal tissue may provide yet another therapeutic avenue. In most cases, the motor effects of these interventions have been emphasized, and the behavioral ramifications have received little exploration, even though the behavioral alterations associated with treatment may provide important insights into the neurobiology of neuropsychological and neuropsychiatric disorders. Behavioral aspects of treatment are emphasized in this volume.

We sincerely hope that our readers will find this compendium useful, that PD patients will be better served by enhanced understanding of the behavioral dimension of their illness, and that new questions and hypotheses will arise from considering the relationship between neurobiological and behavioral alterations in Parkinson's disease.

Kansas City, Kansas   S.J.H.
Los Angeles, California   J.L.C.
July 1991

Acknowledgments

Dr. Huber acknowledges Dr. George Paulson and Dr. Edwin Shuttleworth who provided substantial direction to his interest in Parkinson's disease and behavioral neurology. He would like to thank Dr. Robert Bornstein for his skillful training in both clinical and experimental neuropsychology. The support and collaboration of Dr. William Koller is also gratefully acknowledged.

Dr. Cummings gratefully acknowledges the enduring support of Dr. D. Frank Benson and the leadership of Dr. Robert Collins of the UCLA Department of Neurology. In addition, the enthusiastic collaboration of Dr. William Wirshing of the Brentwood Movement Disorders Laboratory contributed importantly to sustaining Dr. Cummings' interest in Parkinson's disease and other movement disorders.

The authors also thank their wives and families, who make life worthwhile.

Contents

Contributors

RICHARD ABRAMS, M.D.
Department of Psychiatry and Behavioral
  Science
The Chicago Medical Center
University of Health Science/The Chicago
  Medical Schools
North Chicago, IL 60064

WILLIAM W. BEATTY, Ph.D.
Departments of Psychiatry and Behavioral
  Sciences
University of Oklahoma Health Sciences
  Center
Oklahoma City, OK 73190

ROBERT A. BORNSTEIN, Ph.D.
Departments of Psychiatry and Neurology
The Ohio State University College of
  Medicine
Columbus, Ohio 43210

HELENA CHANG CHUI, M.D.
Department of Neurology
University of Southern California
Los Angeles, CA 90033

JEFFREY L. CUMMINGS, M.D.
Departments of Neurology, Psychiatry and
  Behavioral Sciences
UCLA School of Medicine and the
  Behavioral Neuroscience Section
Psychiatry Service, West Los Angeles
  Veterans Affairs Medical Center
Los Angeles, CA 90024-1769

DEAN C. DELIS, Ph.D.
Psychology Service (116B)
Veterans Administration Center
San Diego, CA 92161

BRUNO DUBOIS, M.D.
Clinique de Neurologie et Neuropsychologie
Hôpital de la Salpetriere
47 Bd de l'Hôpital
75651 Paris Cedex 13, France

STEPHEN T. GANCHER, M.D.
Department of Neurology
Oregon Health Sciences University
Portland, OR 97201

SANDER L. GLATT, M.D.
Department of Neurology
The University of Kansas Medical Center
Kansas City, KS 66103

CHRISTOPHER G. GOETZ, M.D.
Department of Neurological Sciences
Rush-Presbyterian/St. Luke's Medical Center
Chicago, IL 60612

DOUGLAS S. GOODIN, M.D.
Department of Neurology
University of California, San Francisco
San Francisco, CA 94143-0114

STEVEN J. HUBER, Ph.D.
Departments of Neurology and Psychiatry
The University of Kansas Medical Center
Kansas City, KS 66103

JOSEPH JANKOVIC, M.D.
Department of Neurology
Baylor College of Medicine
6550 Fannin, Suite 1801
Houston, TX 77030

WILLIAM C. KOLLER, M.D., Ph.D.
Department of Neurology
The University of Kansas Medical Center
Kansas City, KS 66103

BONNIE E. LEVIN, Ph.D.
Department of Neurology (D4-5)
University of Miami, School of Medicine
P.O. Box 016960
Miami, FL 33101

MICHAEL E. MAHLER, M.D.
Department of Neurology
UCLA School of Medicine
Los Angeles, CA 90024-1769

PAUL J. MASSMAN, Ph.D.
Psychology Service (116B)
Veterans Administration Center
San Diego, CA 92161

RICHARD MAYEUX, M.D.
Neurological Institute
Columbia University
New York, NY 10032

LYNN S. PERLMUTTER, Ph.D.
Department of Neurology
University of Southern California
Los Angeles, CA 90033

BERNARD PILLON, M.D.
Clinique de Neurologie et Neuropsychologie
Hôpital de la Salpetriere
47 Bd de l'Hôpital
75651 Paris Cedex 13, France

ALI H. RAJPUT, FRCP
Department of Clinical Neuroscience
University Hospital
Saskatoon, Saskatchewan
Canada, S7N OXO

KEITH G. RASMUSSEN, M.D.
Department of Psychiatry and Behavioral
   Sciences
The Chicago Medical School
North Chicago, IL 60064

GUSTAVO J. REY, Ph.D.
Department of Neurology (D4-5)
University of Miami, School of Medicine
P.O. Box 016960
Miami, FL 33101

DANIEL ROGERS, M.D.
Burden Neurological Hospital
Stoke Lane, Stapleton,
Bristol BS16 1QT
United Kingdom

G. WEBSTER ROSS, M.D.
Department of Neurology
UCLA School of Medicine
Los Angeles, CA 90024-1769

JEAN A. SAINT-CYR, Ph.D.
Playfair Neuroscience Unit
Toronto Western Hospital
Toronto, Ontario, M5T 25B, Canada

MARY SANO, Ph.D.
Neurological Institute
Columbia University
New York, NY 10032

JOAN SANTAMARIA, M.D.
Neurology Service
Hospital Clinic i Provincial de Barcelona
Villarroel, 170
Barcelona 08365, Spain

JONATHAN M. SILVER, M.D.
Columbia University
The Allan Pavilion
New York, NY 10034

MARK STACY, M.D.
Department of Neurology
Baylor College of Medicine
One Baylor Plaza
Houston, TX 77030

SERGIO E. STARKSTEIN, M.D.
Department of Behavioral Neurology
Instituto de Investigaciones Neurologicas
Ayacucho 2166
1112 Buenos Aires
Argentina

GLENN T. STEBBINS, Ph.D.
Department of Neurological Sciences
Rush-Presbyterian/St. Luke's Medical Center
Chicago, IL 60612

CAROLINE M. TANNER, M.D.
Clinical Center for Parkinson's Disease and
   Movement Disorders
San Jose, CA 95128

ANN E. TAYLOR, Ph.D.
Playfair Neuroscience Unit
Toronto Western Hospital
Toronto, Ontario, M5T 258, Canada

EDUARDO TOLOSA, M.D.
Neurology Service
Hospital Clinic i Provincial de Barcelona
c/Villarroel 170
Barcelona 08365, Spain

RACHEL TOMER, Ph.D.
Department of Neurology (D4-5)
University of Miami, School of Medicine
P.O. Box 016960
Miami, FL 33101

STUART C. YUDOFSKY, M.D.
Department of Psychiatry
The University of Chicago
Chicago, IL 60637

I

CLINICAL AND NEUROBIOLOGICAL OVERVIEW

1

The Historical Background
of Behavioral Studies
in Parkinson's Disease

CHRISTOPHER G. GOETZ

Mental function in Parkinson's disease (PD) has received attention since James Parkinson first described the illness in 1817. In his initial study of six patients, only three of whom he had actually examined in detail, Parkinson categorically stated: "The senses and intellect (are) uninjured" (Parkinson, 1817). This assertion remained unchallenged until the era of Charcot in the late 1800s, and since then, a continuing controversy over the frequency and types of mental aberrations in PD has emerged. The introduction of surgical and pharmacological therapies has confounded the controversy, since these interventions by themselves can be associated with mental impairment.

The aim of this introductory chapter is to outline some of the major historical issues related to PD and mentation decline. Of necessity, the chapter does not treat other forms of parkinsonism, specifically, postencephalitic parkinsonism, with its myriad of mental alterations, "atherosclerotic" parkinsonism, a term that has lost and regained favor in passing generations, and parkinsonism associated with multisystem degenerations (e.g., progressive supranuclear palsy, olivopontocerebellar atrophy, Shy-Drager syndrome). The chapter's coverage, for the most part, stops in the late 1960s, just before the introduction of levodopa, since the impact of drug therapy and toxicity is dealt with in detail in other chapters. The citations are not exhaustive but rather are chosen to highlight the historical controversies that set the stage for this book.

DO MENTAL ABERRATIONS OCCUR IN PARKINSON'S DISEASE?

Shortly after his arrival as a junior faculty member at the Salpêtrière hospital in Paris, Charcot joined Vulpian in a systematic categorization of patients with neurological disorders. In a two-part publication (1861–1862), they described patients with PD, extensively detailing motor, autonomic, and other aspects of the clinical presentation. In the same concise and authoritative style as Parkinson himself had used, they concluded "in general, psychic faculties are definitely impaired" (Charcot and Vulpian,

1861–1862). Charcot later added, "at a given point, the mind becomes clouded and the memory is lost."

Subsequently, multiple studies from France reiterated Charcot's claim. Ball reported on seven patients (1882), and Parant among others reported individual case histories (Parant, 1883). The descriptions were varied and suggested that dementia, depression, and other affective, even hallucinatory, disturbances undoubtedly occurred in untreated PD.

Outside France, however, most nineteenth and early twentieth century researchers thought differently and agreed more closely with Parkinson's assertion that mental capabilities were unaffected. Wollenberg (1899), Oppenheim (1911), and Konig (1912), the last reviewing selective past literature and adding his own notes on five patients, concluded that PD was not associated with dementia.

The early studies, both pro and con, all were based on clinical evaluations and observation without formal psychological testing. As was typical for the period, attitudes often polarized along geographical lines, partly because of language barriers that limited circulation of medical information and partly because of nationalistic temperaments and the great personalities in neurology. Undoubtedly, the French school was dominated unilaterally by Charcot, and his influence extended far beyond the walls of the Salpêtrière to influence neurology throughout France. Well known for his overbearing character, Charcot did not encourage disagreement with his views, and his students even mocked themselves for parotting his words (Goetz, 1987). Although the modern reader can find many French citations to mental alterations in PD, it is reasonable to suggest that these were all direct extensions of Charcot's influence and not entirely independent observations. Nevertheless, Charcot was known for his incisive observational skills in clinical neurology, especially in the realm of behavior. Under Janet, he developed a psychology wing within his neurological service at the Salpêtrière. His commitment to the psychological study of PD and other neurological disorders was never cursory, and his position on this issue ultimately proved to be correct. Even though Ball often is regarded as the first authority to recognize the association of PD and dementia, in fact, his senior mentor documented it earlier and distinguished it better from other confusional states.

After the first decade of the twentieth century, there was a 40-year hiatus with very few neurobehavioral studies of PD. Whereas most investigators acknowledged that there was a low but regular coexistence of dementia and PD, such noted authors as Wilson (1940) did not elaborate further. Patrick and Levy (1922) described a large series (140 subjects) in which they found no particular pattern or character of dementia in PD.

Scandinavian investigators contributed two important studies of the prevalence of dementia. Mjones (1949) performed psychological and neurological evaluations of 194 PD patients using limited but systematic test batteries. Eliminating the depressed and delirious patients, he found a prevalence of 3.2 percent of definite cases of senile dementia (termed "senile psychosis"). These results can be compared to the contemporary study by Sjogren (1948) of dementia in the general Swedish population, where it occurred in less than 1 percent.

The only cross-sectional study of dementia prevalence before widespread levodopa availability was conducted by Pollock and Hornabrook (1966). In it, they made the clinical distinction between idiopathic PD and other forms of parkisonism. The cross-sectional design permitted the investigators to resolve limitations found in prior studies, where the prevalence often was believed to reflect a subpopulation (nursing home or psychiatric hospital population). They concluded that dementia occurred in 8 percent of PD patients.

DISTINGUISHING BETWEEN DEMENTIA AND DEPRESSION IN PARKINSON'S DISEASE

In contrast to these studies, Lewy (1923) found that 64 percent of 56 patients had pronounced mental alterations. This study stands out historically for its very high prevalence figure, but, in fact, the author did not distinguish clearly between depression and dementia in many of his patients. In focusing on this distinction, Jackson and colleagues (1923) cited 5 PD patients in a state mental hospital population who were markedly depressed but not demented. They emphasized that depression could be a prominent feature of PD associated with greater disability than the neurological dysfunction, and could precede the motor manifestations of the illness. These patients did not have a characteristic memory problem, and paranoia and hallucinations could accompany the depressive affect.

Interestingly, the distinction between depression and dementia can be sought retrospectively in Parkinson's original essay, where he believed that intelligence was normal but used such words as "melancholy" and "dejected" to describe his patients. Among the early studies, Patrick and Levy (1922) found a 20 percent prevalence of depression, with crying spells and carelessness being dominant symptoms. Within the category of depression without dementia, a further subdivision of pure depression into reactive and endogenous types has raised the issue of whether depression occurs in response to the reality of chronic illness and loss of self-esteem and autonomy, as suggested by Wilson (1940), or whether it is a biochemical aspect of the disorder, intrinsic to the neurodegenerative condition. General assumptions in this paradigm have been that if the depression is reactive, there should be a low prevalence of depression before PD onset, and the depression should clear as motor disability is improved with medication. In fact, Mayeux and associates (1981) found that 43 percent of depressed PD patients were depressed before the appearance of motor signs and that there was no relation between severity of depression and severity of motor disability. This question has been argued in many studies using multiple designs and most recently with positron emission tomography (PET) evaluation of frontal lobe function (Kiyosawa et al, 1990).

In dealing with the overlap between dementia and depression, Mjones (1949) introduced the terms "reactive" and "organic" mental changes, the former being dysphoric and the latter having added memory blunting. This overlap was seen by Brown and Wilson (1972) and later by Lieberman and colleagues (1979), where 25 percent of mildly demented patients also were depressed. Mayeux and associates (1981) even found a correlation between intensity of depression and degree of intellectual impairment, thereby suggesting that the two mental disorders, once confounded, then separated, should be reconsidered as coincident in many patients.

IS BRADYPHRENIA A NEUROLOGICAL ACCOMPANIMENT OF PARKINSON'S DISEASE?

In 1922, Naville introduced the term "bradyphrenia" to describe the slowing of cognitive processing and impairment of concentration seen in parkinsonian patients even in the absence of major dementia. Although most of these patients had postencephalitic parkinsonism, some had PD, and bradyphrenia became a third well-recognized behavioral accompaniment of PD. Bradyphrenia, also known as "psychic akinesia," was introduced as a parallel to the motor slowness of bradykinesia, and whereas reports in the 1930s hypothesized a neurological basis, the next 30 years focused more on psychological explanations for the behavior (Aubrun, 1937; Jelliffe, 1940; Booth, 1948). Coincident with the introduction of levodopa in PD treatment, emphasis returned to organic explanations for the syndrome. Clinical studies have suggested that bradykinesia and bradyphrenia correlate well in patients who have not been given medication (Rogers et al, 1987). Javoy-Agid and Agid (1980) suggested that lesions in mesocorticolimbic dopaminergic systems may be important to both clinical aberrations. Areas of persisting controversy include the relationship of bradyphrenia to depression and the neurochemical basis of the behavioral alteration.

EMERGENCE OF NEUROPSYCHOLOGICAL TESTS IN PARKINSON'S DISEASE

Before the widespread availability of levodopa, very few studies examined mental aberrations in PD with prospectively administered neuropsychological tests. The burgeoning field of neuropsychology developed in the late 1960s and 1970s, and major studies of specific cognitive and affective function tests in PD, therefore, have been at least partly limited by the confounding issue of dopaminergic drug exposure. Through education and dissemination of computerized machinery, there currently are greater standardization of testing tools and more accurate reliability and validity data available. Tests that stress relatively specific anatomical circuits have been developed that can be correlated with improved imaging and biochemical characterizations of PD.

The first studies using standardized tests investigated the effects of dopaminergic therapy on cognitive processes (Beardsely et al, 1971; Garron et al, 1972; Loranger et al, 1973). Typically, these studies assessed patients' IQ with the Wechsler Adult Intelligence Scale or other standardized IQ assessments. Although no long-term improvements in IQ were found with levodopa administration, a marked difference between verbal and visuospatial abilities was found (Loranger et al, 1973). This finding of selective impairment in visuospatial abilities has been replicated many times, although there is controversy about the type and extent of visuospatial deficits in PD (Boller et al, 1984).

Anatomically correlated neuropsychological testing of PD patients also has demonstrated frontal lobe dysfunction, with specific links to aberrations of the mesocortical–limbic–frontal system (Taylor et al, 1986). Further attempts have been made to categorize the cognitive impairments seen in PD as distinct from other disease states, especially Alzheimer's disease. The cognitive impairments associated with PD have been termed "subcortical dementia," and the dementia associated with Alzheimer's disease has been termed "cortical dementia" because of the different location of neuropathological findings in each disease and the presence of aphasia, apraxia, and agnosia in Alzheimer's disease (Benson, 1984). Beyond these broad categories, more specific subcategories are emerging as imaging techniques permit more precise behavioral anatomical correlations.

IS THERE A PARKINSONIAN PERSONALITY OR A PREMORBID BEHAVIORAL PATTERN IN PARKINSON'S DISEASE?

Contemporary theories of a possible latent period of many years between the induction of dopaminergic cell loss and clinical PD have prompted renewed interest in premorbid signs of the condition. Among the many areas of research, personality traits again are being investigated. Charcot stressed the interplay among behavior, hereditary illness, and neurological disorders, but the definition of a specific parkinsonian personality developed from psychoanalytic thinking in the first half of this century. These studies, reviewed by Todes and Lees (1985), described the prototypic patient as introspective, emotionally inflexible, well controlled, and predisposed to depression. Before motoric signs of PD appear, these patients tend to be law-abiding citizens, diligent, trustworthy, and often lacking in self-confidence or willingness to take risks. Studies of twin pairs, one with and one without PD, revealed the affected twin, even as a child, to be the more likely to be self-controlled and a follower. Such findings were adamantly rebuffed by Riklan and colleagues (1959) and by de Ajuriaguerra (1971), but the argument has been rekindled (Poewe et al, 1983).

At a time when strategies for preventive therapy are being developed at an increasing rate, early detection and identification of subjects at high risk are pivotal to early intervention. For these reasons, behavioral attributes of PD have emerged as a new focus for reevaluation.

HAS THE PREVALENCE OF MENTAL CHANGES IN PARKINSON'S DISEASE INCREASED?

This question is raised when one compares the two most complete early studies on population prevalence of dementia in PD with more recent reports from the levodopa era. Mjones (1949) and Pollack and Hornabrook (1966) found the prevalence of dementia to be less than 10 percent, but contemporary studies reveal figures at least twofold higher. Boller (1980) reviewed a large series of articles on prevalence and concluded that almost all recent reports document dementia prevalence at or above 30 percent. Multiple explanations have been offered, including higher indices of suspicion, more careful assessments, and drug exposure. Barbeau (1972) claimed that levodopa-treated PD patients showed more cognitive impairment than did PD patients treated with anticholinergic drugs.

The ability to study the behavioral profile of PD patients who are not receiving symptomatic therapy has been facilitated by projects from the United States and Canada-based Parkinson Study Group (1989), where emphasis has been placed on identification of patients very early in the course of PD when they have never been medically treated for the disease. Prospective examination of such patients will provide clarification of the prevalence of mental changes early in the disease and the evolution of such problems independent of exposure to levodopa, dopamine agonist, or anticholinergic therapies.

REFERENCES

Ajuriaguerra de J. Etude psychopathologique des Parkionsoniens. In: Ajuriaguerra de J, Gauthier G, eds. *Monoamines Noyaux Gris Centraux et Syndrome de Parkinson.* Paris: Masson; 1971:327–351.

Aubrun W. Responses aux emotions-chocs chez les parkinsoniens. *Ann Psychol.* 1937;37:140–171.

Ball B. De l'insanité dans la paralysie agitante. *Encephale J Mal Ment Nerv.* 1882;2:22–32.

Barbeau A. *Dopamine and Mental Function. L-Dopa and Behavior.* New York: Raven Press; 1972:9–33.

Beardsely JV, Puletti F. Personality (MMPI) and cognitive (WAIS) changes after levodopa treatment. *Arch Neurol.* 1971;25:145–150.

Benson DF. Parkinsonian dementia: cortical or subcortical. In: Hassler RG, Christ, JF, eds. *Advances in Neurology: Parkinson-Specific Motor and Mental Disorders. Role of the Pallidum: Pathophysiological, Biochemical, and Therapeutic Aspects.* New York: Raven Press; 1984:289–298.

Boller F. Mental status of patients with Parkinson disease. *J Clin Neuropsychol.* 1980;2:157–172.

Boller F, Passatiume D, Keefe NC, et al. Visuospatial impairments in Parkinson's disease. Role of perceptual and motor factors. Arch Neurol 1984;41:485–490.

Booth G. Psychodynamics in parkinsonism. *Psychom Med.* 1948;10:1–14.

Brown GL, Wilson WP. Parkinsonism and depression. *South Med J.* 1972;65:540–545.

Charcot JM, Vulpian A. De la paralysie agitante. *Gaz Hebdomadaire Med Chir.* 1861;8:765–767; 1862;9:54–59.

Garron DC, Klawans HL, Narin F. Intellectual functioning of persons with idiopathic parkinsonism. *J Nerv Mental Dis.* 1972;154:445–452.

Goetz CG. *Charcot the Clinician: The Tuesday Lessons.* New York: Raven Press; 1987.

Jackson JA, Free GBM, Pike HV. The psychic manifestations in paralysis agitans. *Arch Neurol.* 1923;10:680–684.

Javoy-Agid F, Agid Y. Is the mesocortical dopaminergic system involved in Parkinson disease. *Neurology* 1980;30:1326–1331.

Jelliffe SE. The parkinsonian body posture, some considerations of unconscious hostility. *Review* 1940;27:467–479.

Kiyosawa M, Bosley TM, Kushner M. Middle cerebral artery strokes causing homonymous hemianopia: positron emission tomography. *Ann Neurol.* 1990;28:180–183.

Konig H. Zur psychopathologie der paralysis agitans. *Arch Psychiatr Nervenkrankheit.* 1912;50:285–305.

Lewy FH. Die Lehre Von tonus und der bewegung zugleich systematiche Untersuchinger sur Klinik. In: *Physiologie, Pathologie und Pathogenese der Paralysis Agitans.* Berlin: Springer; 1923.

Lieberman A, Dziatolowski M, Coppersmith M, et al. Dementia in Parkinson's disease. *Ann Neurol.* 1979;6:355–359.

Loranger AW, Goodell H, McDowell FH, et al. Parkinsonism, L-dopa, and intelligence. *Am J Psychiatry.* 1973;130:1386–1389.

Mayeux R, Stern Y, Rosen J, et al. Subcortical dementia: a recognizable clinical syndrome. *Ann Neurol.* 1981;10:100–101.

Mjones H. Paralysis agitans. *Acta Psychiatr Neurol.* 1949;54(suppl):1–195.

Naville F. Les complications et les sequelles mentales de l'encephalite epidemique. *Encephale* 1922;17:369–375, 423–436.

Oppenheim H. *Textbook of Nervous Diseases.* Edinburgh: Otto Schulze and Company; 1911.

Parant V. La paralysie agitant. Examinee comme couase de foile. *Rev. Med Toulouse.* 1883;17:266–280.

Parkinson J. *An Essay on the Shaking Palsy.* London: Sherwood, Neely and Jones; 1817.

Parkinson Study Group. DATATOP: a multi-center clinical trial in early Parkinson's disease. *Arch Neurol.* 1989;46:1052–1060.

Patrick HT, Levy DM. Parkinson's disease: a clinical study of 146 cases. *Arch Neurol Psychiatry.* 1922;7:711–720.

Poewe W, Gerstenbrand F, Ransmayer G, et al. Pre-morbid personality of parkinsonian patients. *J Neurol Trans.* 1983;19(suppl):214–224.

Pollock M, Hornabrook RW. The prevalence, natural history and dementia of Parkinson's disease. *Brain.* 1966;89:429–448.

Riklan M, Weiner H, Diller L. Somato-psychologic studies in Parkinson's disease. 1. An investigation into the relationship of certain disease factors to psychological functions. *J Nerv Ment Dis.* 1959;129:263–272.

Rogers D, Lees AJ, Smith E, et al. Bradyphrenia in Parkinson disease and psychomotor retardation in depressive illness. *Brain.* 1987;110:761–776.

Sjogren T. Genetic, statistical and psychiatric investigations of a west Swedish population. *Acta Psychiatr Neurol Scand.* 1948;52(suppl):1–102.

Taylor AE, Saint-Cyr JA, Lang AE. Frontal lobe dysfunction in Parkinson's disease. The cortical focus of neostriatal outflow. *Brain.* 1986;109:845–833.

Todes CJ, Lees AJ. The pre-morbid personality of patients with Parkinson's disease. *J Neurol Neurosurg Psychiatry.* 1985;48:97–100.

Wilson SAK. *Neurology.* Riverside, NJ: Hafner Publishing Company, Inc; 1940.

Wollenberg R. Paralysis agitans. In: Nothnagel H, ed. *Specielle Pathologie und Therapie.* Wien: Alfred Holder; 1899.

2

Clinical and Neurobiological Aspects of Parkinson's Disease

MARK STACY AND JOSEPH JANKOVIC

HISTORICAL PERSPECTIVE

Our understanding and treatment of Parkinson's disease (PD) have improved greatly since 1817, when James Parkinson published his essay on the "shaking palsy." However, the clinical description of the signs and symptoms originally provided by Parkinson has required little clarification. This chapter gives an overview of the clinical features, etiology, pathology, and treatment of Parkinson's disease.

Similarities between symptoms of parkinsonism and the effects of chronic treatment with reserpine, a monoamine depleting drug, were first noted by Carlsson and colleagues in 1957. After the landmark observation by Ehringer and Hornykiewicz (1960) that striatal dopamine is depleted in the brains of patients with PD, this disorder became the first to be treated with neurotransmitter replacement therapy, levodopa (Birkmayer and Hornykiewicz, 1961; Cotzias et al, 1967). Early enthusiasm about the effectiveness of levodopa in controlling parkinsonian symptoms, however, was dampened by its side effects (e.g., nausea, vomiting, orthostatic hypotension). The discovery of peripheral dopa-decarboxylase inhibitors (carbidopa and benserazide) improved the efficacy and diminished the acute side effects associated with this medication (Bartholini and Pletscher, 1968). Epidemiological comparisons of death rates from PD in the United States from 1950 to 1984 and in Denmark from 1956 to 1985, an interval spanning the pre- and post-levodopa era, have shown a 5-year increase in survival since the introduction of levodopa (Kurtzke and Murphy, 1990).

During the 1970s, the major emphasis in the treatment of parkinsonism has been on optimization of pharmacological therapy to control motor symptoms and on development of strategies to avoid or treat side effects. Dopamine receptor agonists, such as bromocriptine and pergolide, have been shown to enhance the dopaminergic effects of levodopa (Jankovic and Marsden, 1988). Initially used primarily to supplement levodopa and to treat levodopa-induced motor fluctuations, the role of these agents has expanded. They currently are recommended early in the course of antiparkinson therapy to prevent these and other adverse effects associated with chronic levodopa therapy (Cedarbaum et al, 1990).

Extraordinary advances in our knowledge of the mechanisms and treatment of parkinsonism have resulted from the discovery of an association between the meperidine analogue, 1-methyl-4-phenyl-1,2,3,6-tetrahydropyridine (MPTP) and parkinsonism (Langston et al, 1983; Bloem et al, 1990). This compound, a by-product of meperidine synthesis, contaminated an illicit drug supply in northern California and produced persistent parkinsonism in a group of young drug abusers. MPTP-induced parkinsonism in nonhuman primate models has helped to formulate new hypotheses about the etiology, pathogenesis, prevention, and treatment of PD.

FUNCTIONAL ANATOMY

The extrapyramidal system includes the striatum (putamen, caudate), globus pallidus (GP), substantia nigra (SN), subthalamic nucleus (STN), and thalamus (Albin et al, 1989). The caudate and putamen are contiguous and comprise the striatum. The putamen is located lateral to the GP, and the caudate nucleus is ventrolateral to the frontal horns of the lateral ventricles. The SN is a ventral midbrain nucleus which contains dopaminergic, melanin-containing neurons. STN neurons are located inferior to the thalamus, and thalamic nuclei are medial to the GP (Fig. 2–1).

Although multiple parallel circuits are present in the extrapyramidal system, two loops predominate. Excitatory input from various cortical areas, including the prefrontal supplementary motor area (SMA), amygdala, and hippocampus, is topographically distributed to the putamen and caudate (Alexander and Crutcher, 1990). In the

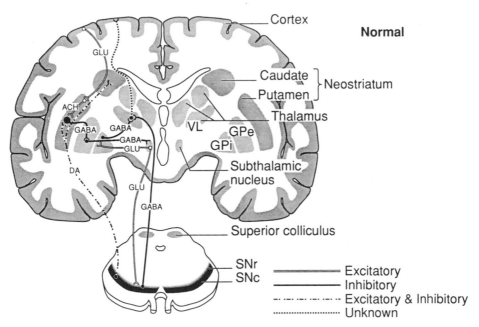

Figure 2–1. Anatomy of the basal ganglia and their connections. GPe, globus pallidus externa; GPi, globus pallidus interna; SNc, substantia nigra pars compacta; SNr, substantia nigra pars reticulata; VL, ventrolateral nucleus of the thalamus; ACH, acetylcholine; DA, dopamine; GABA, gamma-aminobutyric acid; GLU, glutamine. (From Jankovic, In: *Cecil Textbook of Medicine*, 19th ed. Philadelphia: WB Saunders; 1991.)

first loop, the striatum interconnects with neurons in the lateral GP (GPe), which project to the STN. This part of the loop uses the inhibitory neurotransmitter gamma-aminobutyric acid (GABA). In contrast, the STN provides excitatory input via glutamate to the internal segment of the GP (GPi). GPi neurons are GABAergic and synapse in the ventrolateral (VL) nucleus of the thalamus. Thalamic input to the cortex is excitatory.

In the second loop, the putamen interconnects with the SN via striatonigral pars reticulata and nigrostriatal axons. The efferent pallidal neurons (from GPi) are GABAergic, and the afferent input to the striatum (from SN pars compacta) is dopaminergic. Dopaminergic neurons exert both excitatory and inhibitory influence on the striatum. SN destruction in PD ultimately results in an increased striatal input to the GPe and "disinhibition" of the STN. This, in turn, further inhibits the VL thalamus and eventually leads to the development of parkinsonian signs. The major input to the extrapyramidal system through the cortex–putamen–GPe and output through the GPi–thalamus–cortex pathway are modulated by the gatekeeper, the STN (Parent, 1990).

Recent neurophysiological and neurochemical studies have demonstrated clinical correlates of these extrapyramidal pathways. For example, an STN lesion in an experimental animal or in a patient results in contralateral hemiballismus (Dewey and Jankovic, 1989; Shannon, 1990). Furthermore, Bergman and colleagues (1990) have demonstrated amelioration of tremor and bradykinesia with ibotenic acid ablation of the disinhibited STN in MPTP monkeys. In the normal brain, loops 1 and 2 are balanced, and SN dopaminergic modulation of caudatoputaminal (loop 1) output neurons allows smooth motor control. In PD, nigrostriatal (loop 2) neuronal loss causes relative enhancement of the GABAergic pathway (loop 1), and consequent inhibition at GPe functionally disinhibits the STN. Increased STN output causes increased firing of GPi–thalamic cells, inhibition of the thalamus, and decreased firing of motor cortex (Fig. 2–2). Conversely, enhanced dopaminergic (loop 2) activity in the striatum will decrease caudatoputamen GABAergic output. Excessive dopaminergic stimulation, which occurs with dopaminergic overtreatment, may cause dyskinesias clinically similar to other hyperkinetic movement disorders (Nutt, 1990).

The medium-sized spiny neuron is the most common cell type in striatal nuclei and represents the major output pathway of the caudate and putamen (Carpenter and Sutin, 1983). Striatal efferents receive input from cortical (glutaminergic) and SN (dopaminergic) neurons via a rich dendritic network (Smith and Bolam, 1990). SN dopamine receptors are located proximal to the cortical glutamate receptors. This arrangement suggests a modulatory role for striatal dopamine (Graybiel, 1990).

Dopamine receptors are divided into D1, D2, and D3 subtypes. D1 receptors are most abundant. They are linked to one or more G-proteins and, when stimulated, increase adenylate cyclase activity (Anderson et al, 1990). The D2 molecule is also linked to G-proteins, but it is not associated with adenylate cyclase change (Strange, 1990; Mackenzie et al, 1990). Recently, D3 receptor was cloned (Sokoloff et al, 1990). This glycoprotein, which in contrast to D1 and D2 is not linked to G-protein, is found predominantly in the mesolimbic system. Both experimental and clinical evidence suggests that benefit from antiparkinson therapy is mediated chiefly through the D2 receptor (Fleminger et al, 1983). However, D1 stimulation is needed for D2 activation

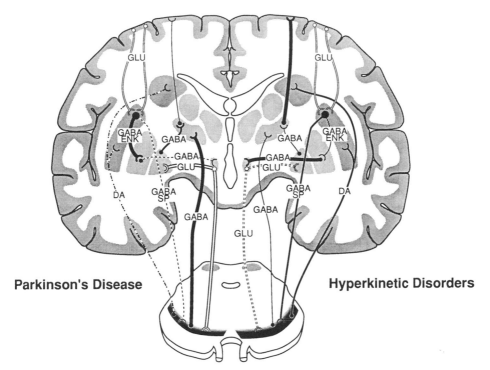

Figure 2–2. Functional organization of the basal ganglia in parkinsonism and hyperkinetic disorders. ACH, acetylcholine; DA, dopamine; ENK, enkephalin; GABA, gammaaminobutyric acid; GLU, glutamine; SP, substance P. (From Jankovic. In: *Cecil Textbook of Medicine,* 19th ed. Philadelphia: WB Saunders; 1991.)

to be expressed (Walters et al, 1987). The function of D3 is similar to that of D2, but its location appears to be distant from the striatum. The significance of this receptor is unknown, but its cortical predominance suggests that D3 activation is associated with behavioral changes. The discovery of the D3 receptor suggests the possibility that pharmacological manipulation using specific D3 antagonists may be useful in the control of psychiatric symptoms without causing parkinsonian side effects and in levodopa-induced psychosis.

Distinct subsets of striatal neurons have been identified by immunohistochemical techniques. Acetylcholinesterase (AChE) staining areas, termed "striosomes," comprise 10 to 20 percent of the volume of the striatum and correspond to afferents from the prefrontal and limbic cortices, whereas AChE-poor areas, matrix, correspond to primary and somatosensory cortex (Albin et al, 1989). Anterograde tracer studies by Gerfen (1989) have demonstrated that corticostriate neurons from cortical areas V and VI project to the striosomes and layers II, III, and V of the cortex terminate in the matrix. D1 receptors are more concentrated in striosomes, whereas the density of D2 receptors is highest in the matrix (Graybiel, 1990). These complex synaptic and topographic relationships may provide the substrate for the diversity of clinical signs and symptoms associated with PD.

CLINICAL FEATURES

Although James Parkinson's localization of the pathological lesions to the medulla was incorrect, his clinical descriptions were quite accurate (Fahn, 1989). In his six cases, he reported tremor, stooped posture, festinating gait, bradykinesia, excessive salivation, and postural instability (Pearce, 1989). However he failed to recognize rigidity, dementia, sensory complaints, and other symptoms and signs associated with the disease.

Traditionally, the parkinsonian findings of tremor and rigidity were considered to be positive signs, believed to be secondary to a release or disinhibition of extrapyramidal neurons by damage to connecting structures in other areas of the brain. The negative signs of bradykinesia and postural instability were thought to result from direct dysfunction of the basal ganglia (Marsden, 1982). This view, however, has been challenged by the recent findings of Bergman and colleagues (1990), who demonstrated improvement in bradykinesia after a chemical lesion in the STN of a parkinsonian monkey.

Tremor is the best recognized feature in PD and half of all PD patients experience this symptom. However, 15 percent do not develop tremor during the course of their illness (Martin et al, 1983). An oscillatory involuntary movement, tremor involves antagonistic muscles and characteristically produces a pill-rolling rest tremor of 4 to 6 Hz frequency. PD tremor often begins unilaterally, increases with stress, and disappears with sleep. Extremities, face, lips, and chin sometimes are involved, but head–neck and voice tremor, typically present in patients with familial essential tremor, are rare in PD. Intraoperative recordings have revealed cyclic repetitive activity in thalamic neurons (Jasper and Bertrand, 1966). Improvement of contralateral tremor by thalamotomy also provides evidence that central mechanisms play a major role in the development of parkinsonian tremor (Kelly et al, 1987). Furthermore, deafferentation of sensory fibers does not arrest tremor in monkeys with ventrotegmental–medial lesions (Lamarre and Joffray, 1979).

PD patients often complain of painful limb stiffness, sometimes misdiagnosed as bursitis or arthritis. The degree of muscle resistance (rigidity) often is proportional to the velocity of movement, the Westphal phenomenon, and probably results from excessive supraspinal drive on intact spinal mechanisms (Lance, 1980). Increased fusimotor drive has been demonstrated in PD patients and may represent increased alpha and gamma motor neuron activity, suggesting an inability for parkinsonian patients to fully relax (Lance, 1980). Rigidity may be increased by stress or contralateral voluntary movement, the so-called Froment's sign. Reduction in rigidity by dorsal root sectioning and by application of local anesthetics suggests a peripheral contribution to increased muscle tone (Abbe-Fessard et al, 1966). However, the improvement seen with thalamotomy and levodopa administration suggests central mechanisms (Beradelli et al, 1983). Striatal dopamine may increase muscle tone by disinhibiting GPi, thus altering suprasegmental activation of intact spinal reflexes. The associated cogwheel phenomenon has been linked to physiological tremor. Both have the same frequencies (Findley et al, 1981).

Whereas rigidity may contribute to slowness of movement, bradykinesia, which in part represents an impairment in motor program retrieval, is primarily responsible for the delayed and slowed execution of movement (Marsden, 1989). One form of akinesia, namely, freezing, is manifested as a delay in the onset of execution of movement. It often occurs at the initiation of movement, for example, when turning or walking through doorways (Jankovic, 1991). Other parkinsonian symptoms and signs may result from similar difficulties in motor program retrieval. Festination may be caused by a delay in the modulation of movement. An inability to execute simultaneous or sequential movements is one of the most fundamental motor disturbances in PD. As a result, PD patients have difficulties if they are turning, walking, and talking at the same time and when performing activities that require simultaneous execution of two or more tasks. The use of visual, auditory, and other sensory cues to overcome freezing suggests that PD patients have an intact motor program but have difficulty accessing the program (Fitzgerald and Jankovic, 1989). The Bereitschaftspotential (BSP), a premovement potential recorded by averaging surface electroencephalographic potentials before self-paced voluntary movements, has been found to be abnormal in some PD patients (Kornhuber and Deecke, 1978; Marsden, 1989). BSP, which represents neuronal transmission delay from the SMA to the basal ganglia, has been shown to diminish when PD patients are treated with levodopa (Dick et al, 1987).

Postural instability, manifested by propulsion and retropulsion, is perhaps the most disabling of all parkinsonian symptoms. Falling is reported in more than one third of parkinsonian patients and often results in a loss of confidence in walking (Koller et al, 1989). The development of pseudoagoraphobia may complicate the diagnosis and treatment of PD. This condition, a fear of falling, particularly interferes with walking in open spaces. Freezing and other gait abnormalities seem to be most frequent in patients with vascular parkinsonism, the so-called lower body parkinsonism (Fitzgerald and Jankovic, 1989).

Originally attributed to damage in the GP (Martin, 1967) and to axial "apraxia" (Lakke, 1985), the mechanism of parkinsonian postural instability is still unknown. Vestibular dysfunction may contribute but probably is not the primary mechanism of postural instability (Reichert et al, 1982). Traub and associates (1980) studied anticipatory compensation in 29 patients with mild and moderate parkinsonism and demonstrated prolonged delay of calf muscle contraction with perturbation and before initiation of voluntary movement. This suggests a centrally mediated mechanism of anticipatory adjustment. In bradykinesia, because of relative inaccessibility to the motor program, the anticipatory adjustments may be delayed. PD patients have been shown to have decreased sensitivity to muscle stretch when compared to a control population.

Other parkinsonian motor abnormalities, such as hypomimia (masked facies), bulbar abnormalities, dysarthria, hypophonia, and sialorrhea, may be secondary to a combination of rigidity and bradykinesia (Hartman and Abbs, 1988; Logemann, 1988). Breathing difficulties may result from rigidity of respiratory muscles but can be related also to levodopa-induced respiratory dyskinesia (Hovestadt et al, 1989). Dystonia, akathisia, and orofacial dyskinesia, although frequently associated with dopaminergic therapy, can be seen also in untreated PD patients.

Although PD is manifested primarily by motor symptoms, sensory disturbances, autonomic dysfunction, and neuropsychological abnormalities are also common. One of the most frequent sensory complaints is shoulder pain, often wrongly attributed to bursitis. Although some sensory symptoms may be attributed to rigidity, certain sensory phenomena, such as burning paresthesias, may result from an involvement of the descending spinal dopaminergic pathways. Analgesia produced by methylphenidate suggests involvement of central neurotransmitters (Cantello et al, 1988).

Autonomic disturbances, although more common in multiple system atrophies, such as the Shy-Drager syndrome, also occur in PD. Korczyn (1990) described prominent gastrointestinal symptoms in 178 patients. He noted constipation in 61 percent and attributed it in part to myenteric plexus involvement. Orthostatic hypotension may be a symptom of PD, but more frequently it is caused by antiparkinsonian medications.

Personality changes may be the earliest sign of PD. Parents of twins noted that from early life, the affected twin seemed to be the follower, to have less confidence, and to be more self-controlled than the unaffected sibling (Ward et al, 1983). Poewe and colleagues (1990) also reported a premorbid personality in their series of 38 patients with a tendency to be pedantic (75 percent), workaholic (71 percent), nonsmoking (66 percent), rigid (50 percent), and depressed (49 percent).

Dementia is estimated to occur in 2 to 77 percent of patients and is more prevalent in parkinsonian patients when compared to age-matched controls (Pirozzolo et al, 1988) (Chapter 10). Mayeux and colleagues (1990) estimated the point prevalence of dementia in a population of PD patients to be 10.9 percent. However, because cognitive decline may affect survival, age-specific incidence may be a more reliable number. In their series of 249 patients, this incidence was calculated to be 69 per 1000 for observed person-years (Mayeux et al, 1990). The mechanisms of cognitive decline may relate to cortical degeneration but also may relate to impaired neurological control of attention (Brown and Marsden, 1988), perhaps through deranged nondopaminergic neuronal systems (norepinephrine and acetylcholine pathways) (Cash et al, 1987; Dubois et al, 1987).

At least two different forms of PD have been proposed, one characterized by predominant bradykinesia, postural instability and gait difficulty (PIGD), and another dominated by tremor (Zetusky et al, 1985). The PIGD form appears to correlate with age, it tends to be associated with cognitive decline, and it is likely to progress rapidly. Tremor appears to be a symptom independent of the other common features in this illness and is associated with younger age, preserved higher cortical function and mobility, and slower progression. These subsets recently have been confirmed by analysis of the clinical correlates in 800 patients with early PD included in the DATATOP study (Jankovic et al, 1990). Four comparisons were performed: early vs late onset, benign vs malignant status, Hoehn-Yahr stage 1 vs stage 2, and tremor vs PIGD types. Patients with young onset PD (mean onset 36 years) appeared to have a slower progression of symptoms than patients with late onset PD (mean age 71). Patients with benign PD (mean Hoehn-Yahr stage 1.8) were younger (mean age 55) and more likely to have tremor (74 percent) than those with malignant PD (mean Hoehn-Yahr stage 2.5), who were older (mean age 68), and only 55 percent had tremor. The malignant group also was more likely to have bradykinesia (55 percent vs 25 percent) and postural instability (45 percent vs 8 percent). When the 233 tremor-dominant patients were compared to the 441 PIGD-dominant patients, the PIGD group had greater occupational disability, depression, intellectual impairment, and motivational problems.

It has been hypothesized that differential damage of subpopulations of neuronal systems is responsible for the diversity of phenotypes seen in PD. Detailed clinical–pathological–biochemical studies will be required to prove or disprove this hypothesis. Original clinical–biochemical studies correlated akinesia with dopamine and homovanillic acid (HVA) loss in the caudate nucleus, whereas tremor was associated with loss of HVA in the pallidum (Bernheimer et al, 1973). Positron emission tomography (PET) in PD patients has demonstrated decreased [^{18}F]-fluorodeoxyglucose uptake in the striatum and accumbens–caudate complex roughly proportional to the degree of bradykinesia (Kuhl et al, 1984; Brooks, 1991). In contrast, memory decline was correlated with impaired uptake in the paraolfactory gyrus–putamen complex.

Quantitative assessment of parkinsonian symptoms and signs is desirable to study underlying physiological mechanisms and to quantitate response to therapeutic interventions. Various computerized techniques have been used, but clinical rating scales seem to provide the most meaningful measure of symptom severity (Henderson et al, 1991). The Unified Parkinson's Disease Rating Scale (UPDRS) is a 42-item assessment that has been validated as a sensitive and reproducible method of measuring mentation, bulbar function, activities of daily living, and motor function (Fahn et al, 1987). Each item is rated on a 0 to 4 scale, with a higher score indicating poorer function. Historical information is used to rate intellectual impairment, hallucinations, motivation, depression, salivation, swallowing, handwriting, cutting food, dressing, performing daily hygiene activities, turning over in bed, walking, freezing, falling, and sensory symptoms. The other items, such as speech, facial expression, tremor, rigidity, rapid alternating movements, postural stability, gait, and body bradykinesia, are rated by the examiner. Levodopa-related fluctuations, dyskinesia, dystonia, and on/off function also are rated.

The Hoehn-Yahr scale is a convenient 5-point staging system to categorize patients by their global motor and ambulatory ability. Stage 0 = asymptomatic, 1 = unilateral involvement, 2 = bilateral symptoms without balance impairment, 3 = bilateral symptoms with some postural instability, 4 = severe disability but able to walk or stand unassisted, and 5 = wheelchair-bound or bedridden unless aided (Hoehn and Yahr, 1967). The Schwab and England Activities of Daily Living Scale provides a useful measure of overall functional ability (Schwab and England, 1969). Patients are asked to rate their functional abilities from 100 percent (completely independent) to 0 percent (bedridden).

ETIOLOGY AND PATHOGENESIS

Much of our current understanding of the possible etiology and pathogenesis of PD is derived from studies of the MPTP model of parkinsonism (Bloem et al, 1990). An autopsy report from a patient with MPTP parkinsonism showed degeneration of the SN (Davis et al, 1979). Subsequent studies of 22 MPTP patients with less severe parkinsonism further document the similarities with PD (Tetrud et al, 1989), although MPTP patients seemed to have more cognitive and emotional disability, as well as difficulties with salivation and gait instability. Tremor was less prominent in the MPTP group. The more severely affected patients reported by Langston and colleagues (1983) were similar to young onset PD patients and demonstrated marked levodopa sensitivity and levodopa-related fluctuations. The similarities in clinical and pathological features between MPTP and idiopathic parkinsonism provide support for the environmental hypothesis of PD. Models using prolonged exposure to lower doses of MPTP in older monkeys have demonstrated Lewy body-like inclusions in both the SN and the locus ceruleus (Forno et al, 1986). This suggests that aging increases the vulnerability of pigmented neurons to the toxic effects of MPTP, although age cannot be the only risk factor for increased susceptibility to PD.

Some population studies have supported the role of aging in the pathogenesis of PD, but other studies have concluded that aging plays only a minor role, if any. Prevalence of PD has been reported to range from 44 to 347 per 100,000 in the general population (Tanner and Langston, 1990). In populations older than age 60, however, the prevalence has been estimated to be 758 per 100,000 (Kurland, 1958). An increase in incidence of PD with age has been reported in some studies (Calne et al, 1986), but other surveys have shown peaks in age-specific incidence in the seventh decade and decline thereafter (Rajput et al, 1984; Koller et al, 1986). If age were to play a significant role in the pathogenesis of PD, increased concordance would be expected in twins because of their identical ages, but twin studies have failed to demonstrate such concordance (Ward et al, 1983; Marttila et al, 1988).

In vivo and autopsy studies of age-related decline in the concentration of dopamine (DA), DA receptors, and dopaminergic neurons have provided conflicting evidence for the role of aging in the pathogenesis of PD (Carlsson and Winblad, 1976). Based on postmortem examinations of normal brains, the annual decline in caudate DA has been estimated at 13 percent after age 45 (Riederer and Wuketich, 1979). At this rate, DA concentration would reach 35 percent of baseline levels at age 95. Since the onset of PD symptoms usually is in the sixth decade, when there should be about 80 percent DA depletion, other causes besides aging must be considered in the pathogenesis of the disease. However, no age-related decline in striatal DA, as measured by L-6-^{18}Fluorodopa uptake with PET scans, was found in 26 healthy volunteers between the ages of 27 and 76 (Sawle et al, 1990), suggesting that aging alone cannot explain the neuronal loss in PD. Furthermore, the frequently quoted figure of 80 percent DA depletion, which is based on postmortem analyses of PD brains, has been challenged by in vivo studies using PET scans. In one study, L-6-^{18}Fluorodopa regional uptake, a measure of regional levodopa metabolism in striatal dopaminergic nerve terminals was coupled with PET imaging of [^{11}C]nomifensine, an index of striatal monoaminergic (principally dopaminergic) reuptake (Leenders et al, 1990). To the extent that these techniques measure the integrity of dopaminergic nerve terminals, this study showed that these cellular elements were reduced to only 40 percent in the putamens of PD patients as compared to normal controls. This suggests that nigrostriatal decline in PD patients is not as severe as previous autopsy studies had indicated.

Using tritiated alpha-dihydrotetrabenazine as a ligand to presynaptic storage vesicles in 57 parkinsonian and 49 control brains, Scherman and associates (1989) found an age-dependent linear reduction in striatal dopamine of about 7.4 percent per decade in the control brains when extrapolated to baseline levels at birth. This corresponds to the estimated 6.9 percent age-dependent linear decline of dopaminergic neurons in SN (McGeer et al, 1977). In contrast, an exponential rate of decrease in the binding of alpha-dihydrotetrabenazine was found in the caudate nucleus of PD brains, although the rate remained relatively constant when the disease lasted 20 years or longer. The rate of reduction in dopaminergic striatal terminals was estimated to be at least twice as rapid in PD patients as in normal subjects. Since it was the same in brains of patients whose symptoms began before and after age 60, Scherman and colleagues (1989) concluded that aging did not play a major role in the pathogenesis of PD. These new findings from studies of autopsied brains, coupled with those based on in vivo PET data (Leenders et al, 1990), suggest that perhaps only 50 percent to 60 percent DA depletion is needed for PD symptoms to appear. Although nigrostriatal dopaminergic function may be relatively preserved with aging, there seems to be an age-related decline in the density of both D1 and D2 dopamine receptors (Rinne et al, 1989; De Keyser et al, 1990).

Although environmental causes, based primarily on hypotheses generated by the MPTP model, are currently favored by many experts, no environmental toxins have been identified that can be implicated specifically in the genesis of PD. Enzyme abnormalities causing impairment of toxin metabolism (e.g., cytochrome P450) have been suggested as playing a role in the pathogenesis of PD, but Barbeau's initial findings (1986) have not been verified (Poirier et al, 1987; Steventon et al, 1989). Epidemiological studies have drawn attention to some interesting trends. Parkinson's disease appears to be more prevalent in rural areas (Barbeau et al, 1986), and its occurrence has been correlated with the use of well water (Koller et al, 1990) or exposure to herbicides and pesticides (Ho et al, 1989; Barbeau, 1986). Extensive chemical analyses of well water in areas of high PD prevalence in Israel failed to identify any potential neurotoxins (Goldsmith et al, 1990), however. The inverse correlation between PD and smoking has now been attributed to a nonsmoking personality in PD patients rather than protective effects of tobacco (Golbe, 1990; Baron, 1986). In an attempt to define risk factors, Golbe et al (1990b) compared PD patients to their spouses (as a control group) and noted a comparatively low incidence of PD in spouses who had consumed foods high in vitamin E (e.g., peanut butter and salads) during childhood.

In the 1970s hospital-based surveys estimated the prevalence of PD to be four times higher in caucasian than in black populations (Kessler, 1972; Paddison and Griffith, 1974). This led investigators to postulate that melanin may have a neuroprotective function (Lerner and Goldman, 1987). Some have suggested that cutaneous melanin binds potential toxins, like neuronal melanin binds MPTP, before crossing the blood–brain barrier and thereby prevents substantia nigra damage (D'Amato et al, 1987). Because these studies assess only patients seeking medical care, the prevalence statistics may be biased and, therefore, difficult to interpret. The door-to-door population-based survey of PD in Copiah County, Mississippi, a demographically similar population with respect to race, found a similar prevalence in whites and blacks (Schoenberg et al, 1985). In addition, population-based studies in Nigeria (Osuntokun, 1971) and China (Li et al, 1985) also reported similar frequencies of PD prevalence in the white and nonwhite population.

The search for genetic mechanisms in PD has been inconclusive. Concordance among monozygotic twins has been documented rarely (Jankovic and Reches, 1986). Ward and associates (1983) reported concordance in only 1 set of 43 pairs of monozygotic twins, and a Finnish study found no concordance in 18 pairs of monozygotic siblings (Marttila et al, 1988). Although these data seem to argue against the possibility of heritable factors in PD, recent reanalysis of the twin study challenged these conclusions and renewed interest in genetic theories for at least some forms of idiopathic parkinsonism (Johnson et al, 1990; Golbe, 1990). Roy et al (1983) have described 10 families with akinetic rigid PD that fit an autosomal recessive pattern of inheritance. In addition, two large kindreds with dominantly inherited, autopsy-proven PD have been reported (Golbe et al, 1990a). An association between PD and familial essential tremor (Geraghty et al, 1985) and the occurrence of autosomal dominant dopa-responsive dystonia (Nygaard et al, 1990) has been proposed as further evidence for the role of genetic factors in the pathogenesis of PD.

Recent studies have explored the possibility of mitochondrial inheritance in PD. Because maternal mitochondria are distributed randomly, a nonmendelian transmission is possible (Golbe, 1990a; Mizuno et al, 1990). Some support for mitochondrial involvement is provided by MPTP studies. MPTP, a lipophilic protoxin that readily crosses the blood–brain barrier, is converted rapidly by MAO-B to 1-methyl-4-phenylpyridium (MPP+), its active metabolite (Chiba et al, 1984). MPP+ is concentrated in the mitochondrial matrix, perhaps by passive transport via an energy-dependent transmembrane potential (Heikkila et al, 1984), resulting in the depletion of ATP (Scotcher et al, 1990) and, ultimately, neuronal destruction.

A selective deficiency in the mitochondrial complex I, with a mean reduction of 42 percent of NADH CoQ reductase activity, was noted in the substantia nigra of seven PD brains by Schapira and associates (1990a). The deficiency seems to be region-specific (the activity of this enzyme was normal in caudate, cerebral cortex, and GP), apparently is not related to levodopa therapy, and has not been found in brains of patients with multiple system atrophy. The same mitochondrial enzyme defect has been found in platelets of PD patients (Parker et al, 1989). The specificity of this finding and its relationship to the pathogenesis of the disease, however, are unknown. Thirty-five percent reduction of complex I activity also was found in platelets of patients with Huntington's disease (Parker et al, 1990). It has been suggested that because of lack of a histone coat, the mitochondrial DNA is particularly susceptible to the damaging (mutagenic) effects of free radicals (Schapira et al, 1990b). Mitochondrial DNA may be more vulnerable to mutation due to its absence of histone coat and its lack of mitochondrial DNA repair mechanisms.

The search for endogenously generated toxic molecules, though inconclusive, has found some potential candidates for nigral neuronal destruction. Melanin is formed through oxidative metabolism of catecholamines. Its by-products include hydrogen peroxide, superoxide anions, and hydroxyradicals (Hirsch et al, 1989). These oxidative products play an important role in the development of PD, and support the *free radical* hypothesis as a model for parkinsonism (Ceballos et al, 1990; Halliwell, 1989). Free radicals, through interaction with membrane lipids, cause lipid peroxidation and membrane disruption, which may lead to cell death (Olanow, 1990). Elemental iron also increases the formation of free radicals in the nervous system, and this element is increased in brains of PD patients (Olanow, 1990). Hemoglobin and elemental iron may serve as endogenous toxins responsible for the pathological changes of PD (Youdim et al, 1990).

Strong support for an environmental hypothesis for PD is provided by the observation that numerous environmental agents can cause parkinsonism. These include carbon monoxide, manganese, carbon disulfide, and cyanide (Jankovic, 1989). Parkinsonian symptoms can result also from head trauma (Jordon, 1987; Krul and Wokke, 1987), cerebrovascular disease (FitzGerald and Jankovic, 1989; Murrow et al, 1990), hydrocephalus (Jankovic et al, 1986), hypoparathyroid abnormalities (Berger

Table 2-1. Classification of Parkinson's Disease

Primary Parkinson's disease
Secondary parkinsonism
A. Drugs (Dopamine blocking or depleting drugs, alpha-methyl dopa, lithium, diazoxide, flunarizine, cinnarizine)
B. Vascular (multi-infract, Binzwanger's)
C. Toxins (MPTP, manganese, carbon monoxide, carbon disulfide, cyanide, mercury, ethanol)
D. Metabolic (parathyroid, acquired hepatocerebral degeneration, GM1 gangliosidosis, Gaucher's disease)
E. Viral/postencephalitic (slow virus, human immunodeficiency virus, von Economo's encephalitis)
F. Tumor/paraneoplastic
G. Trauma and pugilistic encephalopathy
H. Hydrocephalus
Multiple system degenerations
A. Sporadic
   1. Progressive supranuclear palsy
   2. Shy-Drager syndrome
   3. Olivopontocerebellar atrophy
   4. Striatonigral degeneration
   5. Parkinsonism-dementia-amyotrophic lateral sclerosis complex of Guam
   6. Corticobasal degeneration
   7. Alzheimer's disease with parkinsonism
B. Inherited
   1. Huntington's disease
   2. Hallervorden-Spatz disease
   3. Wilson's disease
   4. Familial parkinsonism dementia syndrome
   5. Familial basal ganglia calcification
   6. Neuroacanthocytosis
   7. Spinocerebellar-nigral degeneration
   8. Glutamine dehydrogenase deficiency

and Ross, 1981), paraneoplastic degeneration (Golbe et al, 1989), and many other causes (Table 2-1). Infectious causes include encephalitis (most notably, 1917–1925 Von Economo's encephalitis) (Krusz et al, 1987), slow virus-associated infections (Brown et al, 1986), and human immunodeficiency virus (HIV)-associated infections (Nath et al, 1987). The parkinsoninsm-amyotrophic lateral sclerosis complex of Guam was once attributed to ingestion of cycad flour and the excitatory neurotoxin, 2-amino-methylamino-propanoic acid (BMMA) (Spencer et al, 1987). Recent studies contradict this association (Duncan et al, 1990).

PATHOLOGY

There is disagreement over the pathological criteria for diagnosis of PD. At autopsy, depigmentation, neuronal loss, and gliosis of the SN, particularly the pars compacta and locus ceruleus, are noted. Neuronal degeneration also is present in the dorsal nucleus of the vagus and in the substantia inominata (Barbeau, 1986; Jellinger 1990). Using an unbiased stereological method in seven PD patients at autopsy, Pakkenberg et al (1991) found a 66 percent reduction in the pigmented neurons in the SN from a normal count of 550,000 and a 24 percent reduction in the nonpigmented neurons from the normal 260,000.

Cytoplasmic inclusions, the Lewy and pale bodies, typically are encountered in the brains of patients with PD (Gibb et al, 1991). Lewy bodies are round eosinophilic inclusions, 7 to 20 nm in diameter, composed of microfilament subunits, tubulin, and microtubule-associated protein 1 and 2, but they are not related to tau protein (Galloway et al, 1988). The presence of Lewy bodies in two 7-μm hemisections of the midbrain (SN) and the preservation of significant numbers of intact pigmented neurons are required for the pathological diagnosis of PD (Gibb and Lees, 1989). Lewy bodies are found also in the basal nucleus of Meynert, the locus ceruleus, the sympathetic ganglia, the dorsal vagal nucleus, and even the myenteric plexus (Gibb, 1989). They are present in 5 to 10 percent of the brains of normal elderly persons but are most numerous in the SN of PD patients (Duvoisin and Golbe, 1989). In a retrospective analysis of 78 brains from patients who met the clinical criteria for PD, Lewy bodies were present in 73 (Gibb, 1990). Lewy bodies are increased also in patients with other neurodegenerative diseases, dementia, Hallervorden-Spatz disease, ataxia telangiectasia, progressive supranuclear palsy, and corticobasal ganglionic atrophy (Gibb, 1990). Pale bodies are found in some PD brains, particularly in the SN and locus ceruleus, and always are associated with Lewy bodies (Gibb et al, 1991). Pale bodies are less numerous than Lewy bodies and are less reliable in confirming the diagnosis of PD (Gibb et al, 1991).

PATHOPHYSIOLOGY

Studies with MPTP monkeys have provided information about the neurophysiological mechanisms of PD symptoms. Crossman (1990) contends that the medial (GPi) and lateral segments of the GP (GPe) respond differently to dopaminergic input, and Clarke et al (1989) demonstrated increased activity of the putaminopallidal projections to GPe and decreased input to the GPi in an MPTP primate. The resulting imbalance is believed responsible for aberrant motor responses. In early PD, dopaminergic agents restore this relative imbalance, and there is a therapeutic response. With progression, preferential stimulation of the GPe with dopaminergic drugs causes inhibition of the STN. This ameliorates the parkinsonian symptoms, but if excessive dosages are used, dyskinesias can occur. Recently, Bergman and associates (1990) observed improvement in two parkinsonian monkeys after stereotaxic ablation of the STN. These animals developed akinesia, rigidity, tremor, postural instability, and drooling 5 days after treatment with systemic MPTP. When these symptoms stabilized, ibotenic acid was injected stereotactically into one STN. Almost instantly, the animals demonstrated improved function and marked reduction of tremor in the contralateral extremities. Necropsy revealed bilateral reduction of SN dopaminergic cells, neuronal loss, and gliosis confined to the STN.

TREATMENT

Despite many advances in the treatment of PD, levodopa remains the most effective antiparkinsonian drug. It is metabolized both peripherally and in the brain by aromatic amino acid decarboxylase to DA (Boomsma et al, 1989). Peripheral DA is largely responsible for some of the levodopa-induced side effects, such as nausea, vomiting, and orthostatic hypotension. Levodopa is absorbed in the small intestine via the aromatic and branched-chain L amino acid carrier system and competes with other amino acids for carrier protein sites (Nutt and Fellman, 1984). Recent evidence suggests that similar carrier systems in the blood–brain barrier may play a role in levodopa-related motor fluctuations (Nutt et al, 1989). In the elderly, gastric emptying may be delayed, and thus the onset of action may be blunted. Gastric emptying may be slowed by the use of dopaminergic and anticholinergic medications (Baruzzi et al, 1987). Antacids and metoclopramide, a D2 receptor antagonist, may facilitate gastric emptying, although metoclopromide blocks the striatal DA receptors and, therefore, should be avoided in PD patients. Domperidone is a peripheral dopamine receptor antagonist with excellent antiemetic effects that does not block the central effect of levodopa (Parkes, 1986). Levodopa is metabolized by decarboxylation, oxidation, O-methylation, and transamination. Because of rapid peripheral metabolism, only 1 percent of the total dose reaches the striatum (Jankovic and Marsden, 1988).

Long-term side effects, such as dyskinesia, in the form of chorea, dystonia, and myoclonus are seen in 50 percent of patients after 5 years of levodopa therapy and 70 percent of patients after 10 years of treatment (Jankovic and Marsden, 1988). Delaying the use of levodopa preparations may allow patients to function longer without development of embarrassing and sometimes painful dyskinesias. Whether levodopa is introduced soon after the onset of symptoms or delayed until the symptoms become socially or occupationally disturbing does not seem to influence the mortality rate in PD patients (Scigliano et al, 1990). Initially, patients report prolonged benefit from levodopa, requiring dosing only three times daily. The benefit may last several days after the medication is discontinued. With progression of the underlying disease and with chronic levodopa treatment, more severe motor fluctuations may occur. The predictable wearing-off phenomenon is later replaced by more complex fluctuations, characterized by sudden, unpredictable changes in motor function (the on/off response). Sinemet CR, a new, controlled-release form of carbidopa/levodopa prolongs plasma levodopa levels and improves motor fluctuations (Cedarbaum et al, 1989).

Of the two dopamine agonists available in the United States, bromocriptine stimulates D2 and inhibits D1, and pergolide activates both D1 and D2 receptors (Calne et al, 1984; Jankovic and Marsden, 1988). Bromocriptine requires the concurrent use of levodopa for maximum effectiveness, but pergolide may show therapeutic effect even in de novo patients not treated with levodopa. Other dopamine agonists that are used include apomorphine and lisuride. With the discovery of the D3 receptor, it is possible that future pharmacological therapy will be tailored to avoid or to treat drug-induced psychosis.

The most recent medication to be added to the armamentarium for PD is deprenyl, a potent MAO-B inhibitor. Depenyl has been used in Europe since 1964, but its full potential was not realized until recently. Besides improving clinical symptoms, deprenyl may be useful in slowing progression of the disease (Parkinson Study Group, 1989). DATATOP, the Deprenyl and Tocopherol Antioxidative Treatment of Parkinson's Disease study, was designed to test the hypothesis that antioxidant agents, such as deprenyl, have a protective effect and favorably alter the natural progression of PD.

This placebo-controlled trial of 800 patients confirmed the findings of an earlier and smaller study (Tetrud and Langston, 1989) that deprenyl delays the progress of symptoms.

Interest in surgical therapy for PD has increased since Madrazo et al (1987) reported marked improvement in two patients with intractable PD who underwent autologous adrenal medullary transplantation to the putamen. However, a multicenter trial duplicating the procedures outlined by Madrazo and associates in 19 patients showed improvement in only selected areas of motor function (average percentage on-time and percentage on without chorea) and potentially serious complications. One patient developed a persistent vegetative state (Goetz et al, 1989). In an 18-month follow-up study, the improvement observed at 6 months in this population of 18 patients had returned to baseline (Olanow et al, 1990). Because of the significant number of complications that resulted from abdominal surgery, implantation of human fetal mesencephalic dopamine cells has been attempted in a number of patients. Freed et al (1990) report a 42 percent improvement in contralateral hand speed and 40 percent improvement in drug therapy 12 months after transplantation in a 52-year-old man. This patient also had a 17 percent increase in walking speed, and on-time increased from 69 percent to 86 percent. Madrazo et al (1990) report a 53 percent to 85 percent improvement in the UPDRS scores in 7 patients 6 to 19 months after implantation into the caudate nucleus of fetal ventral mesencephalon (4 patients) and fetal adrenal tissue (3 patients). However, because of many methodological problems, including the use of spontaneously aborted fetuses of gestational age 12 to 14 weeks, the results of this report are difficult to interpret. No graft survival was seen at autopsy 6 weeks (Waters et al, 1990), 4 months (Hirsch et al 1990; Peterson et al, 1989), and 8 months (Jankovic et al, 1990) after an autologous adrenal implant. One patient, who died 4 months after surgery without detectable clinical improvement, was found to have evidence of sprouting of striatal dopaminergic fibers in the vicinity of the necrotic graft (Hirsch et al, 1990).

REFERENCES

Abbe-Fessard D, Arfel G, Guiot G, et al. Electrophysiologic studies of some deep cerebral structures in man. *J Neurol Sci.* 1966;3:37–51.

Albin RL, Young AB, Penney JB. The functional anatomy of basal ganglia disorders. *Trends Neuro Sci.* 1989;12:366–375.

Alexander GE, Crutcher MD. Functional architecture of basal ganglia circuits: neural substrates of parallel processing. *Trends Neuro Sci.* 1990;13:266–271.

Andersen PH, Gingrich JA, Bates MD, et al. Dopamine receptor subtypes: beyond D1/D2 classification. *Trends Pharmacol Sci.* 1990;11:231–236.

Barbeau A. Parkinson's disease: clinical features and etiopathology. In: Vinken PJ, Bruyn GW, Klawans HL, eds. *Handbook of Clinical Neurology.* Amsterdam: Elsevier; 1986;5:85–152.

Barbeau A, Roy M, Cloutier T, et al. Environmental and genetic factors in Parkinson's disease. In: Yahr MD, Bergmen KJ, eds. *Parkinson's Disease. Adv Neurol.* New York: Raven Press; 1986;45:299–306.

Baron JA. Cigarette smoking and Parkinson's disease. *Neurology.* 1986;36:1490–1496.

Bartholini G, Pletscher A. Cerebral accumulation and metabolism of C14-dopa after selective inhibition of peripheral decarboxylase. *J Pharmacol Exp Ther.* 1968;161:14–20.

Baruzzi A, Contin M, Riva R, et al. Influence of meal ingestion time on pharmacokinetics of orally administered levodopa in parkinsonian patients. *Clin Neuropharmacol.* 1987;10:527–537.

Beradelli A, Sabra AF, Hallet M. Physiologic mechanisms of rigidity in Parkinson's disease. *J Neurol Neurosurg Psychiatry.* 1983;46:45–53.

Berger JR, Ross DB. Reversible Parkinson syndrome complicating postoperative hypoparathyroidism. *Neurology.* 1981;31:881–882.

Bergman H, Wichman T, DeLong MR. Reversal of experimental parkinsonism by lesion of the subthalamic nucleus. *Science.* 1990;249:1436–1438.

Bernheimer H, Birkmayer W, Hornykiewicz O, et al. Brain dopamine and the syndromes of Parkinson and Huntington: clinical, morphological and neurochemical correlations. *J Neurol Sci.* 1973;20:415–455.

Birkmayer W, Hornykiewicz O. Der L-3,4-dioxyphenylalanin (L-dopa)—Effekt bei der Parkinson-Akinese. *Wein Klin Wochenschr.* 1961;73:787–788.

Bloem BR, Irwin I, Buruma OJS, et al. The MPTP model: versatile contributions to the treatment of idiopathic Parkinson's disease. *J Neurol Sci.* 1990;97:273–293.

Boomsma F, Meerwaldt JD, Man In't Veld AJ, et al. Induction of aromatic-L-amino acid decarboxylase by decarboxylase inhibitors in idiopathic parkinsonism. *Ann Neurol.* 1989;25:624–628.

Brooks DJ. PET: its clinical role in neurology. *J Neurol Neurosurg Psychiatry.* 1991;54:1–4.

Brown P, Cathala F, Castigne P, Gajdusek DC. Creutzfeldt-Jacob disease: clinical analysis of consecutive series of 230 neuropathologically verified cases. *Ann Neurol.* 1986;20:597–602.

Brown RG, Marsden CD. Internal versus external cues and the control of attention in Parkinson's disease. *Brain.* 1988;111:323–345.

Calne DB, Burton K, Beckman J, et al. Dopamine agonists in Parkinson's disease. *Can J Neurol Sci.* 1984;11:221–224.

Calne DB, Eisen A, McGeer E, Specer P. Alzheimer's disease, Parkinson's disease, and motor neuron disease: Abiotrophic interaction between aging and environment? *Lancet.* 1986;2:1067–1070.

Cantello R, Aguggia M, Gilli M, et al. Analgesic action of methylphenidate on parkinsonian sensory symptoms. *Arch Neurol.* 1988;45:973–976.

Carlsson A, Winblad B. Influence of age and time interval between death and autopsy on dopamine and 3-methoxytyramine levels in the human basal ganglia. *J Neurol Transm.* 1976;38:271–276.

Carlsson A, Lindqvist M, Magnusson T. 3,4-Dihydroxyphenalanine and 5-hydroxytryptophan as reserpine antagonists. *Nature.* 1957;180:1200.

Carpenter MB, Sutin J. *Human Neuroanatomy.* Baltimore: Williams & Wilkins; 1983;579–611.

Cash R, Dennis T, L'Heureux R, et al. Parkinson's disease and dementia: norepinephrine and dopamine in locus ceruleus. *Neurology.* 1987;37:42–46.

Ceballos I, Lafon M, Javoy-Agid F, et al. Superoxide dismutase in Parkinson's disease. *Lancet.* 1990;335:1035–1036.

Cedarbaum JM, Silvestri M, Clark M, et al. L-Deprenyl, levodopa pharmacokinetics, and response fluctuations in Parkinson's disease. *Clin Neuropharm.* 1990;13:29–35.

Cedarbaum JM, Kutt H, McDowell FH. A pharmacokinetic and pharmacodynamic comparison of Sinemet CR (50/200) and standard Sinemet 25/100. *Neurology.* 1989;39(suppl 2):45–52.

Chiba K, Trevor A, Castagnoli N. Metabolism of the neurotoxic tertiary amine, MPTP, by brain monoamine oxidase. *Biochem Biophys Res Commun.* 1984;120:574–578.

Clarke CE, Boyce S, Robertson RG, et al. Drug-induced dyskinesia in primates rendered hemiparkinsonian by intracarotid administration of 1-methyl-4-phenyl-1,2,3,6-tetrahydro-pyridine (MPTP). *J Neurol Sci.* 1989;90:307–314.

Cotzias GC, Van Woert MH, Schiffer LM. Aromatic amino acids and modification of parkin-sonism. *N Engl J Med.* 1967;276:374–379.

Crossman AR. A hypothesis on the pathophysiological mechanisms that underlie levodopa or dopamine agonist-induced dyskinesia in Parkinson's disease: implications for future strategies in treatment. *Mov Disord.* 1990;5:100–108.

D'Amato RJ, Alexander GM, Schwartzman RJ, et al. Evidence for neuromelanin involvement in MPTP-induced neurotoxicity. *Nature.* 1987;327:324–327.

Davis GC, Williams AC, Markey SP, et al. Chronic parkinsonism secondary to injection of meperidine analogues. *Psychiatry Res.* 1979;1:249–254.

De Keyser J, Ebinger G, Vaughelin G. Age-related changes in the human nigrostriatal dopami-nergic system. *Ann Neurol.* 1990;27:157–161.

Dewey RB, Jankovic J. Hemiballism–hemichorea. *Arch Neurol.* 1989;46:862–867.

Dick PJR, Cantello R, Buruma O, et al. The Bereitschaftspotential, L-dopa and Parkinson's dis-ease. *Electroencephalogr Clin Neurophysiol.* 1987;66:263–274.

Dubois B, Danze, Pillon B, et al. Cholinergic-dependent cognitive deficits in Parkinson's disease. *Ann Neurol.* 1987;22:26–30.

Duncan MW, Steel JC, Kopin IJ, Markey SP. 2-Amino-3 (methylamino)-propanoic acid (BMAA) in cycad flour: an unlikely cause of amyotrophic lateral sclerosis and parkin-sonism–dementia complex of Guam. *Neurology.* 1990;40:767–772.

Duvoisin RC, Golbe LI. Toward a definition of Parkinson's disease. *Neurology.* 1989;39:746.

Ehringer H, Hornykiewicz O. Verteilung von Noreadrenalin und Dopamin (3-Hydroxytyra-min) im Gehirn des Menschen und ihr Verhalten bei Erkrankungen des extrapyrami-dalen Systems. *Wein Klin Wochenschr.* 1960;38:1236–1239.

Fahn S. The history of parkinsonism. *Mov Disord.* 1989;4(suppl 1):S2–S10.

Fahn S, Elton RL. Members of the UPDRS Development Committee. Unified Parkinson's dis-ease rating scale. In: Fahn S, Marsden CD, Calne DB, Lieberman A, eds. *Recent Devel-opments in Parkinson's Disease.* Florham Park, NJ: Macmillan Health Care Informa-tion; 1987;2:153–163.

Findley LJ, Gretsty MA, Halnmagyi GM. Tremor, the cogwheel phenomenon and clonus in Parkinson's disease. *J Neurol Neurosurg Psychiatry.* 1981;44:534–546.

FitzGerald PM, Jankovic J. Lower body parkinsonism: evidence for vascular etiology. *Mov Disord.* 1989;4:249–260.

Fleminger S, Rupniak MJ, Hall MD, et al. Changes in apomorphine-induced stereotypy as a result of subacute neuroleptic treatment correlates with increased D-2 receptors, but not with increased D-1 receptors. *Biochem Pharmacol.* 1983;32:2921–2927.

Forno LS, Langston JW, DeLanney LE, et al. Locus ceruleus lesions and eosinophilic inclusions in MPTP-treated monkeys. *Ann Neurol.* 1986;20:449–455.

Freed CR, Breeze RE, Rosenberg NL, et al. Transplantation of human fetal dopamine cells for Parkinson's disease. *Arch Neurol.* 1990;47:505–512.

Galloway PG, Bergeron C, Perry G. The presence of tau distinguishes Lewy bodies of diffuse Lewy body disease from those of idiopathic Parkinson's disease. *Neurosci Lett.* 1989;100:6–10.

Geraghty JJ, Jankovic J, Zetusky WJ. Association between essential tremor and Parkinson's dis-ease. *Ann Neurol.* 1985;17:329–333.

Gerfen CR. The neostriatal mosaic: striatal patch–matrix organization is related to cortical lam-ination. *Science.* 1989;246:385–388.

Gibb WRG. Neuropathology in movement disorders. *J Neurol Neurosurg Psychiatry.* 1989:(suppl):55–67.

Gibb WRG. The Lewy body. *Curr Opin Neurol Neurosurg.* 1990;3:346–349.

Gibb WRG, Lees AJ. The significance of the Lewy body in the diagnosis of idiopathic Parkinson's disease. *Neuropathol Appl Neurobiol.* 1989;15:27–44.

Gibb WRG, Scott T, Lees AG. Neuronal inclusions in Parkinson's disease. *Mov Disord.* 1991;6:2–11.

Goetz CG, Olanow W, Koller WC, et al. Multicenter study of autologous adrenal medullary transplantation to the corpus striatum in patients with advanced Parkinson's disease. *N Eng J Med.* 1989;320:337–341.

Golbe LI. The genetics of Parkinson's disease: a reconsideration. *Neurology.* 1990;40(suppl 3):7–14.

Golbe LI, Di Iorio G, Bonavita V, et al. A large kindred with autosomal dominant Parkinson's disease. *Ann Neurol.* 1990a;27:276–282.

Golbe LI, Farrell TM, Davis PH. Follow-up study of early-life protective and risk factors in Parkinson's disease. *Mov Disord.* 1990b;5:66–70.

Golbe LI, Miller DC, Duvoisin R. Paraneoplastic degeneration of the substantia nigra with dystonia and parkinsonism. *Mov Disord.* 1989;4:147–152.

Goldsmith JR, Herishanu Y, Abarbanel JM, Weinbaum Z. Clustering of Parkinson's disease points to environmental etiology. *Arch Environ Health.* 1990;45:88–94.

Graybiel AM. Neurotransmitters and neuromodulators in the basal ganglia. *TINS.* 1990;13:244–253.

Halliwell B. Oxidants and the central nervous system: some fundamental questions. *Acta Neurol Scand.* 1989;126:23–33.

Hartman DE, Abbs JH. Dysarthrias of movement disorders. In: Jankovic J, Tolosa E, eds. *Facial Dyskinesias. Adv Neurol.* New York: Raven Press; 1988;49:289–306.

Heikkila RE, Manzino L, Cabbat FS, Duvoisin RC. Protection against the dopaminergic toxicity of 1-methyl-4-phenyl tetrahydropyridine by monoamine oxidase inhibitors. *Nature.* 1984;311:467–469.

Henderson L, Kennard C, Crawford TJ, et al. Scales for rating motor impairment in Parkinson's disease: studies of reliability and convergent validity. *J Neurol Neurosurg Psychiatry.* 1991;54:18–24.

Hirsch EC, Graybiel AM, Agid Y. Selective vulnerability of pigmented dopaminergic neurons in Parkinson's disease. *Acta Neurol Scand.* 1989;126:19–22.

Hirsch EC, Duyckaerts C, Javoy-Agid F, et al. Does adrenal graft enhance recovery of dopminergic neurons in Parkinson's disease? *Ann Neurol.* 1990;27:676–682.

Ho SC, Woo J, Lee CM. Epidemiologic study of Parkinson's disease in Hong Kong. *Neurology.* 1989;39:1314–1318.

Hoehn MM, Yahr MD. Parkinsonism: onset, progression and mortality. *Neurology.* 1967;17:427–442.

Hovestadt A, Bogaard JM, Meerwaldt JD, van der Meche FGA. Pulmonary function in Parkinson's disease. *J Neurol Neurosurg Psychiatry.* 1989;52:329–333.

Hurtig H, Joyce J, Sladek JR, Trojanowski JQ. Postmortem of adrenal medulla-to-caudate autograft in a patient with Parkinson's disease. *Ann Neurol.* 1989;25:607–614.

Jankovic J. Clinical aspects of Parkinson's disease. In: Marsden CD, Fahn S, eds. *New Trends in the Treatment of Parkinson's Disease.* Carnforth, England: Parthenon Publishing; 1991.

Jankovic J. The relationship between Parkinson's disease and other movement disorders. In: Calne DB, ed. *Handbook of Experimental Pharmacology.* Berlin: Springer-Verlag; 1989;88:227–270.

Jankovic J, Marsden CD. Therapeutic strategies in Parkinson's disease. In: Jankovic J, Tolosa E, eds. *Parkinson's Disease and Movement Disorders.* Baltimore: Urban & Schwarzenberg; 1988;95–120.

Jankovic J, Reches A. Parkinson's disease in monozygotic twins. *Ann Neurol.* 1986;19:405–408.

Jankovic J, Newmark M, Peter P. Parkinsonism and acquired hydrocephalus. *Mov Disord.* 1986;1:59–64.

Jankovic J, McDermott M, Carter J, et al. Variable expression of Parkinson's disease: a base-line analysis of the DATATOP cohort. *Neurology.* 1990;40:1529–1534.

Jasper HH, Bertrand G. Recording from microelectrodes in stereotactic surgery for Parkinson's disease. *J Neurol.* 1966;24:219–221.

Jellinger K. New developments in the pathology of Parkinson's disease. In: *Parkinson's Disease: Anatomy, Pathology, and Therapy. Adv Neurol.* New York: Raven Press; 1990;53:1–16.

Johnson WG, Hodge SE, Duvoisin R. Twin studies and the genetics of Parkinson's disease—a reappraisal. *Mov Disord.* 1990;5:187–194.

Jordon BD. Neurologic aspects of boxing. *Arch Neurol.* 1987;44:453–459.

Kelly PJ, Ahlskog JE, Goerss SJ, et al. Computer-assisted stereotactic ventralis lateralis thalamotomy with microelectrode recording control in patients with Parkinson's disease. *Mayo Clin Proc.* 1987;62:655–664.

Kessler II. Epidemiologic studies of Parkinson's disease. III. A community-based study. *Am J Epidemiol.* 1972;96:242–254.

Koller WC, Glatt S, Vetere-Overfield B, Hassanein R. Falls in Parkinson's disease. *Clin Neuropharmacol.* 1989;12:98–105.

Koller WC, Ohara R, Weiner W, et al. Relationship of aging to Parkinson's disease. In: Yahr MD, Bergmann KJ, eds. *Parkinson's Disease. Adv Neurol.* New York: Raven Press; 1986;45:317–321.

Koller WC, Vetere-Overfield B, Gray C, et al. Environmental risk factors in Parkinson's disease. *Neurology.* 1990;40:1218–1221.

Korczyn AD. Autonomic nervous system disturbances in Parkinson's disease. In: *Parkinson's Disease: Anatomy, Pathology, and Therapy. Adv Neurol.* New York: Raven Press; 1990;53:463–468.

Kornhuber HH, Deecke L. An electrical sign of participation of the mesial supplementary motor cortex in human voluntary finger movement. *Brain Res.* 1978;159:473–476.

Krul JMJ, Wokke JHJ. Bilateral subdural hematoma presenting as subacute parkinsonism. *Clin Neurol Neurosurg.* 1987;89:107–109.

Krusz JC, Koller WC, Ziegler DK. Historical review: abnormal movements associated with epidemic encephalitis lethargica. *Mov Disord.* 1987;2:137–141.

Kuhl DE, Metter EJ, Riege WH. Patterns of local cerebral glucose utilization in Parkinson's disease by the [18F] fluorodeoxyglucose method. *Ann Neurol.* 1984;15:419–424.

Kurland LT. Epidemiology: incidence, geographic distribution and genetic considerations. In: Field W, ed. *Pathogenesis and Treatment of Parkinsonism.* Springfield, IL: Charles C Thomas; 1958;5–43.

Kurtzke JF, Murphy FM. The changing patterns of death rates in parkinsonism. *Neurology.* 1990;40:42–49.

Lakke JPWF. Axial apraxia in Parkinson's disease. *J Neurol Sci.* 1985;69:37–46.

Lamarre Y, Joffray AJ. Experimental tremor in monkey: activity of thalamic and precentral cortical neurons in the absence of peripheral feedback. In: Poirier LJ, Sourkes TL, Bedard PJ, ed. *The Extrapyramidal System and its Disorders. Adv Neurol.* New York: Raven Press; 1979;24:109–122.

Lance JW. The control of muscle tone, reflexes, and movement: Robert Wartenberg lecture. *Neurology.* 1980;30:1303–1313.

Langston JW, Ballard PA, Tetrud JW, Irwin I. Chronic parkinsonism in humans due to a product of meperidine analogue synthesis. *Science.* 1983;219:979–980.

Leenders KL, Salmon EP, Tyrrell P, et al. The nigrostriatal dopaminergic system assessed in vivo by positron emission tomography in healthy volunteer subjects and patients with Parkinson's disease. *Arch Neurol.* 1990;47:1290–1298.

Lerner MR, Goldman RS. Skin colour, MPTP and Parkinson's disease. *Lancet.* 1987;1:212.

Li SC, Schoenberg BS, Wang CC, et al. A prevalence survey of Parkinson's disease and other movement disorders in the People's Republic of China. *Arch Neurol.* 1985;42:655–657.

Logemann JA. Dysphagia in movement disorders. In: Jankovic J, Tolosa E, eds. *Facial Dyskinesias. Adv Neurol.* New York: Raven Press; 1988;49:307–316.

Mackenzie RG, Kebabian JW, Roa D. Molecular biology of the D2 dopamine receptor. *Curr OP Neurol Neurosurg.* 1990;3:544–547.

Madrazo I, Drucker-Colin R, Diaz V, et al. Open microsurgical autograft of the adrenal medulla to the right caudate nucleus in two patients with intractable Parkinson's disease. *N Engl J Med.* 1987;316:831–834.

Madrazo I, Franco-Bourland R, Ostrosky-Solis F, et al. Fetal homotransplants (ventral mesencephalon and adrenal tissue) to the striatum of human subjects. *Arch Neurol.* 1990;47:1281–1285.

Marsden CD. Slowness of movement in Parkinson's disease. *Mov Disord.* 1989;4(suppl 1):S26–S37.

Marsden CD. The mysterious motor function of the basal ganglia: the Robert Wartenberg lecture. *Neurology.* 1982;32:514–539.

Martin JP. *The Basal Ganglia and Posture.* London: Pitman Medical Publishing Company; 1967.

Martin WE, Loewenson RB, Resch JA, Baker AB. Parkinson's disease: a clinical analysis of 100 patients. *Neurology.* 1983;23:783–390.

Marttila RJ, Kaprio J, Kostenvuo MD, Rinne UK. Parkinson's disease in a nationwide twin cohort. *Neurology.* 1988;38:1217–1219.

Mayeux R, Chen J, Mirabello E, et al. An estimate of the incidence and prevalence of dementia in idiopathic Parkinson's disease. *Neurology.* 1990;40:1513–1516.

McGeer PL, McGeer EG, Suzuki JS. Aging and extrapyramidal function. *Arch Neurol.* 1977;34:33–35.

Mizuno Y, Ohta S, Tanaka M, et al. Deficiencies in complex 1 subunits of the respiratory chain in Parkinson's disease. *Biochem Biophys Res Commun.* 1990;163:1450–1455.

Murrow RW, Schweiger GD, Kepes JJ, Koller WC. Parkinsonism due to a basal ganglia lacunar state: clinicopathologic correlation. *Neurology.* 1990;40:897–900.

Nath A, Jankovic J, Pettigrew C. Movement disorders and AIDS. *Neurology.* 1987;37:37–41.

Nutt JG. Levodopa-induced dyskinesia: review, observations, and speculations. *Neurology.* 1990;40:340–345.

Nutt JG, Fellman JH. Pharmacokinetics of levodopa. *Clin Neuropharmacol.* 1984;7:35–49.

Nutt JG, Woodward WR, Carter JH, Trotman TL. Influence of fluctuations of plasma large neutral amino acids with normal diets on the clinical response to levodopa. *J Neurol Neurosurg Psychiatry.* 1989;52:481–487.

Nygaard TG, Trugman JM, de Yebeemes, Fahn S. Dopa-responsive dystonia. The spectrum of clinical manifestations in a large North American family. *Neurology.* 1990;40:60–69.

Olanow W. Oxidation reactions in Parkinson's disease. *Neurology.* 1990;40(suppl 3):32–37.

Olanow W, Koller W, Goetz CG, et al. Autologous transplantation of adrenal medulla in Parkinson's disease. *Arch Neurol.* 1990;47:1286–1289.

Osuntokun BO. The pattern of neurological illness in tropical Africa: experience at Ibadan, Nigeria. *J Neurol Sci.* 1971;12:417.

Paddison RM, Griffith RP. Occurrence of Parkinson's disease in black patients at Charity Hospital in New Orleans. *Neurology.* 1974;24:688.

Pakkenberg B, Moller A, Gundersen HJG, et al. The absolute number of nerve cells in substantia nigra in normal subjects and in patients with Parkinson's disease estimated with an unbiased stereological method. *J Neurol Neurosurg Psychiatry.* 1991;54:30–33.

Parent A. Extrinsic connection of the basal ganglia. *TINS.* 1990;13:254–258.

Parker WD, Boyson SJ, Luder AS, Parks JK. Evidence for a defect in NADH: ubiquinone oxidoreductase (complex I) in Huntington's disease. *Neurology.* 1990;40:1231–1234.

Parker WD, Boyson SJ, Parks JK. Abnormalities of the electron transport chain in idiopathic Parkinson's disease. *Ann Neurol.* 1989;26:719–723.

Parkes JD. Domperidone and Parkinson's disease. *Clin Neuropharm.* 1986;89:517–532.

Parkinson Study Group. Effect of deprenyl on the progression of disability in early Parkinson's disease. *N Engl J Med.* 1989;321:1364–1371.

Pearce JMS. Aspects of the history of Parkinson's disease. *J Neurol Neurosurg Psychiatry.* 1989;(special suppl):6–10.

Peterson DI, Price ML, Small CS. Autopsy findings in a patient who had adrenal-to-brain transplant for Parkinson's disease. *Neurology.* 1989;39:235–238.

Pirozzolo FJ, Swilhart AA, Rey G, et al. Cognitive impairments associated with Parkinson's disease and other movement disorders. In: Jankovic J, Tolosa E, eds. *Parkinson's Disease and Other Movement Disorders.* Baltimore: Urban & Schwarzenberg; 1988:425–439.

Poewe W, Daramat E, Kemmler GW, Gerstenbrand F. The premorbid personality of patients with Parkinson's disease: a comparative study with healthy controls and patients with essential tremor. In: *Parkinson's Disease: Anatomy, Pathology, and Therapy. Adv Neurol.* New York: Raven Press; 1990;53:339–342.

Poirier J, Roy M, Campenella G, et al. Ecogenetics of Parkinson's disease. *Lancet.* 1987;2:1213–1216.

Rajput AH, Offord KP, Beard CM, Kurlan LT. Epidemiology of parkinsonism: incidence, classification, and mortality. *Ann Neurol.* 1984;16:278–282.

Reichert WH, Dolittle J, McDowell FM. Vestibular dysfunction in Parkinson's disease. *Neurology.* 1982;32:1133–1138.

Riederer P, Wuketich S. Time course of nigrostriatal degeneration in Parkinson's disease. *J Biol Med.* 1979;247:3170–3175.

Rinne JO, Lonnberg P, Marjamaki P. Age-dependent decline in human brain dopamine D1 and D2 receptors. *Brain Res.* 1989;508:349–352.

Roy M, Boyer L, Barbeau A. A prospective study of 50 cases of familial Parkinson's disease. *Can J Neural Sci.* 1983;10:37–42.

Sawle GV, Colebatch JG, Shah A, et al. Striatal function in normal aging: implications for Parkinson's disease. *Ann Neurol.* 1990;28:799–804.

Schapira AHV, Cooper JM, Dexter D, et al. Mitochondrial complex I deficiency in Parkinson's disease. *J Neurochem.* 1990a;54:823–827.

Schapira AHV, Holt IJ, Sweeney M, et al. Mitochondrial DNA analysis in Parkinson's disease. *Mov Disord.* 1990b;5:294–297.

Scherman D, Desnos C, Darche F, et al. Striatal dopamine deficiency in Parkinson's disease. *Ann Neurol.* 1989;26:551–557.

Schoenberg BS, Anderson DW, Haerer AF. Prevalence of Parkinson's disease in the biracial population of Copiah County, Mississippi. *Neurology.* 1985;35:841.

Schwab RS, England AC. Projection technique for evaluating surgery in Parkinson's disease. In: Gillingham FJ, Donaldson MC, eds. *Third Symposium on Parkinson's Disease.* Edinburgh: E & S Livingston; 1969.

Scigliano G, Musicco M, Soliveri P, et al. Mortality associated with early and late levodopa therapy initiation in Parkinson's disease. *Neurology.* 1990;40:265–269.

Scotcher KP, Irwin I, Delaney LE, et al. Effects of 1-methyl-4-phenyl-1,2,3,6-tetrahydropyridine and 1-methyl-4-phenylpyridinium ion on ATP levels of mouse and brain synaptosomes. *J Neurochem.* 1990;54:1295–1301.

Shannon K. Hemiballismus. *Clin Neuropharm.* 1990;13:413–425.

Smith AD, Bolam JP. The neural network of the basal ganglia as revealed by the study of synaptic connection of identified neurons. *TINS.* 1990;13:259–265.

Sokoloff P, Giros B, Martres M, et al. Molecular cloning of a novel dopamine receptor (D3) as a target for neuroleptics. *Nature.* 1990;347:146–151.

Spencer PS, Nunn PB, Hugon J, et al. Guam amyotrophic lateral sclerosis–parkinsonism–dementia linked to a plant excitant neurotoxin. *Science.* 1987;237:517–522.

Steventon GB, Heafield MTE, Waring RH, Williams AC. Xenobiotic metabolism in Parkinson's disease. *Neurology.* 1989;39:883–887.

Strange PG. Aspects of the structure of the D2 receptor. *TINS.* 1990;13:373–378.

Tanner CM, Langston JW. Do environmental toxins cause Parkinson's disease? A critical review. *Neurology.* 1990;(suppl 3):17–31.

Tetrud JW, Langston JW, Garbe PL, Ruttenber AJ. Mild parkinsonism in persons exposed to 1-methyl-4-phenyl-1,2,3,6-tetrahydropyridine (MPTP). *Neurology.* 1989;39:1483–1487.

Traub MM, Rothwell JC, Marsden CD. Anticipatory postural reflexes in Parkinson's disease and other akinetic–rigid syndromes and cerebellar ataxia. *Brain.* 1980;103:393–412.

Walters JW, Bergstrom DA, Carlsson JM, et al. D1 dopamine receptor activation required for postsynaptic expression of D2 agonist effects. *Science.* 1987;236:719–722.

Ward CD, Duvoisin RC, Ince S, et al. Parkinson's disease in 65 pairs of twins and in a set of quadruplets. *Neurology.* 1983;33:815–824.

Waters C, Itabashi HH, Apuzzo MLJ, Weiner LP. Adrenal to caudate transplantation—postmortem study. *Mov Disord.* 1990;5:248–251.

Youdim MBH, Ben-Shachar D, Yehuda S, Riederer P. The role of iron in the basal ganglion. In: Striefler M, Korczyn AD, Melamed E, Youdim MBH, eds. *Parkinson's Disease: Anatomy, Pathology and Therapy. Adv Neurol.* New York: Raven Press; 1990;53:155–162.

Zetusky WJ, Jankovic J, Pirozzolo F. The heterogeneity of Parkinson's disease: clinical and prognostic implications. *Neurology.* 1985;35:522–526.

3

Neuropsychological Evaluation of Parkinson's Disease

STEVEN J. HUBER AND ROBERT A. BORNSTEIN

The consistent message in this volume is that neurobehavioral changes are common in patients with Parkinson's disease (PD). Research related to the neurobehavioral features of PD is of both theoretical and practical importance. From a theoretical perspective, this line of investigation has provided new insights into the role of subcortical structures or related projection systems in human cognitive and emotional functions (Chapters 11 and 25). Information derived from basic clinical research is also of practical importance, since behavioral symptoms are a common cause of disability in PD. Proper clinical management thus entails evaluation of these symptoms to determine their potential impact on overall disability, to assess possible side effects of antiparkinsonian medications (Chapters 21 through 23), and to evaluate the effectiveness of specific treatment modalities (Chapters 18 and 19).

There is compelling evidence that memory, visuospatial skills, executive functions, bradyphrenia, and depression are the most common areas of neurobehavioral abnormality associated with PD. The fact that these deficits have been demonstrated using a variety of neuropsychological procedures emphasizes the pervasiveness of the problems and the reliability of the observations. However, the lack of consistency in the measures used restricts comparison among studies.

This chapter focuses on dementia (Part III) and depression (Part IV), which are the main areas where variations in methodology have contributed to inconsistencies in the research literature. Emphasis is placed on specific methodological differences among previous reports, difficulties unique to the evaluation of dementia and depression in PD, and recommendations for standardized research approaches to the diagnosis of dementia and staging of its severity. The final section outlines a set of neuropsychological tests that could facilitate communication among researchers and provide a standardized method of assessing the behavioral abnormalities of PD.

DEPRESSION

Depression is common in PD, but there is little agreement about its specific aspects. It has been estimated that 30 percent to 90 percent of PD patients have depressive symptoms (Gotham et al, 1986; Huber et al, 1988a; Levin et al, 1988). The specific manifestations of depression in PD have not been clearly established (Gotham et al, 1986; Huber et al, 1990a). The relationship between severity of motor symptoms and depressive symptoms also is controversial. Some investigators report a roughly parallel relationship (Gotham et al, 1986; Huber et al, 1988b; Mayeux et al, 1981), whereas others suggest that the severity of depression is independent of disease severity (Horn, 1974; Marsh and Markham, 1973; Robins, 1976).

Methodological differences in the assessment of depression have contributed to the divergent results of previous studies. The most commonly used scales are the Beck Depression Inventory (BDI) (Beck et al, 1961) and the Hamilton Depression Rating Scale (Hamilton, 1960). Total scores derived from these scales may be difficult to interpret because of overlapping somatic features of depression and those related to PD (Gotham et al, 1986; Levin et al, 1988). Further, specific features of depression in PD vary as a function of disease severity (e.g., somatic features), whereas other features (e.g., mood) do not. Thus, the relationship between depressive and motor changes might be evident for some aspects of depression and not for others.

In a recent study, we examined the relationship between disease severity and features of depression as measured by the BDI (Huber et al, 1990a). Items from the BDI were divided into those related to mood, self-reproach, vegetative, and somatic features of depression. As can be seen in Table 3–1, three distinct patterns were observed. Symptoms related to mood and self-reproach were significantly higher in the PD patients compared with controls, but the magnitude of the elevated symptoms did not vary as a function of disease severity. Significant elevations of vegetative symptoms were evident only in patients with relatively more severe disease. Finally, patients with mild disease had significant elevations of somatic symptoms that increased as a function of disease severity.

Since the severity of specific features of depression varies with respect to advancing PD, depression appears to be more complicated than the simple reactive/endogenous dichotomy would imply. In addition, the question of which features of depression are most common may depend on the specific stage of disease. Symptoms related to mood and self-reproach do not appear to vary with disease severity, whereas symptoms related to somatic and vegetative features covary with disease severity. Thus, the use of total scale scores may overestimate the incidence of depression in PD. Evaluation

Table 3–1. Average scores (SD) on Beck Depression Inventory (BDI) for normal controls, patients with mild Parkinson's disease (PD), and patients with advanced PD. Patterns of post hoc comparisons are indicated $(=, <, >)$

BDI	Controls $(n = 47)$		Mild PD $(n = 53)$		Advanced PD $(n = 50)$	Kruskal-Wellis ANOVA
Total	4.1 (2.9)	<	8.1 (6.6)	<	11.5 (5.8)	<0.0001
Mood	0.8 (1.0)	<	2.1 (2.4)	=	2.4 (2.2)	<0.0004
Self-reproach	0.3 (0.6)	<	1.5 (2.1)	=	2.0 (2.2)	<0.0001
Vegetative	1.5 (1.4)	=	1.6 (1.8)	<	3.2 (2.1)	<0.0001
Somatic	1.5 (1.4)	<	2.9 (2.0)	<	3.9 (1.8)	<0.0001

From Huber et al.: The pattern of depressive symptoms varies with progression of Parkinson's disease. J Neurol Neurosurg Psychiatry 1990; 53:275–278.

of symptoms that do not vary with disease severity (i.e., mood and self-reproach) may provide the best indicators for estimating the prevalence of depression.

DEMENTIA

Dementia refers to an acquired and persistent impairment of cognitive function that represents a departure from the previous level of function (Cummings and Benson, 1983). It is generally acknowledged that dementia can occur in PD, but there is little agreement about its incidence, nature, or severity. For example, estimates of the prevalence of dementia in PD have varied from 4 percent to 93 percent (Cummings et al, 1988). This extreme divergence is due primarily to the lack of standardized criteria of definition and variation in the methodologies for assessing it (Brown and Marsden, 1984; Cummings et al, 1988; Huber et al, 1990b). Controversies related to dementia in PD extend beyond frequency estimates (Chapter 10). The lack of standardized criteria has contributed to inconsistencies in the literature with respect to the clinical, radiological, pathological, biochemical, and electrophysiological correlates of dementia (Chapters 11 through 15).

Diagnosis of dementia in PD is complicated by the range and distribution of the overall cognitive disturbance. As illustrated by the work of Pirozzolo and associates (1982), the range of cognitive disturbances is normally distributed (Fig. 3–1). That is, a minority of patients show no deficits or are very mildly impaired, and a minority has very severe cognitive dysfunction. The majority of patients fall between these extremes. Since the spectrum of cognitive impairment in PD is continuous and there are no clearly defined patient groups with respect to severity, establishing a cutoff for dementia is an arbitrary approach to definition. This issue is further complicated by the likelihood that there are several types of dementia occurring in PD, with different etiologies contributing to the mild, moderate, and severe cognitive deficits (Cummings, 1988).

For research purposes, development of clearly defined methods of evaluation and criteria for dementia in PD are essential. Application of common methods and criteria will improve the similarity of patient samples among studies and will make the results more comparable.

Research Criteria for Dementia in Parkinson's Disease

In this section, we review the two most popular standardized criteria for the diagnosis of dementia. Special attention is paid to their appropriateness for use in PD and the methodology necessary to evaluate the criteria.

One set of criteria (Table 3–2) to diagnose dementia is outlined in the *Diagnostic and Statistical Manual of Mental Disorders,* Third Edition, Revised (DSM IIIR) (American Psychiatric Association, 1987). The appropriateness of these widely used criteria may depend on the specific patient population to be studied. For example, these criteria can be used in a relatively straightforward manner in patients with presumed Alzheimer's disease, since significant impairment of social or occupational function is a direct reflection of the degree of cognitive impairment. This determination, however, is not so straightforward in patients with PD since the movement dis-

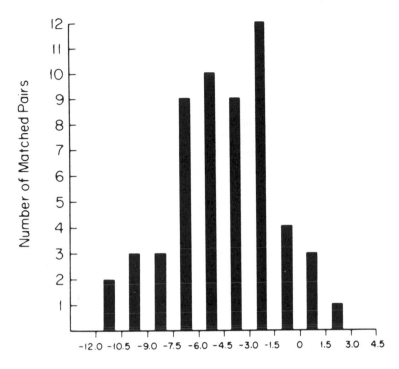

Discriminant Difference Scores

Figure 3-1. Frequency distribution of matched-pair difference scores on the derived five-variable discriminant function predicting group membership. Difference scores of greater than zero reflect patients performing better than their matched control, and conversely scores less than zero reflect worse performance by patients. The absolute size of the signed difference score is related to the magnitude of performance differential. Solid bars refer to the number of matched pairs falling within each 1.5-unit interval demarcated by numbered cut points. Only 56 matched pairs were utilized in this analysis due to failure of 4 patients to complete the Digit Symbol test. (From Pirozzolo et al., *Brain Cognition.* 1982;1:71–83.)

Table 3-2. Criteria for dementia defined in DSM IIIR

1. Memory impairment
2. One of the following
   a. Impaired abstraction
   b. Impaired judgment
   c. Aphasia
   d. Apraxia
   e. Agnosia
   f. Constructional difficulty
   g. Personality change
3. The impairment of (1) and (2) is sufficient to impair social or occupational function
4. Alert state of consciousness

order can also affect social or occupational impairment (Growdon and Corkin, 1986; Huber et al, 1990b; Mayeux et al, 1983). The potential confound represented by the motor component in PD and the difficulty in separating the contribution of motor and cognitive factors related to social and occupational impairment introduce interrater variability that is problematic for research.

The criteria for dementia defined by Cummings and Benson (1983) are presented in Table 3–3. To meet these criteria for dementia, there must be impairment in at least three of the five neurobehavioral areas listed. We believe that the Cummings and Benson approach is preferable for patients with PD because these criteria can be implemented in a straightforward objective manner, and they avoid the subjective assessment related to social and occupational function incorporated into the DSM IIIR approach. In addition, since the Cummings and Benson approach can be applied to various dementing disorders because of its strictly objective method of evaluation, we believe that this procedure should be adopted for use in comparative studies of dementing disorders. One useful application would be in evaluating the distinction between cortical and subcortical dementia syndromes (Chapter 11). Comparison of these disorders requires standardized and appropriate methodology to diagnose dementia, since this is not a universal finding in patients with predominantly subcortical disorders, including PD.

Diagnosis and Staging Dementia in Parkinson's Disease

We describe here a specific set of guidelines to implement the Cummings and Benson criteria for the diagnosis of dementia in PD. Because of the broad spectrum of cognitive impairments in PD, an objective method is presented to define the severity of dementia. The three primary methodological issues involve the selection of appropriate neuropsychological procedures, guidelines to define what constitutes significant impairment for any of the five areas of cognitive dysfunction defined in these criteria, and an objective method to stage dementia severity. The next section of this chapter describes neuropsychological procedures that we believe are appropriate for use in PD, including tests related to each of the five categories defined in the dementia criteria.

Impairment on any assessment procedure can be determined by converting the raw scores to standardized T scores using age- and education-matched control samples. This conversion is desirable when evaluating multiple areas of cognitive function, since T scores provide a common metric that allows direct comparison of performance levels among the various assessment procedures required for the diagnosis of dementia. Statistical significance is traditionally defined by a p value of less than 0.05. Since T scores usually are based on an average score of 50 with a standard deviation of 10,

---

Table 3–3.   Criteria for dementia defined by Cummings and Benson (1983)

Significant impairment in at least three of these areas is required
1. Language
2. Memory
3. Visuospatial skills
4. Personality/mood
5. Cognition (executive function)

---

this level of statistical significance corresponds to a T score of 30 or less (2 standard deviations or more below the mean).

When evaluating the question of an isolated impairment (e.g., memory), a p value of 0.05 is used almost universally to define statistical significance. However, for the evaluation of dementia where multiple areas of impairment are required for the diagnosis, this statistical definition may be too conservative. The use of such a conservative approach may require the presence of severe dementia in order to meet the criteria. This may be problematic for the evaluation of patients with predominantly subcortical disorders, including PD, since the dementia syndrome typically is associated with relatively mild but generalized cognitive dysfunction.

We recommend that in the evaluation of dementia, a T score of 40 or less may be a more commonsense metric to define impairment in individual areas of cognitive function. If the average performance in procedures under any one of the five areas results in a mean T score of less than 40 or performance on a single procedure from the area has a T score of less than 30, significant impairment for that area can be inferred. If this occurs in three or more areas, the criteria for dementia are met.

A dichotomous approach to the diagnosis of dementia defined by strict guidelines, however, has limited clinical use. There is probably little impact on daily life function as a consequence of cognitive impairment between patients just meeting criteria for dementia and those falling just shy of meeting criteria. This approach may present problems for research applications as well, since patients who meet criteria for dementia may vary in overall severity of cognitive dysfunction.

A staging system to define the severity of dementia is presented in Table 3–4. This system is similar to the Clinical Dementia Rating (CDR) scale developed by Berg and associates (1982), with the primary exception being that severity of dementia is based on objective rather than subjective criteria. In fact, a recent study of interrater reliability using the CDR found only moderate agreement among clinicians (Lopez et al, 1990). This underscores the difficulty in applying subjective ratings of dementia.

The major value of an objective system to grade dementia is for research purposes. When comparing the qualitative features of various dementia syndromes, a necessary

Table 3–4. Classification of dementia severity based on application of Cummings and Benson criteria (1983)

Normal mental status
   A mean T score of above 40 and no single test with a T score below 35 for each of the five areas of cognitive function
Borderline impairment
   A mean T score of less than 40 or a T score of less than 30 on a single test in 1 or 2 areas of cognitive function
Levels of dementia
Mild
   At least 3 of the 5 areas with a mean T score of less than 40 or a single test from an area with a T score of 30 or less (criteria for dementia); none of the five areas have a mean T score of less than 30
Moderate
   Meets criteria for dementia, and 1 or 2 of the areas have a mean T score below 30
Severe
   Meets criteria for dementia, and at least 3 areas have mean T scores below 30

part of the methodology is to match the patient groups for overall severity of cognitive impairment. Comparisons of possible qualitative differences among dementing disorders are meaningful only if the patient groups are similar with respect to overall cognitive impairment. The method outlined in Table 3-4 to determine the severity of cognitive dysfunction has an advantage over single measures, such as the Mini Mental State Examination (Folstein et al, 1975), because it is based on a much more comprehensive examination.

NEUROPSYCHOLOGICAL EXAMINATION IN PARKINSON'S DISEASE

This section describes a battery of neuropsychological procedures that we use for the behavioral evaluation of patients with PD. Five specific criteria were used to select the most appropriate neuropsychological tests (Table 3-5). First, we used information provided by contributors to this volume to derive a set of procedures that is most sensitive to the impairments commonly associated with PD. Second, the battery was designed to limit total administration time to approximately 3 hours. For clinical purposes, this reduces the possible influence of fatigue, which is common in aged patients. Third, procedures were chosen to provide a comprehensive examination of each cognitive function when possible. For example, procedures were selected to examine verbal, nonverbal, and contextual memory. Fourth, there was an emphasis on selecting tests developed using knowledge derived from basic clinical research examining cog-

Table 3–5. Proposed neuropsychological procedures for evaluation of patients with Parkinson's disease

Memory
　California Verbal Learning Test (Delis et al, 1987)
　Continuous Visual Memory Test (Trahan and Larrabee, 1988)
　Logical Memory (Wechsler, 1987)
Visuospatial skills
　Raven's Standard Progressive Matrices (Raven, 1958)
Language
　Verbal Fluency (Benton, 1968)
　Boston Naming Test (Kaplan et al, 1983)
Executive functions
　Wisconsin Card Sorting Test (Heaton, 1981)
　Verbal Concept Attainment Test (Bornstein, 1983)
Attention and concentration
　Digit Span Forward and Backwards (Wechsler, 1987)
　Visual Span Forward and Backwards (Wechsler, 1987)
Bradyphrenia
　Simple Reaction Time
　Choice Reaction Time
Depression
　Beck Depression Inventory (Beck et al, 1961)
Global cognitive function
　Mattis Dementia Rating Sacle (Mattis, 1976)

nitive processing deficits responsible for impaired performance. Whenever possible, procedures were chosen that provide not only a quantitative estimate of performance level but also qualitative information related to the nature of the underlying cognitive deficits. This approach provides maximal overlap between clinical and research data. Finally, we have attempted to incorporate tests that have age-related norms that can be useful also for repeated measures over time.

Memory

Memory abnormalities are among the cognitive symptoms seen most commonly in patients with PD (Huber et al, 1989; Pirozzolo et al, 1982; Pillon et al, 1986; Sahakian et al, 1988). Previous studies suggest that PD patients may have deficits in recent verbal, nonverbal, and contextual memory. Several measures have been introduced or refined that would appear to be potentially useful in evaluating these deficits. These tests include the California Verbal Learning Test (CVLT) (Delis et al, 1987), the Selective Reminding Test (Buschke and Fuld, 1974), the Rey Auditory Verbal Learning Test (Lezak, 1983), and the Continuous Visual Memory Test (Trahan and Larrabee, 1988).

The CVLT examines many constructs derived from experimental neuropsychological research that have been shown to influence memory performance (Delis et al, 1989). Twenty-six parameters are derived from this procedure based on age- and sex-adjusted normative data. These parameters include type of recall (e.g., immediate, delayed, and recall consistency), acquisition strategies (e.g., semantic clustering, serial position), interference effects (e.g., proactive and retroactive inhibition), and error analysis (e.g., intrusions and perseverations). Analysis of the nature of the underlying cognitive concepts responsible for memory failures can be of clinical significance as well as providing useful research data (Butters, 1984).

In addition to verbal list learning tasks (e.g., CVLT) based on noncontextual material, it is important to evaluate contextual memory. This aspect of memory is assessed in our battery by the Logical Memory Subtest of the Wechsler Memory Scale Revised (WMS-R), which entails immediate and delayed recall of short paragraphs (Weschler, 1987). Although many components of the WMS-R have been criticized (Chelune et al, 1989, 1990; Bornstein and Chelune, 1988; Loring, 1989), the Logical Memory Subtest has explicit scoring and normative data that are advantageous for both clinical and research applications. In addition, there are few other tests available for assessment of contextual memory.

Memory for these two types of information differs in several important ways. Acquisition and retrieval of the story's contextual information requires more elaborate encoding, which involves both syntactic and semantic properties. Since the amount of information to be retained exceeds the storage capacity of working memory, an active decision process is required to determine which of the presented ideas are most important (Delis et al, 1990).

In addition to measures of verbal learning and memory, we believe it is also necessary to examine memory for nonverbal material. Many nonverbal memory tests, including Benton's Visual Retention Test (1974) and the Visual Reproduction Test (VRT) from the WMS-R (Wechsler, 1987), entail reproduction of geometric designs from memory. It has been suggested that the visually presented information in the VRT is susceptible to verbal mediation (Delis et al, 1990; Bornstein and Chelune, 1988), and the scoring procedures emphasize drawing accuracy so heavily that it diminishes its usefulness as a measure of memory (Chelune et al, 1990). For patients with PD, it can be especially difficult to determine whether poor performance on such measures is the result of a memory or a drawing impairment secondary to motor limitations. The Continuous Visual Memory Test (Trahan and Larrabee, 1988) provides a measure of nonverbal memory with no motor component. The task requires the recognition of previously presented geometric designs from an array that contains the target and several distractor items. This procedure examines both immediate and delayed memory performance. Performance level is derived using a signal detection analysis to control for response biases. In addition, a spatial analysis subtest is provided to determine whether poor performance reflects a memory or a perceptual impairment.

Visuospatial Skills

Numerous studies have demonstrated that spatial abilities are impaired in PD (Pirozzolo et al, 1982; Boller et al, 1984; Brown and Marsden, 1986). These studies suggest that the deficits cannot be attributed completely to motor slowing (Boller et al, 1984). Nevertheless, motor or cognitive slowing may be a confounding factor because most tests of visuospatial abilities typically involve a motor task or are scored on the basis of time to completion (e.g., Block Design from the Wechsler Adult Intelligence Scale-Revised (WAIS-R)). Both of these factors represent potentially confounding factors for patients with PD. Raven's Progressive Matrices (Raven, 1958) provides an appropriate test of visuospatial skills in PD patients, since it does not have a motor component and is not timed. This test measures both simple perceptual matching and more complex visuospatial reasoning skills.

Language

Disorders of language and comprehension are rare in patients with PD (Cummings et al, 1988). The most common disturbances involve naming and verbal fluency (Matison et al, 1982; Lees and Smith, 1983; Huber et al, 1989). Several comprehensive language batteries are available that incorporate evaluation of a wide range of language abilities, such as the Boston Diagnostic Aphasia Examination (Goodglass and Kaplan, 1972) and the Western Aphasia Battery (Kertesz, 1979). Because language deficits are relatively uncommon in PD and because of the time required to administer the entire battery, we do not believe these comprehensive language assessments need to be given in their entirety. Rather, since naming difficulties are the most prominent symptoms, a test such as the Boston Naming Test (Kaplan et al, 1983) directed toward evaluation of confrontation naming ability is preferred.

Several studies have demonstrated impairment in the ability to generate words according to some predetermined criteria (e.g., letters or semantic categories). The Controlled Oral Word Association Test (FAS) (Benton, 1968) is the most commonly used measure of verbal fluency. Performance on these tests may be related to language factors or dysarthria and may also be secondary to impairment of executive function.

Executive Functions

Research reviewed in Chapter 6 suggests that impairment of executive function is a prominent feature in PD, even in its earliest stages (Lees and Smith, 1983). Therefore, it is important to provide a thorough examination of these abilities. A number of procedures have been employed, including the Category Test (Halstead, 1947), Trail Making Tests (Reitan and Davison, 1974), the Wisconsin Card Sorting Test (Heaton, 1981), and the Verbal Concept Attainment Test (Bornstein, 1983; Bornstein and Leason, 1985). The Category Test is used widely in neuropsychological assessment, but it is time consuming and does not provide any information about specific aspects of executive function (e.g., perseverative errors or maintenance of response set). The Trail Making Test requires, among other things, the ability to shift between two lines of thought. This test is scored on the basis of time to completion, which raises the potential confounding of motor slowing in PD patients. In contrast, the Wisconsin Card Sorting Test (Heaton, 1981) provides a number of indices, including the number of concepts acquired, ability to maintain response set, and the number of perseverative errors. This procedure measures nonverbal concept formation, and verbal abstracting and reasoning abilities can be assessed using the Verbal Concept Attainment Test (Bornstein, 1983; Bornstein and Leason, 1985).

Attention and Concentration

Attention and concentration can be assessed using the digit-span and visual-span subtests of the WMS-R (Wechsler, 1987). These procedures use both auditory verbal and visual information.

Bradyphrenia

Bradyphrenia refers to the slowness of mental processes and traditionally has been considered to be the cognitive correlate of slowness of movement or bradykinesia. It is this very slowness of movement, however, that makes bradyphrenia difficult to study in PD. If the procedure used to study bradyphrenia requires a motor response, it can be difficult to determine whether poor performance is the result of slowed motoric or slowed cognitive processing.

Some of the newer reaction time (RT) procedures can independently measure motor and mental processing latencies. In a measure of simple RT, the task is to depress one lever and to depress a second lever when a randomly timed light flashes. The time from when the response light comes on to the release of the depressed lever is the decision time, and the time to depress the second lever once the decision has occurred is the movement time. In a choice RT paradigm, the task is to depress one lever when a predetermined color appears or a second lever when the alternate colored light appears. The difference in latency between the choice and simple RT tasks provides a measure of cognitive processing speed independent of motoric influences.

Depression

The Beck Depression Inventory (BDI) (Beck et al, 1961) is a self-rated depression scale that provides a brief and objective method for assessing depressive symptoms. It has been assumed that the use of such scales may be problematic when assessing PD patients because of overlapping somatic features of depression and symptoms of PD. Levin et al (1988) examined whether the somatic items diminish the usefulness of this procedure in PD, and their results indicate that the BDI is a reliable and valid measure of depression in PD and that the depression in PD is not only somatic. Our results (Huber et al, 1990a) also suggest that depressive symptoms other than somatic features are significantly elevated in PD and the pattern of these symptoms varies with disease severity. The BDI has received the most research attention in studying PD and it appears to provide a valid assessment of the quantitative and qualitative aspects of depression in the disease.

Global Cognitive Function

The set of procedures described earlier to diagnose and stage the severity of dementia provides a measure of cognitive status based on a comprehensive examination. In many situations, however, such as research related to a single cognitive function (e.g., memory), a brief method is desirable. Some description of overall cognitive status is necessary to compare results among different studies. This section discusses the two most widely used brief procedures of overall cognitive status in terms of their applicability to PD.

The Mini Mental State (MMS) Exam (Folstein et al, 1975) is the most widely used global assessment procedure. The MMS may be most useful for detection of severe and generalized cognitive deficits and may not be sensitive to mild cognitive deficits. In PD, there is a wide range of cognitive impairment (Fig. 3–1), and in the majority of cases, the compromise is mild and restricted to one or a few discrete domains. Even when the impairment was severe enough to meet Cummings and Benson's criteria for dementia (1983), only 46 percent of the demented PD patients scored below the traditional cutoff score of 24 on the MMS (Huber et al, 1990b). This test is insensitive to mild cognitive deficits in PD because more than half of the points are derived from measures of orientation and language, which are typically spared even in PD patients with moderately severe cognitive impairment (Chapter 11).

The Dementia Rating Scale (DRS) developed by Mattis (1976) is more appropriate than the MMS for use in PD. The DRS has a wider range of measurements (144 vs 30 possible points), and broader areas of cognitive function are examined, including attention, initiation/perseveration, construction, conceptualization, and memory. Thus, this procedure would appear to be potentially more sensitive to the wide range of cognitive status changes among patients with PD.

SUMMARY

The primary purpose of this chapter was to discuss methodological issues related to neuropsychological assessment in PD. The second section discusses methodology and criteria for the diagnosis of dementia in PD. Research related to the clinical, radiological, pathological, biochemical, and electrophysiological correlates sometimes has produced conflicting results. Controversies in the literature will persist unless standardized methods and criteria to diagnose dementia in PD are developed. We believe that the Cummings and Benson criteria for dementia are preferable for use in PD research because of the more objective method of evaluation. Methods of applying these criteria in PD and an objective system to stage the severity of dementia were presented.

Important issues related to PD including the natural history of neurobehavioral symptoms, remain unresolved. It has been suggested that specific cognitive functions do not change in a uniform fashion with progression of PD (Huber et al, 1991), and the same may be true of specific symptoms related to depression (Huber et al, 1990a). These studies, however, used prospective comparisons of patient groups in different stages of disease. An adequate evaluation of the natural history of neurobehavioral symptoms in PD patients requires multicenter longitudinal studies using standardized methods of assessment, such as those presented in this chapter.

REFERENCES

American Psychiatric Association. *Diagnostic and Statistical Manual of Mental Disorders.* 3rd ed, Revised. Washington, DC: American Psychiatric Association; 1987.

Beck AT, Ward CH, Mendelson M, et al. An inventory for measuring depression. *Arch Gen Psychiatry.* 1961;4:561–571.

Benton AL. Differential behavioral effects in frontal lobe disease. *Neuropsychologia.* 1968;5:53–60.

Benton AL. The Revised Visual Retention Test. 4th ed. New York: The Psychological Corporation; 1974.

Berg L, Hughes CP, Coben LA, et al. Mild senile dementia of Alzheimer type: research diagnostic criteria, recruitment, and description of a study population. *J Neurol Neurosurg Psychiatry.* 1982;45:962–968.

Boller F, Passatiume D, Keefe NC, et al. Visuospatial impairments in Parkinson's disease. *Arch Neurol.* 1984;41:485–490.

Bornstein RA. Verbal Concept Attainment Test: cross validation and validation of a booklet form. *J Clin Psychiatry.* 1983;39:743–745.

Bornstein RA, Chelune GJ. Factor structure of the Wechsler Memory Scale-revised. *Clin Neuropsychologist.* 1988;2:107–115.

Bornstein RA, Leason M. Effects of localized lesions on the Verbal Concept Attainment Test. *J Clin Exp Neuropsych.* 1985;7:421–429.

Brown RG, Marsden CD. How common is dementia in Parkinson's disease? *Lancet.* 1984;1:1262–1265.

Brown RG, Marsden CD. Visuospatial function in Parkinson's disease. *Brain.* 1986;109:987–1002.

Buschke H, Fuld PA. Evaluating storage, retention, and retrieval in disordered memory and learning. *Neurology.* 1974;11:1019–1025.

Butters N. The clinical aspect of memory disorders: contribution from experimental studies of amnesia and dementia. *J Clin Exp Neuropsych.* 1984;6:17–36.

Chelune GJ, Bornstein RA, Prifitera A. The Wechsler Memory Scale-Revised. In: McReynolds P, Rosen JC, Chelune GJ, eds. *Advances in Psychological Assessment,* vol 7. New York and London: Plenum Press; 1990;65–99.

Chelune GJ, Goormastic M, Naugle RI. Construct validity of the Wechsler Memory Scale-Revised (WMS-R) within the context of a neuropsychological battery for seizure patients. *J Clin Exp Neuropsych.* 1989;11:63.

Cummings JL. Intellectual impairment in Parkinson's disease: clinical, pathological, and biochemical correlates. *J Geriatr Psychiatry Neurol.* 1988;1:24–36.

Cummings JL, Benson DR. *Dementia: A Clinical Approach.* Stoneham, Mass: Butterworth Publishers Inc; 1983.

Cummings JL, Darkins A, Mendez M, et al. Alzheimer's disease and Parkinson's disease: comparison of speech and language alterations. *Neurology.* 1988;38:680–684.

Delis DC, Kaplan E, Ober BA. *The California Verbal Learning Test.* New York: The Psychological Corporation; 1987.

Delis DC, Kramer JH, Fridlund AJ, Kaplan E. A cognitive science approach to neuropsychological assessment. In: McReynolds P, Rosen JC, Chelune GJ, eds. *Advances in Psychological Assessment,* vol 7. New York and London: Plenum Press; 1990;65–99.

Folstein MF, Folstein SE, McHugh PR. Mini mental state: a practical guide for grading the mental state of patients for the clinician. *J Psychiatr Res.* 1975;12:189–198.

Goodglass H, Kaplan E. *The Assessment of Aphasia and Related Disorders.* Philadelphia: Lea and Febiger; 1972.

Gotham AM, Brown RC, Marsden CD. Depression in Parkinson's disease. A qualitative analysis. *J Neurol Neurosurg Psychiatry.* 1986;49:381–389.

Growdon JH, Corkin S. Cognitive impairments in Parkinson's Disease. In: Yahr MD, Bergman KJ, eds. *Advances in Neurology,* vol 45. New York: Raven; 1986.

Halstead WC. *Brain and Intelligence.* Chicago: University of Chicago Press; 1947.

Hamilton M. A rating scale in depression. *J Neurol Neurosurg Psychiatry.* 1960;23:56–62.

Heaton RK. *Wisconsin Card Sorting Test Manual.* Oderson, Florida: Psychological Assessment Resources; 1981.

Horn S. Some psychological factors in Parkinsonism. *J Neurol Neurosurg Psychiatry.* 1974;37:27–21.

Huber SJ, Christy JA, Paulson GW. Cognitive heterogeneity associated with clinical subtypes of Parkinson's disease. *Neuropsychol Neuropsychiatry Behav Neurol.* 1991;4:147–157.

Huber SJ, Paulson GW, Shuttleworth EC. Depression in Parkinson's disease. *Neuropsych Behav Neurol.* 1988a;1:47–51.

Huber SJ, Paulson GW, Shuttleworth EC. Relationship of motor symptoms, intellectual impairment, and depression in Parkinson's disease. *J Neurol Neurosurg Psychiatry.* 1988b;51:855–858.

Huber SJ, Shuttleworth EC, Christy JA, Rice RR. A brief scale of dementia of Parkinson's Disease. *J Neuropsych Clin Neurosci.* 1990b;2:183–188.

Huber SJ, Freidenberg DL, Paulson GW, Shuttleworth EC, Christy JA. The pattern of depressive symptoms varies with progression of Parkinson's disease. *J Neurol Neurosurg Psychiatry.* 1990a;53:275–278.

Huber SJ, Freidenberg DL, Shuttleworth EC, et al. Neuropsychological impairments associated with severity of Parkinson's disease. *J Neuropsych Clin Neurosci.* 1989;1:154–158.

Kaplan E, Goodglass H, Weintraub S. *The Boston Naming Test.* Philadelphia: Lea and Febiger; 1983.

Kertesz A. *Aphasia and Associated Disorders.* New York: Grune and Stratton; 1979.

Lees AJ, Smith E. Cognitive deficits in the early stages of Parkinson's disease. *Brain.* 1983;106:257–270.

Levin BE, Llabre MM, Weiner WJ. Parkinson's disease and depression: psychometric properties of the Beck Depression Inventory. *J Neurol Neurosurg Psychiatry.* 1988;51:1401–1404.

Lezak MD. *Neuropsychologic Assessment.* 2nd ed. New York: Oxford University Press; 1983.

Lopez OL, Swihart AA, Becker JT, et al. Reliability of NINCDS-ADRDA clinical criteria for the diagnosis of Alzheimer's disease. *Neurology.* 1990;40:1517–1522.

Loring DW. The Wechsler Memory Scale-Revised, or the Wechsler Memory Scale-Revisited? *Clin Neuropsychologists.* 1989;3:59–69.

Marsh GG, Markham CH. Does Levodopa alter depression and psychopathology in Parkinsonism patients? *J Neurol Neurosurg Psychiatry.* 1973;36:925–935.

Matison R, Mayeux R, Rosen J, et al. "Tip-of-the-tongue" phenomenon in Parkinson's disease. *Neurology.* 1982;32:567–570.

Mattis S. Mental status examination for organic mental syndrome in the elderly patient. In: Bellack L, Karasu TB, eds. *Geriatric Psychiatry.* New York: Grune and Stratton; 1976;77–121.

Mayeux R, Stern Y, Rosen J, et al. Depression, intellectual impairment, and Parkinson's Disease. *Neurology.* 1981;31:645–650.

Mayeux R, Stern Y, Rosen J, Benson DF. Is subcortical dementia a recognizable clinical entity? *Ann Neurol.* 1983;14:278–283.

Pillon B, Dubois B, Lhermitte F, Agid Y. Heterogeneity of cognitive impairment in progressive supranuclear palsy, Parkinson's disease, and Alzheimers' disease. *Neurology.* 1986;36:1179–1185.

Pirozzolo FJ, Hansch EC, Mortimer JA, et al. Dementia in Parkinson's disease: a neuropsychological analysis. *Brain Cognition.* 1982;1:71–83.

Raven JC. *Standard Progressive Matrices.* New York: Psychological Corp; 1958.

Reitan RM, Davison LA. Clinical neuropsychology: current status and application. Washington: Winston; 1974.

Robins AH. Depression in patients with Parkinsonism. *Br J Psychiatry.* 1976;128:141–145.

Sahakian BJ, Morris RG, Evenden JL, et al. A comparative study of visuospatial memory learning in Alzheimer-Type dementia and Parkinson's disease. *Brain.* 1988;111:695–718.

Trahan DE, Larrabee GJ. *Continuous Visual Memory Test.* Odessa, Fla: Psychological Assessment Resources, Inc.; 1988.

Wechsler D. *Wechsler Memory Scale-Revised.* New York: Harcourt Brace Jovanovich Publishers; 1987.

II

COGNITIVE IMPAIRMENTS

4

Memory Disturbances in Parkinson's Disease

WILLIAM W. BEATTY

It is now widely acknowledged that disturbances in memory are among the most common of the cognitive deficits experienced by patients with Parkinson's disease (PD). This chapter summarizes current knowledge of the nature of anterograde and retrograde memory disturbances in PD. Although I do not address directly the question of whether PD is a subcortical or a cortical dementia (Chapter 11), it will be evident that memory disturbances associated with PD are similar to those that occur in such subcortical disorders as Huntington's disease and multiple sclerosis and distinct (both quantitatively and qualitatively) from the memory deficits that occur in cortical dementias, such as Alzheimer's disease. In addition to memory disturbances, patients with PD, Huntington's disease, or multiple sclerosis are likely to exhibit deficits in problem solving and on other tests of executive functions (Chapter 6). The extent to which such deficits contribute to memory impairments in PD is an important issue that is under active investigation by a number of researchers. Finally, it is important to realize that memory impairments, like other cognitive deficits, are not seen in all PD patients (El-Awar et al, 1987).

ANTEROGRADE MEMORY

Deficits in learning and remembering new information are well documented in PD. Most studies have examined explicit memory tasks, in which subjects consciously attempt to recall or recognize as much information as they can. Only recently has implicit memory, which does not require conscious recollection, been studied.

Explicit Verbal Memory

When asked to recall newly learned verbal information, PD patients often exhibit deficits. Comparable impairments have been reported for word lists (Beatty et al, 1989d; Taylor et al, 1986; Villardita et al, 1982), paired associates (El-Awar et al, 1987; Huber et al, 1986b; Pirozzolo et al, 1982), and brief prose passages (Pirozzolo et al, 1982; Taylor et al, 1986). By contrast, when verbal memory is tested by recognition methods, deficits are small and may not be evident at all.

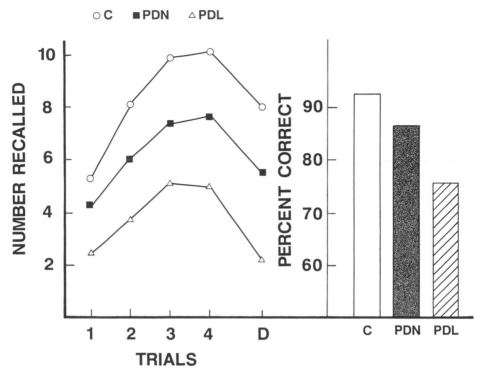

Figure 4-1. Acquisition, delayed recall, and delayed recognition of a 14-word list by controls (C), PD patients of normal mental status (PDN), and PD patients of lower than normal mental status (PDL). (Redrawn from data reported in Beatty et al., 1989d.)

Figure 4-1 illustrates the typical findings. In this study (Beatty et al, 1989d), PD patients were divided into two groups based on their performance on the Mini-Mental State Exam (Folstein et al, 1975). One group (PDN) scored within the range of normal controls (28–30), whereas the other group (PDL) scored lower than the normal range (22–27). In addition, the PDL group exhibited deficits in problem solving, naming, and visuospatial perception that were not evident in PDN patients.

All subjects received four presentation-recall trials of a 14-word list of 7 high and 7 low imagery words. Thirty minutes after the fourth trial, delayed recall was tested. Immediately afterward, delayed (yes–no) recognition was measured.

On the immediate recall trials, both PD groups exhibited deficits on the first recall trial but improved over trials at a nearly normal rate. Deficits varied with global mental status, but even the PDN patients were significantly impaired. In studies with multiple sclerosis (Beatty et al, 1988a; 1989b) and Huntington's disease (Beatty and Butters, 1986) patients using the same materials and procedures, the same pattern was observed.

On delayed memory tests, differences between the PDN and PDL groups were evident also. Rates of forgetting for the PDN and control groups were similar, but the PDL patients forgot at a faster rate than the other subjects. Because of the differences in performance on trial 4, forgetting was measured as a percentage savings score. (Number recalled on delay/number recalled on trial 4) × 100.)

The PDN patients attained nearly normal savings scores (70 percent vs 78 percent for controls), and they also performed normally on the recognition memory test. Normal rates of forgetting and nearly normal recognition memory were observed for multiple sclerosis patients on the same test (Beatty et al, 1988a; 1989b).

PDL patients exhibited lower than normal savings (42 percent) and impaired recognition memory. On these measures, their performance was intermediate between that of the PDN patients and a group of Alzheimer's disease patients studied earlier (Beatty et al, 1986). The Alzheimer's disease patients averaged 10 percent savings and 62 percent correct on delayed recognition.

The differential sensitivity of recall and recognition measures of verbal memory appears to hold for PD patients over a broad range of mental status. Among patients of normal mental status, even those so recently diagnosed that they are not receiving medication, recall of verbal material is impaired, but recognition is not (Taylor et al, 1986; Weingartner et al, 1984). Among patients with dementia (such as the PDL patients described previously), deficits are evident on recognition tests, but they are less severe than on recall. When PD and Alzheimer's disease patients were matched for intelligence (a measure of dementia severity) and verbal recall, the PD patients recognized significantly more items than did the Alzheimer's disease patients (Helkala et al, 1988).

The fact that verbal memory is impaired on the first learning trial raises the possibility that PD patients suffer some deficit in encoding information. In support of this possibility, Tweedy and associates (1982) reported mild deficits by PD patients in release from proactive interference (PI) following a shift in the semantic category of the stimuli. On this test, subjects receive a series of short-term memory trials in which three words from the same class (e.g., tools) are presented. Performance deteriorates over trials until, without warning, the semantic class of the words is changed. Improvement in memory on the trials after the shift in semantic class is termed release from PI. Failure to show release from PI as reported by Tweedy et al (1982) implies impaired semantic encoding. However, Beatty et al (1989d) were unable to replicate these results. They reported that both nondemented and mildly demented PD patients showed normal release from PI. Further, PD patients exhibited the normal pattern of better recall of high than of low imagery words in the experiment described earlier (Beatty et al, 1989d). Similar findings have been reported for Huntington's disease (Beatty and Butters, 1986) and multiple sclerosis (Beatty et al, 1989b) patients. Taken together, these observations suggest that PD, Huntington's disease, and multiple sclerosis patients retain the capacity for normal semantic encoding although they may not be able to use this ability as efficiently as normal controls because of their difficulties in processing information rapidly (Beatty et al, 1989a; Huber and Paulson, 1987; Huber et al, 1989).

Explicit Nonverbal Memory

On recall measures that involve reproducing complex designs (Bowen, 1976; Riklan et al, 1976) or learning the locations of places on maps (Beatty et al, 1989d), both demented and nondemented PD patients exhibit deficits that are similar to those observed with multiple sclerosis patients (Beatty et al, 1988a). On recognition measures, however, the impairments of PD patients may be more severe for nonverbal than for verbal material.

Although Flowers and associates (1984) reported that PD patients performed normally on both verbal and nonverbal recognition memory tests, Taylor et al (1986) found deficits among nondemented PD patients on the spatial position component of the Delayed Recognition Test (Albert and Moss, 1984). Recognition memory for words and geometric designs was normal. Sahakian and colleagues (1988) observed deficits on both spatial and visual pattern recognition memory using matching to sample and nonmatching to sample procedures. None of their patients were demented, and the deficits were more severe for medicated than for nonmedicated patients (who were so early in the course of their disease that they did not require medication). Interestingly, the pattern recognition memory deficits were evident even with no delay and were equal in magnitude at all delays tested. Sullivan and Sagar (1989) found deficits in memory for abstract designs among both demented and nondemented PD patients. Overall the demented patients were more severely impaired, but both patient groups showed poorer memory at short than at long retention intervals.

Sullivan and Sagar (1989) suggested that the normal performance of the PD patients observed by Flowers and associates (1984) might have arisen because those researchers used relatively long retention intervals (1–45 minutes) and, therefore, may have missed deficits in visual short-term memory. Sullivan and Sagar (1989) argued that impairments in short-term memory in association with relative sparing of long-term memory might be related to the clinical phenomenon of bradyphrenia (Chapter 7). A comparable pattern of relatively greater deficits on short-term than on long-term memory tests has been observed at times for verbal material in PD (Sagar et al, 1988b; Taylor et al, 1986), but this finding is by no means universal. Recent work by Bradley and associates (1989) suggests that speed of information processing deficits by PD patients may be especially prominent on visuospatial tasks. Thus, bradyphrenia may be more of a problem for these patients on nonverbal than on verbal tests.

Implicit Memory

Amnesic subjects perform poorly when asked to recall or recognize information experienced since the onset of the event that triggered their amnesia, but they often perform normally if memory can be displayed implicitly, without engaging conscious attempts at recollection. For example, on various types of priming tasks, a prior experience biases subsequent performance in a way that indicates that some fragment of the experience has been retained.

Heindel and colleagues (1989) studied pursuit rotor learning and lexical priming in PD, Huntington's disease, and Alzheimer's disease patients. The Huntington's disease patients showed normal priming but severely impaired pursuit rotor learning, and the Alzheimer's disease patients showed normal pursuit rotor learning but severely impaired priming. PD patients who performed normally on a mental status examination performed normally on both tasks, but mildly demented PD patients showed impaired priming and pursuit rotor learning. Unfortunately, Beatty and Monson (in press) were unable to replicate these findings with PD patients. They found that both demented and nondemented PD patients primed normally and showed normal pursuit rotor learning. In the same study, both groups of patients exhibited deficits on measures of explicit memory when they were asked to recognize words used on the priming task or facts about the pursuit rotor task acquired incidentally.

Saint-Cyr and associates (1988) compared the performance of PD, Huntington's disease, and amnesic patients on a cognitive task, the Tower of Toronto (TT), which they consider to be a measure of implicit procedural learning. On the TT, subjects must learn to rebuild a tower of four discs in the minimum number of moves allowed by the task rules. The PD patients performed normally on several measures of explicit recall and recognition memory but were impaired in learning the TT task. The amnesic patients were impaired on the explicit memory tasks but performed normally on the TT. Of the patients who were early in the course of Huntington's disease, there were two subgroups: one group resembled the PD patients, and the other resembled the amnesics. Despite this complication, Saint-Cyr and associates concluded that their results supported "the hypothesis that the neostriatum and associated structures belong to a circuit essential for the normal acquisition of cognitive procedures" (1988, p 951). Although this idea is not without appeal, the inconsistencies in the existing data preclude any firm conclusions about the role of the neostriatum in procedural learning or implicit memory. Instead, it may be useful to consider alternative explanations for the PD patients' difficulties on the TT. One possibility assumes that the TT is, in part, a test of spatial reasoning. If so, the deficits Saint-Cyr and colleagues (1988) observed in their nondemented PD patients may reflect disturbances in the same cognitive operations that lead to deficits on such tasks as Raven's Matrices, which have been observed consistently in demented PD patients (Huber et al, 1986b, 1989) and have not been considered failures of procedural learning.

ACCESS TO ESTABLISHED MEMORIES

Remote Memory

Most studies of remote memory in patients with subcortical diseases have used versions of the Albert Remote Memory battery, which requires identification of famous people from photographs and recall or recognition of past public events. With one exception (Sagar et al, 1988a), results have been remarkably consistent. Patients with PD (Freedman et al, 1984; Huber et al, 1986a), Huntington's disease (Albert et al, 1981; Beatty et al, 1988b), or multiple sclerosis (Beatty et al, 1988a, 1989b) exhibit remote memory deficits that are equally severe for all past decades. By contrast, Alzheimer's disease patients show marked overall impairments that are relatively less severe for knowledge of the distant past (Beatty et al, 1988b; Sagar et al, 1988a). Figure 4–2 illustrates typical findings for PD patients.

All studies are in agreement that deficits in remote memory are related to mental status. For PD patients, impairments are observed only if patients are mildly demented (Freedman et al, 1984; Huber et al, 1986a; Sagar et al, 1988a), but for multiple sclerosis patients, moderate remote memory deficits are evident even among patients of normal mental status (Beatty et al, 1988a, 1989b).

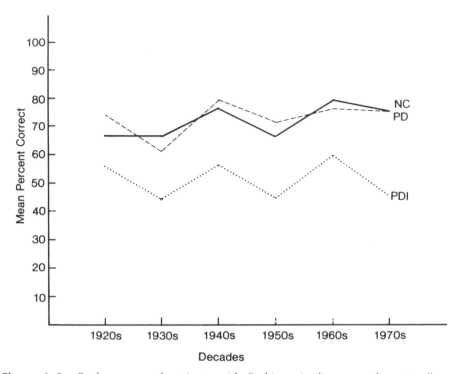

Figure 4–2. Performance of patients with Parkinson's disease without intellectual impairment (PD) and with intellectual impairment (PDI) and of normal controls (NC) on famous faces test. (From Huber et al., 1986a.)

Semantic Memory

Like patients with multiple sclerosis (Beatty et al, 1988a, 1989b) or Huntington's disease (Beatty et al, 1986), PD patients do not produce as many correct words as normal controls on verbal fluency tasks (e.g., name as many animals as possible in 1 minute). Such deficits are very mild among nondemented PD patients but are more severe if patients are mildly demented (Beatty et al, 1989d; Lees and Smith, 1983; Matison et al, 1982; Taylor et al, 1986).

Since verbal fluency tests measure the ability to access overlearned knowledge, deficits on such tests are likely to arise from difficulty in retrieving information. The flat temporal gradient of retrograde amnesia exhibited by PD patients on remote memory tests, retained capacity for normal semantic encoding, and the tendency to perform better on recognition than on recall tests of anterograde memory are consistent with the idea that the memory difficulties of PD patients are largely the result of retrieval failure.

In an influential article, Taylor and associates (1986) argued that the cognitive deficits in PD arise from impaired ability to generate efficient strategies when forced to rely on self-directed task-specific planning, which they attributed to disturbances in the flow of information between the neostriatum and the prefrontal cortex. With specific reference to memory functions, this hypothesis, in effect, maintains that PD patients are unable to formulate and deploy efficient strategies for memory retrieval.

Beatty and colleagues (1989c) tested this hypothesis by asking PD patients and controls to name as many items as possible that might be found in a supermarket. The instructions were designed to encourage the subjects to use the spatial arrangement of departments (e.g., fruits, meats) in a supermarket as the basis of an efficient search strategy. That is, high search efficiency would occur if a subject named various different fruits, then moved on to meats, and so on.

As expected, PD patients generated fewer correct items and searched less efficiently than did controls. However, search efficiency scores for the patients were related to measures that reflect access to semantic memory (i.e., letter and category fluency, naming) and not to measures of problem solving (i.e., categories achieved, perseverative responding on the Wisconsin Card Sorting Test). Thus, low search efficiency by PD patients appeared to be a consequence of impaired access to semantic memory and not the result of an inability to formulate and deploy an effective retrieval strategy. Similar results were obtained for multiple sclerosis patients in the same study (Beatty et al, 1989c).

Temporal Memory

Sagar and colleagues have shown that PD patients have particular difficulty making temporal judgments about events in memory. Such deficits have been observed for dating events in remote memory (Sagar et al, 1988b) as well as for relatively recent judgments involving both verbal and nonverbal stimuli (Sagar et al, 1988b; Sullivan and Sagar, 1989). These deficits in temporal memory may be secondary to a general impairment in both motor and cognitive sequencing, which has been demonstrated in PD (Beatty and Monson, unpublished observations; Sullivan et al, 1989). For PD patients, both motor and cognitive sequencing impairments were associated with difficulties on the Wisconsin Card Sorting Test (WCST) but not with performance of nonsequential motor acts or neurological measures of disability. Hence, the anatomical substrates for movement and sequencing appear to be different, and these systems may not be affected homogeneously in PD (Beatty and Monson, unpublished observations).

SUMMARY

The patterns of memory failure in PD, Huntington's disease, and multiple sclerosis are quite similar. On multitrial learning tasks, impairments are evident on the first acquisition trial, but patients generally improve at a nearly normal rate. On delayed recall, forgetting rates usually are normal and deficits on delayed recognition are typically modest, at least in comparison to the recall impairments. Because these characteristics are observed in PD patients who vary widely in overall mental status, the results encourage the view (Cummings, 1988; Huber et al, 1989) that cognitive disturbances in the dementias of PD and Alzheimer's disease can be differentiated. Since there is little evidence that encoding mechanisms are compromised in PD, multiple sclerosis, or Huntington's disease, the available evidence suggests that some sort of retrieval difficulty is responsible for the observed memory deficits in these diseases. The flat temporal gradient of retrograde amnesia observed on tests of remote memory also is consistent with this conclusion.

Because the pattern of memory disturbances and other cognitive changes is similar in PD, Huntington's disease, and multiple sclerosis, it is tempting to search for a common neurobiological mechanism. Dysfunction in the circuits that interconnect the midbrain, neostriatum, and areas of prefrontal cortex is one obvious possibility, and Taylor and colleagues (1986) have suggested that disturbances in frontal striatal function can account for all of the intellectual changes that occur early in the course of PD.

At present, attempts to test this and other similar hypotheses depend on comparisons in the neuropsychological performances of PD patients and patients with focal lesions of the frontal cortex (usually resulting from neurosurgical removal of tumors or seizure foci). Such patients vary enormously in the location and extent of their lesions as well as with respect to the nature and duration of the brain pathology that occasioned neurosurgical intervention (Stuss and Benson, 1986). Populations of patients with focal frontal lesions are not available to all investigators studying cognition in PD, precluding direct comparison of patient groups.

In the absence of such direct comparisons, investigators are forced to rely on tests, such as the WCST, to provide a benchmark of frontal lobe dysfunction. There are a number of serious difficulties with this strategy: (1) patterns of impairment on the WCST by patients with diffuse brain injury resemble those of patients with frontal lesions (Heaton, 1981), and, hence, poor performance on the WCST is not a specific sign of frontal dysfunction, (2) performance on the WCST by normal elderly people is highly variable (Heaton, 1981), which may be responsible for the fact that (3) patterns of impairment on the WCST and similar tests by nondemented PD patients vary from one study to another (see Beatty et al, 1989d, for review).

These considerations preclude any serious attempt to localize memory or other cognitive deficits in PD at present, especially since the pathophysiology of the disease is quite complicated (Cummings, 1988). However, rapid advances in neuroimaging techniques offer exciting possibilities for future studies (Chapter 12).

REFERENCES

Albert M, Butters N, Brandt J. Development of remote memory loss in patients with Huntington's disease. *J Clin Neuropsychol.* 1981;3:1–12.

Albert MS, Moss M. The assessment of memory disorders in patients with Alzheimer's disease. In: Squire LR, Butters N, eds. *Neuropsychology of Memory.* New York: Guilford Press; 1984;236–246.

Beatty WW, Butters N. Further analysis of encoding in patients with Huntington's disease. *Brain Cognition.* 1986;5:387–398.

Beatty WW, Butters N, Janowsky DS. Patterns of memory failure after scopolamine treatment: implications for cholinergic hypothesis of dementia. *Behav Neural Biol.* 1986;45:196–211.

Beatty WW, Goodkin DE, Beatty PA, Monson W. Frontal lobe dysfunction and memory impairment in patients with chronic progressive multiple sclerosis. *Brain Cognition.* 1989a;11:73–86.

Beatty WW, Goodkin DE, Monson N, Beatty PA. Cognitive disturbances in patients with relapsing remitting multiple sclerosis. *Arch Neurol.* 1989b;46:1113–1119.

Beatty WW, Goodkin DE, Monson N, et al. Anterograde and retrograde amnesia in patients with chronic progressive multiple sclerosis. *Arch Neurol.* 1988a;45:611–619.

Beatty WW, Monson N. Lexical priming and pursuit rotor learning in patients with Parkinson's disease. *Int J Clin Neuropsychol.* (in press).

Beatty WW, Monson N, Goodkin DE. Access to semantic memory in Parkinson's disease and multiple sclerosis. *J Geriatr Psychiatry Neurol.* 1989c;2:153–162.

Beatty WW, Salmon DP, Butters N, et al. Retrograde amnesia in patients with Alzheimer's disease or Huntington's disease. *Neurobiol Aging.* 1988b;9:181–186.

Beatty WW, Staton RD, Weir WS, et al. Cognitive disturbances in Parkinson's disease. *J Geriatr Psychiatry Neurol.* 1989d;2:22–33.

Bowen FP. Behavioral alterations in patients with basal ganglia lesions. In: Yahr ed. *The Basal Ganglia.* New York: Raven Press; 1976;169–184.

Bradley VA, Welch JL, Dick DJ. Visuospatial working memory in Parkinson's disease. *J Neurol Neurosurg Psychiatry.* 1989;52:1228–1235.

Cummings JL. Intellectual impairments in Parkinson's disease: clinical pathologic, and biochemical correlates. *J Geriatr Psychiatry Neurol.* 1988;1:24–36.

El-Awar M, Becker JT, Hammond KM, et al. Learning deficit in Parkinson's disease: comparison with Alzheimer's disease and normal aging. *Arch Neurol.* 1987;44:180–184.

Flowers KA, Pearce I, Pearce JMS. Recognition memory in Parkinson's disease. *J Neurol Neurosurg Psychiatry.* 1984;47:1174–1181.

Folstein MF, Folstein SE, McHugh PR. Mini-Mental State: A practical method for grading the cognitive state of patients for the clinician. *J Psychiatr Res.* 1975;12:189–198.

Freedman M, Rivoira P, Butters N, et al. Retrograde amnesia in Parkinson's disease. *Can J Neurol Sci.* 1984;11:297–301.

Heaton RK. *Wisconsin Card Sorting Test Manual.* Oderson, Florida: Psychological Assessment Resources; 1981.

Heindel WC, Salmon DP, Shults CW, et al. Neuropsychological evidence for multiple implicit memory systems: a comparison of Alzheimer's, Huntington's and Parkinson's disease patients. *J Neurosci.* 1989;9:582–587.

Helkala E-V, Laulumaa V, Soininen H, Riekkinen P. Recall and recognition memory in patients with Alzheimer's and Parkinson's diseases. *Ann Neurol.* 1988;24:214–217.

Huber SJ, Paulson GW. Memory impairments associated with progression of Huntington's disease. *Cortex.* 1987;23:275–283.

Huber SJ, Shuttleworth EC, Freidenberg DL. Neuropsychological differences between the dementias of Alzheimer's and Parkinson's diseases. *Arch Neurol.* 1989;46:1287–1291.

Huber SJ, Shuttleworth EC, Paulson GW. Dementia in Parkinson's disease. *Arch Neurol.* 1986a;43:987–990.

Huber SJ, Shuttleworth EC, Paulson GW, et al. Cortical vs subcortical dementia: neuropsychological differences. *Arch Neurol.* 1986b;43:392–394.

Lees AJ, Smith E. Cognitive deficits in the early stages of Parkinson's disease. *Brain.* 1983;106:257–270.

Matison R, Mayeaux R, Rosen J, Fahn S. "Tip-of-the-tongue" phenomenon in Parkinson's disease. *Neurology.* 1982;32:567–570.

Pirozzolo FJ, Hansch EC, Mortimer JA, et al. Dementia in Parkinson's disease: a neuropsychological analysis. *Brain Cognition.* 1982;1:71–83.

Riklan M, Whelihan W, Cullinan T. Levodopa and psychometric test performance in Parkinsonism—five years later. *Neurology.* 1976;26:172–179.

Sagar HJ, Cohen NJ, Sullivan EV, et al. Remote memory function in Alzheimer's disease and Parkinson's disease. *Brain.* 1988a;111:185–206.

Sagar HJ, Sullivan EV, Gabrieli JDE, et al. Temporal ordering and short-term memory deficits in Parkinson's disease. *Brain.* 1988b;111:525–539.

Sahakian BJ, Morris RG, Evenden JL, et al. A comparative study of visuospatial memory and learning in Alzheimer-type dementia and Parkinson's disease. *Brain.* 1988;111:695–718.

Saint-Cyr JA, Taylor AE, Lang AE. Procedural learning and neostriatal dysfunction in man. *Brain.* 1988;111:941–959.

Stuss DT, Benson DF. *The Frontal Lobes.* New York: Raven Press; 1986.

Sullivan EV, Sagar HJ. Non-verbal recognition and recency discrimination deficits in Parkinson's and Alzheimer's disease. *Brain.* 1989;112:1503–1517.

Sullivan EV, Sagar HJ, Gabrieli JDE, et al. Different cognitive profiles on standard behavioral tests in Parkinson's disease and Alzheimer's disease. *J Clin Exp Neuropsychol.* 1989;11:799–820.

Taylor AE, Saint-Cyr JA, Lang AE. Frontal lobe dysfunction in Parkinson's disease: The cortical focus of neostriatal outflow. *Brain.* 1986;109:845–883.

Tweedy JR, Langer KG, McDowell FH. The effect of semantic relations on the memory deficit associated with Parkinson's disease. *J Clin Neuropsychol.* 1982;4:235–247.

Villardita C, Smirni P, LePira F, et al. Mental deterioration, visuoperceptive disabilities and constructional apraxia in Parkinson's disease. *Acta Neurol Scand.* 1982;66:112–120.

Weingartner H, Burns S, Diebel R, LeWitt PA. Cognitive impairments in Parkinson's disease: distinguishing between effort-demanding and automatic cognitive processes. *Psychiatry Res.* 1984;11:223–235.

5

Visuospatial Abnormalities in Parkinson's Disease

JEFFREY L. CUMMINGS AND STEVEN J. HUBER

Humans exist in space, and survival depends on effective movement within a sensory space. The brain forms spatial maps using sensory information to guide activity. All exterosensory systems—visual, auditory, tactile—contribute to the construction of these maps. Humans have become particularly dependent on their sense of vision. Deficits of visuospatial abilities have a disproportionate impact on daily functions, and tests of visuospatial skills provide a telling means of detecting spatial compromise. Visuospatial abilities are complex, requiring integration of occipital, parietal, and frontal lobe functions as well as contributions from subcortical structures. Investigation of visuospatial skills in Parkinson's disease (PD) provides an avenue for gaining insight into subcortical and frontal–subcortical contributions to these activities.

In this chapter, a classification of visuospatial abilities is introduced, special issues in the evaluation of visuospatial skills in Parkinson's disease (PD) are summarized, evidence for visuospatial dysfunction in PD is reviewed, relationships between visuospatial changes and alterations in other cognitive and motor abilities are discussed, and the response of visuospatial abnormalities to treatment is described.

CLASSIFICATION OF VISUOSPATIAL ABILITIES

Table 5–1 presents a classification of visuospatial abilities. To provide a format for discussing visuospatial functions, they have been divided into visual sensory abilities, visual perceptual skills (discrimination and recognition), visuomotor abilities, visuospatial attention, visuospatial cognition, and body–spatial orientation. A classification of this type is necessarily somewhat arbitrary, introducing divisions of convenience into a seamless neurophysiological process. Nevertheless, all the domains identified require slightly different combinations of visual, motor, and cognitive abilities, and each is tested with different instruments. In addition, PD commonly affects some of these activities while leaving others intact.

METHODOLOGICAL ISSUES IN EVALUATION OF VISUOSPATIAL SKILLS IN PARKINSON'S DISEASE

Investigation and understanding of visuospatial abilities in PD have been hampered by a number of definitional, conceptual, and methodological problems. The most daunting of these issues has been the inevitable contamination of any test requiring a motor response by the PD motoric abnormalities. Visuomotor failures in PD may be attributed to the elementary motor difficulties or to an associated visuospatial deficit. When a motor response is a part of the test requirement, the patient's treatment, time since last dose, and relationship to the on/off phenomenon (if present) must be considered in the test interpretation. Recently, a number of investigators developed motor-free tasks either requiring no motor response or minimizing the dexterity, speed, and coordination demands of the task. These tests provide insight into the existence of visuospatial disturbances free of motor confounds. In addition, statistical techniques can be used to explore relationships between motor and visuospatial deficits and can help determine if spatial deficits are consistent in magnitude with or in excess of those attributable to motor abnormalities.

A related methodological issue concerns psychomotor slowing in PD. The performance subtests of the Wechsler Adult Intelligence Scale (WAIS, or revised form, WAIS-R) frequently are used to assess visuospatial abilities (Lezak, 1976). The performance subtests of the WAIS are timed, whereas the verbal subtests are not. Thus, PD patients may be penalized for slowness despite intact accuracy in visuospatial task responses. Timeliness of response is a crucial aspect of visuospatial ability and requires

Table 5–1.   Classification of visuospatial abilities

Visual sensory abilities
  Visual acuity
  Color vision
  Depth perception
Visuoperceptual abilities
  Discrimination
    Line orientation
    Facial matching (including facial
      expression matching)
    Embedded figures
  Recognition
    Right–left orientation
    Familiar faces
    Familiar places
Visuomotor abilities
  Drawing
  Figure reproduction
Visuospatial attention
  Spatial search
Visuospatial cognition
  Spatial anticipation
  Mental figure rotation and folding
  Visuospatial sequencing
  Prism adaptation
  Visual organization of parts to form a whole
  Perceptial abstraction
Body–spatial orientation
  Route finding
  Postural knowledge
  Body part identification

investigation, but untimed tests must be administered to allow a comprehensive evaluation of visuospatial skills in PD patients.

The presence of dementia is another important issue in the interpretation of visuospatial abnormalities in PD. Do visuospatial deficits characterize a distinct subgroup of PD patients with disproportionate or isolated impairment in this domain, or do they occur as part of a more generalized syndrome of multifaceted, if mild, cognitive deficits? As discussed in other chapters (3 and 11), dementia has been defined in a variety of ways, and different definitions include different populations of patients. Some patients exhibiting the syndrome of subcortical dementia (Cummings, 1986) may not meet all the criteria for dementia required by the revised third edition of the *Diagnostic and Statistical Manual of Mental Disorders* (DSM IIIR)(American Psychiatric Association, 1987). Thus, investigators implementing the concept of subcortical dementia might exclude specific individuals from studies concentrating on nondemented patients, whereas researchers adhering to DSM IIIR criteria might include them as nondemented. It is likely that some of the patients included as nondemented in studies of visuospatial deficits in PD manifested the syndrome of subcortical dementia.

PD dementia has several possible etiologies. Intellectual changes may be associated primarily with dopamine deficiency, cognitive alterations may stem from combined transmitter losses including dopamine and acetylcholine, and some patients may have mixed PD and Alzheimer's disease. There is currently no validated means of identifying these separate syndromes in the PD patient with cognitive compromise. Interpretation of the pathophysiological basis of visuospatial changes in PD patients with dementia must incorporate these contingencies.

Depression is also common in PD and mood changes might affect the speed, accuracy, and motivation to perform visuospatial tests. Assessment of mood changes as possible confounds to be included in interpretation of test performance is an important methodologic consideration in PD studies.

Parkinson's disease is a gradually progressive disorder, and new cognitive and visuospatial deficits might be expected to develop over the course of the illness just as motor system disturbances become more severe. Most studies have used average test scores derived from patient samples of mixed severity to investigate visuospatial function. This approach obscures the possible developmental pattern of visuospatial deficits in PD. Use of mixed severity samples may account for some of the discrepancies in the literature. Samples with more mildly affected patients may produce results differing from studies including a larger number of more advanced patients.

Finally, studies of normal individuals suggest that age, gender, handedness, and aspects of cognitive style (e.g., field dependence vs field independence) influence visuospatial task performance (Beaton, 1985; Bryden, 1982) and might be anticipated to affect studies of PD patients. There have been few investigations of these issues.

STUDIES OF VISUOSPATIAL PROCESSING IN PARKINSON'S DISEASE

Table 5–2 summarizes the most consistently reported abnormalities in the visuospatial test performance of PD patients. Performance abilities usually found to be normal also are noted.

Table 5–2. Summary of visuospatial tests applied in evaluation
of Parkinson's disease and results most consistently reported

Parameter	Result
Visual sensory abilities	
Visual acuity	Normal
Color vision	Normal
Depth perception	Normal
Electroretinography	Mildly delayed
Contrast sensitivity	Mildly abnormal
Visuoperceptual abilities	
Discrimination	
Rod orientation	Impaired
Line orientation	Impaired
Facial matching	Impaired
Detection of embedded figures	Impaired
Pattern matching	Impaired
Mosaic discrimination	Impaired
Recognition	
Right–left orientation	Normal
Familiar faces	Normal
Familiar places	Normal
Visuomotor abilities	
Figure drawing	Impaired
Figure copying	Impaired
Object assembly	Impaired
Block design	Impaired
Visuospatial attention	
Cancellation	Impaired
Line bisection	Impaired
Orienting response to cues	Impaired
Visuospatial cognition	
Perceptual abstraction (matrices)	Impaired
Mazes	Impaired
Picture arrangement	Impaired
Picture completion	Impaired
Visual organization	Mixed reports
Figure rotation	Impaired
Prism adaptation	Impaired
Body–spatial orientation	
Route finding	Impaired
Map reading	Impaired
Rod alignment judgment	Impaired
Body part identification	Impaired

Visual Sensory Function

Visual sensory function is normal in PD. Visual acuity, color perception, and depth
appreciation are unaffected. Electroretinography is normal or demonstrates mildly
increased response latencies (Jaffe et al, 1987; Kupersmith et al, 1982). Contrast sensitivity, a subtle measure of spatial vision, is disturbed. The abnormalities are insuffi-
cient to compromise acuity but conceivably could contribute subtly to the visuoper-

ceptual findings of PD (Mestre et al, 1990). Neuroophthalmological abnormalities, including decreased upgaze, hypometric saccades, and impaired convergence, have been documented in PD patients (Corin et al, 1972; White et al, 1988). These disturbances might slow visual search and produce diplopia on near vision but would not otherwise compromise visuospatial abilities.

Visual Perception

Visual perception may be divided into discrimination skills (the ability to analyze novel stimuli) and recognition skills (the ability to identify familiar visual stimuli). Visual recognition tasks involve memory for previously learned visual information as well as accurate visual perception and interpretation. Visual recognition skills are preserved in PD in the absence of overt dementia. Patients do not exhibit visual recognition deficits, such as agnosia, prosopagnosia, or environmental agnosia. Identification of famous faces is normal in nondemented PD patients, although it is impaired in PD patients with overt dementia (Freedman et al, 1984). Right–left orientation, another type of recognition task, is also intact in PD (Brown and Marsden, 1986).

Visual discrimination is compromised in PD. Boller and colleagues (1984) in a comprehensive assessment of visuospatial deficits demonstrated that PD patients with normal Verbal IQs manifested a variety of visuospatial deficits, including pattern matching-to-sample tests and line orientation tests. Goldenberg and associates (1986) also identified line orientation test abnormalities in PD patients. Girotti and co-workers (1988b) reported that when PD patients were divided into those with and those without dementia, the line orientation test was one of the few tasks that distinguished the nondemented PD patients from controls, whereas many tests differentiated the demented patients from controls. Levin and colleagues (1989, 1990), however, did not identify line orientation abnormalities in their mildly and moderately affected PD patients but did observe disturbances in facial discrimination and embedded figure tests. Patients with advanced disease failed the line orientation test. Thus, the line orientation test is often abnormal in PD but may be normal in patients with less advanced disease.

A variety of other visuospatial discrimination abnormalities have been noted in PD. Hovestadt and colleagues (1987) developed a rod orientation test that is particularly sensitive to visuoperceptual disturbances in PD. Forty-three of 44 early PD patients who had not yet been treated with levodopa were impaired on the test. Villardita and colleagues (1982) demonstrated that PD patients performed more poorly than controls on tests of figure-ground discrimination, perception of spatial positions, perception of constancy of shape and size, and perception of spatial relationships. No difference was found between PD patients with and without dementia on these tasks. PD patients have difficulty identifying which of several mosaics differs from others with closely related designs (Mohr et al, 1990) and perform abnormally on tests requiring them to match complex designs (Huber et al, 1986a,b; Pirozzolo et al, 1982). Similarly, PD patients have difficulty identifying specific figures embedded in more complex patterns (Levin et al, 1990). Facial discrimination (matching photographs of unfamiliar persons obtained at different camera angles) is impaired in PD (Hovestadt et al, 1987; Levin, 1990).

Visuomotor Abilities

Visuomotor skills depend on a motor response in the test situation. The tests usually require analyzing a visual stimulus and then reproducing it using motor executive (especially copying) skills. Riklan and Diller (1961) observed abnormalities on the Bender Gestalt drawing test in PD patients referred for thalamotomy. They attributed the abnormalities to visuospatial deficits rather than motor disturbances but did not adopt strategies to limit the potential impact of motor dysfunction. Villardita and co-workers (1982) documented more abnormalities in the drawings of PD patients than in those of controls. Qualitative evaluations of the drawings revealed that the patients exhibited distortions, misplacements, perseveration, rotations, omissions, and size errors not ascribable entirely to motor system disturbances. Globus and colleagues (1985) found that composite scores on drawing and copying tasks were lower in PD patients than in normal controls. Mohr and associates (1990) and Ogden and colleagues (1990) found that mildly cognitively impaired and nondemented PD patients performed more poorly than controls when copying the Rey-Osterrieth Complex Figure.

The performance subtests of the WAIS have been used frequently to assess visuomotor abilities. Block Design and Object Assembly require visuomotor skills. Hietanen and Teravainen (1988) found that patients with both early and late onset PD (onset under or over age 60 years, respectively) differed from age-matched controls on Block Design performance. Mohr and colleagues (1990) documented impairment on the Object Assembly subtest of the WAIS-R and noted that performance on this test was more abnormal than that of patients with Alzheimer's disease with similar overall severity of dementia. Levin and colleagues (1990) reported that even when the motor demands of the Block Design subtest were minimized and time constraints were removed, PD patients in the middle and late phases of the disease continued to perform more poorly than controls. Huber and co-workers (1990) also reported that untimed performance on the Block Design subtest of the WAIS-R was significantly impaired in PD patients compared to age-matched controls, and Brown and Marsden (1988) found PD patients to be significantly more impaired on Block Design than controls matched for performance on the Vocabulary subtest of the WAIS-R. Girotti and associates (1988b) reported significant differences between nondemented PD patients and controls on Block Design and Object Assembly subtests. A few studies failed to identify Block Design abnormalities in PD. Asso (1969) and Morris and colleagues (1988) reported no difference between PD patients and established norms or control performance for the WAIS Block Design subtest. The latter investigators, however, found abnormalities in the Object Assembly subtest in PD patients. Thus, a majority of investigations have shown deficits in Block Design in PD even when the motor demands and time constraints of the task were minimized. Similarly, drawing tests frequently reveal abnormalities in PD although these results may be more affected by motor disturbances.

Visual Attention

Visual attention refers to the active surveillance of visual space. A few studies have found that patients with left hemi-PD (right brain dysfunction) or bilateral PD tend to neglect the left side of space (Levin, 1990; Villardita et al, 1983). Ransmayr and colleagues (1987), however, were not able to demonstrate visual neglect in their PD patients.

Zazzo's test is a means of assessing visual attention by having patients cancel all items corresponding to two model figures in a specified period of time. Girotti and colleagues, in two separate studies (1986, 1988b), found nondemented PD patients to be significantly impaired on the task compared with normal controls.

Yamada and co-workers (1990) and Wright and colleagues (1990) demonstrated abnormalities in response to preparatory visual cues in PD patients engaged in visual search tasks.

Visuospatial Cognition

Visuospatial cognition requires an active mental manipulation of a visual stimulus in order to produce an accurate test response. The tasks are more complex than the more elementary matching tasks of visual discrimination or the copying response of the visuomotor tasks. The Picture Completion and Picture Arrangement subtests of the WAIS-R are used frequently to assess this type of intellectual ability. Asso (1969) and Reitan and Boll (1971) were among the first to report that Picture Arrangement was significantly impaired in PD compared to expected levels of performance. Mohr and colleagues (1990) found that PD patients (most of whom had mild cognitive impairment on tests of intelligence) exhibited deficits on Picture Completion and Picture Arrangement subtests. Hietanen and Teravainen (1988) found that patients with early-onset PD differed from age-matched controls the Picture Completion subtests of the WAIS-R, and late-onset PD patients were significantly more impaired on Picture Arrangement than were early-onset patients. Beatty and Monson (1990) developed a simplified picture arrangement test and were still able to demonstrate a difference between PD patients and normal controls in the ability to sequence the pictures correctly to produce a coherent story. The cognitive abilities involved in sequencing a group of pictures into a logical series appear to be compromised in PD and the test is particularly well suited to detecting the visuospatial–cognitive disturbances of PD patients.

Mental rotation and reconstruction tasks require that patients mentally visualize how an object or shape would appear if it were rotated or folded. The tests require no motor response. Oyebode and co-workers (1986) found that a visuospatial imagery test requiring patients to mentally reconstruct a three-dimensional image from a line drawing was performed more poorly by PD patients than by controls. Ransmayr and colleagues (1987) administered the Rybakoff Figure Test, a task requiring mental rotation and reconstruction, to PD patients and found them to be significantly impaired compared to control subjects. These observations are particularly compelling because the PD patients were matched to controls for other types of visuospatial abilities. Ogden and colleagues (1990) reported that PD patients were as accurate as controls on a mental folding test, but it took them significantly longer to complete the task.

Spatial anticipation tests require the patient to fill in missing elements of complex patterns. The task has motor as well as spatial forecast elements. Stern and co-workers (1983, 1984) found that PD patients had more difficulty than controls on the test and that the test was more closely related to constructional than motor abnormalities.

Della Sala and co-workers (1986), however, were not able to demonstrate abnormalities in PD patients using a similar directional forecast test.

Raven's Progressive Matrices require the patient to choose a pattern from among several alternatives that will complete a specified spatial array. The test is not timed and requires no motor response. Piccirilli and colleagues (1984) reported an age relationship with performance on Progressive Matrices in PD. They found that 32 percent of patients 49 to 59 years of age, 37 percent of PD patients 60 to 69 years of age, and 60 percent of patients age 70 to 79 years old failed the test. Similarly, Dubois and colleagues (1990) noted that patients with onset of PD after age 65 years were more impaired on Raven's Matrices than were those whose disease began before age 45 years. Both groups were more impaired than age-matched controls. Huber and associates (1986b) demonstrated that PD patients performed significantly worse than matched controls on the test. There was no difference between the performance of PD patients meeting criteria for dementia and those who did not.

The Hooper Visual Organization Test is used to assess the ability of patients to mentally synthesize visual components into a complete figure. Use of this test in PD patients has produced variable results. Boller and colleagues (1984) found no difference between PD and control subjects on the Hooper Visual Organization Test, although Globus and associates (1985) observed that PD patients were significantly more impaired than normal controls. In the latter study, 14 of 48 PD patients met criteria for dementia. Levin and colleagues (1990) reported visual organization abnormalities in middle and late stage patients but not in those in the early phases of their disease.

A variety of other tests have been designed to assess visuospatial cognition. PD patients performed more poorly than controls when reading a standardized street map (Mohr et al, 1990). Beatty and Monson (1989) found that nondemented PD patients had more difficulty locating cities on United States maps compared to controls and demented PD patients were impaired on attempts to locate United States cities, regional cities, and gross geographical features. Canavan and co-workers (1990) demonstrated that PD patients took significantly longer to adapt to prism glasses that distorted perception than did age-matched controls. Their performance resembled that of patients with right frontal lobe lesions, and the test scores correlated with frontal tests, such as the Wisconsin Card Sort Test. A more complex result was reported by Stern and colleagues (1988) in their tests of prism adaptation in PD. They found that patients adapted as readily as controls, but there was a more rapid loss of adaptation aftereffects in PD patients. Dubois and colleagues (1990) found that PD patients were significantly more impaired on a test requiring identification of 15 superimposed images compared with controls, and those with onset of PD after age 65 were more impaired than were those whose disease began before age 45. Taylor and colleagues (1986) likewise found that PD patients took significantly longer to disambiguate superimposed figures than did normal controls, although the accuracy of their responses was normal.

Taken together, these observations indicate that visuospatial cognition is abnormal in PD and that these disturbances can be demonstrated in motor-free tasks. Picture Arrangement, mental rotation, Raven's Matrices, and map-reading tests are the instruments most likely to demonstrate these deficits.

Body–Spatial Orientation

Body–spatial orientation refers to the special class of abnormalities described in PD in which the patient's personal orientation in the environment is compromised. Parkinson's disease patients have difficulty determining when a rod is vertical if they are in a darkened room. This abnormality has been shown both in patients seated in a chair that is tilted to the right or left (Proctor et al, 1964; Levin, 1990) and in patients who are upright (Danta and Hilton, 1975). This test is failed also by patients with frontal lobe lesions. Route-walking guided by a map has been shown to be impaired in PD patients (Bowen et al, 1972). Moreover, the test is selectively sensitive to those with bilateral and right brain dysfunction (left hemi-PD) and not those with left brain dysfunction. Likewise, patients with right brain dysfunction and bilateral disease did significantly worse than controls and PD patients with left brain dysfunction on a test of body scheme identification (Bowen et al, 1976).

RELATIONSHIP OF VISUOSPATIAL ABNORMALITIES TO OTHER ASPECTS OF PARKINSON'S DISEASE

Correlations between visuospatial deficits and severity of motor abnormalities, Hoehn and Yahr stage, and predominant side of motor disturbance have been examined. With regard to severity of motor impairments, Riklan and Diller (1961) found that scores on the Bender Gestalt drawing test were worse in patients with greater tremor, rigidity, bradykinesia, autonomic nervous system involvement, and mental impairment (excluding overt dementia). In a more rigorous study, Riklan and co-workers (1962) found statistically significant correlations between rigidity and several scored aspects of human figure drawings. Danta and Hilton (1975) observed relationships between the rod alignment test and degree of patient rigidity and tremor but not with bradykinesia. Mortimer and colleagues (1982) found a significant correlation between both timed and untimed visuospatial test performance and bradykinesia. There were no correlations with tremor or rigidity and the correlations remained significant after controlling for age and age at onset of PD. Goldenberg and associates (1986) identified correlations between performance on the Picture Completion subtest of the WAIS-R and overall severity of motor disability. Girotti and co-workers (1988a) found significant correlations between reaction and movement times and scores on the Block Design and Object Assembly subtests of the WAIS-R. When adjusted for reaction times, differences between subtest scores of PD patients and controls were no longer significant. Hovestadt and colleagues (1987, 1988) found no correlation between performance on their rod orientation test and age, length of illness, Verbal IQ, Hoehn and Yahr stage, motor scale score, or disability score before levodopa treatment. Moreover, no improvement occurred after initiation of therapy. Ransmayr and associates (1987) identified no differences in figure rotation or line cancellation performance among patients with akinetic–rigid, tremor dominant, or combined types of PD. Globus and colleagues (1985) observed no correlation between cerebral blood flow and neuropsychological deficits, including visuospatial alterations, in PD. Levin and co-workers (1990) found a progressive evolution of visuospatial deficits, with mildly affected patients performing abnormally on embedded figure and facial discrimination tests. Moderately affected patients failed the visual organization tests, Block Design subtest, facial discrimination, and embedded figures tests, and patients with advanced disease failed on all these measures plus the line orientation test. Thus, correlations between visuospatial and motor deficits have been inconsistent. Bradykinesia is the abnormality most often associated with disturbances in visuospatial performance.

Similarly, patients in more advanced Hoehn and Yahr stages usually have been found to have more evident visuospatial deficits. Boller and colleagues (1984) found that patients in Hoehn and Yahr stage 3 did more poorly on motor-free visuospatial tasks than did patients in stage 1 or 2. Huber and associates (1989a) found that PD patients in Hoehn and Yahr stages 1 and 2 had mean Block Design subtests scores indistinguishable from controls but that patients in stages 3 and 4 demonstrated significant impairment on the test. No time constraints were imposed on the performance.

Unilateral onset and asymmetry in severity of PD are not unusual, and it might be predicted that patients with greater left-sided PD (more right brain dysfunction) would have more visuospatial deficits than patients with right-sided PD and left brain involvement. Bowen and colleagues (1972) found support for this hypothesis, noting that patients with left-sided or bilateral PD performed abnormally on a map-reading and route-walking test, whereas those with right-sided PD performed at control levels. Direnfeld and associates (1984) also identified supporting data in their study of asymmetrical PD. Using a composite score of copying, drawing, and visual organization tests, they found that patients with left hemi-PD performed significantly worse than those with right-sided PD. Spicer and colleagues (1988), however, observed no difference between patients with left and right-sided PD on tests of facial discrimination or line orientation. Similarly, Blonder and associates (1989) reported that both left-sided and right-sided PD patients were impaired on line orientation and Block Design tests, but there was no significant difference in the level of impairment. Huber and co-workers (1989b) found no difference on Block Design or Progressive Matrices scores between patients with left or right unilateral PD, and no difference between patients with bilateral but right-predominant or left-predominant PD. Several studies of line bisection have shown that patients with left-dominant PD may show mild left-sided spatial neglect (Levin, 1990; Starkstein et al, 1987; Villardita et al, 1983).

Treatment with levodopa has been found to have no or only modest effects on visuospatial function in PD. Where effects were found, they usually involved visuomotor functions and may be attributable to improved motor performance. Meier and Martin (1970) documented significant improvement in maze performance after treatment with levodopa. Beardsley and Puletti (1971) reported significant improvement in Block Design, Picture Arrangement, and Object Assembly subtests of the WAIS 1 and 6 months after treatment compared with pretreatment performance levels. Fisher and Findley (1981) also reported improved Block Design performance 6 months and 2 years after initiation of levodopa treatment compared with baseline values. Levin and colleagues (1990) found higher scores on line orientation, embedded figures, and Block Design in patients treated with anitcholinergic agents. Levodopa treatment has little impact on the speed of visuospatial task performance in PD. Pillon and associates (1989) documented correlations between performance on a 15-item overlapping figure test and severity of disability in PD. No changes were observed when the patients were tested on and off levodopa.

COMMENT

Abnormalities of visuospatial function are common in PD. Although not all studies yield identical results, the majority of investigations provide evidence of dysfunction in several domains of visuospatial ability. In some cases, these alterations reflect the motor disorder of PD, but visuospatial deficits are demonstrable also on motor-free tasks. The lack of consistent relationships between visuospatial and motor distur-bances also supports the hypothesis that the deficits are not entirely motoric in origin. The presence of frontal systems disturbances and bradyphrenia in PD (see chapters 6 and 7) suggests that some of the visuospatial performance deficits can be ascribed to poor strategy and planning and psychomotor retardation. This may be particularly true for visuomotor abnormalities, visual cognitive failures, and deficits on tests with time constraints. The existence of disturbances on elementary untimed tests, such as the line orientation test and matching-to-sample tasks, however, indicates that vis-uoperceptual abnormalities may also contribute to the visuospatial compromise of PD.

A pattern of progression of visuospatial deficits emerges from review of the existing studies. Rod orientation tests may show the earliest abnormalities and be most sensi-tive to mild visuospatial deficits. In the middle phases of the illness, line orientation, Block Design, and Picture Arrangement tests are failed. In the final stages, facial dis-crimination also is impaired. Not all abilities are affected simultaneously, and some skills (such as right–left orientation) are spared throughout most of the disease course.

A spectrum of severity of compromised visuospatial function has been demon-strated. The deficits do not correlate well with motor function. Some abnormalities (e.g., rod orientation) are evident early in the disease before treatment, and others are consistently more apparent in patients in more advanced stages of the illness. Identi-fication of visuospatial deficits has not been shown to predict prognosis or treatment response. Evidence for a distinct subgroup of PD patients with a prominent visuospa-tial syndrome is not compelling at present.

Some patients with PD and dementia are suffering from co-occurring Alzheimer's disease (Gaspar and Gray, 1984). There is currently no widely accepted means of iden-tifying this subgroup of patients. Visuospatial investigations may help investigators recognize this important subtype of mixed dementias. Huber and colleagues (1989c), for example, observed that patients with Alzheimer's disease had significantly poorer Block Design performance and better Progressive Matrices scores than PD patients, whereas the reverse pattern was observed in PD patients (better Block Design and worse Progressive Matrices than Alzheimer's disease patients). This may reflect the more severe posterior hemispheric changes in Alzheimer's disease and the more severe frontal systems involvement in PD. Examination of the relationship between tasks requiring frontal systems planning and parietal constructional skills may provide insight into the type of disease present.

The lack of response of visuospatial deficits to dopamine replacement therapy, the general absence of correlations between motor and visuospatial function, and the failure of visuospatial performance to change during on and off episodes all suggest that the dopamine deficit in PD is not primarily responsible for the visuospatial abnormalities or that the dopamine deficit is combined with other pathological or neurochemical changes to produce this class of deficits.

Assessment of visuospatial dysfunction in PD reveals an important domain of cognitive dysfunction, indicates an important role for frontal systems in visuospatial skills, and may help identify patients with combined PD and Alzheimer's disease.

ACKNOWLEDGMENTS

This project was supported by the Department of Veterans Affairs.

REFERENCES

American Psychiatric Association. *Diagnostic and Statistical Manual of Mental Disorders,* revised 3rd ed. Washington, DC: American Psychiatric Press; 1987.

Asso D. WAIS scores in a group of Parkinson patients. *Br J Psychiatry.* 1969;115:555–556.

Beardsley JV, Puletti F. Personality (MMPI) and cognitive (WAIS) changes after levodopa treatment. *Arch Neurol.* 1971;25:145–150.

Beaton A. *Left Side Right Side. A Review of Laterality Research.* New Haven, CT: Yale University Press; 1985.

Beatty WW, Monson N. Geographical knowledge in patients with Parkinson's disease. *Bull Psychonomic Soc.* 1989;27:473–475.

Beatty WW, Monson N. Picture and motor sequencing in Parkinson's disease. *J Geriatr Psychiatry Neurol.* 1990;3:192–197.

Blonder LX, Gur RE, Gur RC, et al. Neuropsychological functioning in hemiparkinsonism. *Brain Cogn.* 1989;9:244–257.

Boller F, Passafiume D, Keefe NC, et al. Visuospatial impairment in Parkinson's disease. Role of perceptual and motor factors. *Arch Neurol.* 1984;41:485–490.

Bowen FP, Burns MM, Brady EM, Yahr MD. A note on alterations of personal orientation in parkinsonism. *Neuropsychologia.* 1976;14:425–429.

Bowen FP, Hoehn MM, Yahr MD. Parkinsonism: alterations in spatial orientation as determined by a route-walking test. *Neuropsychologia.* 1972;10:355–361.

Brown RG, Marsden CD. Internal versus external cues and the control of attention in Parkinson's disease. *Brain.* 1988;111:323–345.

Brown RG, Marsden CD. Visuospatial function in Parkinson's disease. *Brain.* 1986;109:987–1002.

Bryden MP. *Laterality. Functional Asymmetry in the Intact Brain.* New York: Academic Press; 1982.

Canavan AGM, Passingham RE, Marsden CD, et al. Prism adaptation and other tasks involving spatial abilities in patients with Parkinson's disease, patients with frontal lobe lesions and patients with unilateral temporal lobectomies. *Neuropsychologia.* 1990;28:969–984.

Corin MS, Elizan TS, Bender MB. Oculomotor function in patients with Parkinson's disease. *J Neurol Sci.* 1972;15:251–265.

Cummings JL. Subcortical dementia. Neuropsychology, neuropsychiatry, and pathophysiology. *Br J Psychiatry.* 1986;149:682–697.

Danta G, Hilton RC. Judgment of the visual vertical and horizontal in patients with parkinsonism. *Neurology.* 1975;25:43–47.

Della Sala S, De Lorenzo G, Giodano A, Spinnler H. Is there a specific visuo-spatial impairment in Parkinsonians? *J Neurol Neurosurg Psychiatry.* 1986;49:1258–1265.

Direnfeld LK, Albert ML, Volicer L, et al. Parkinson's disease. The possible relationship of laterality to dementia and neurochemical findings. *Arch Neurol.* 1984;41:935–941.

Dubois B, Pillon B, Sternic N, Lhermitte F, Agid Y. Age-induced cognitive disturbances in Parkinson's disease. *Neurology.* 1990;40:38–41.

Fisher K, Findley L. Intellectual changes in optimally treated patients with Parkinson's disease. In: Rose FC, Capildeo R, eds. *Research Progress in Parkinson's Disease.* Tunbridge Wells, England: Pitman Medical; 1981:53–60.

Freedman M, Rivoira P, Butters N, et al. Retrograde amnesia in Parkinson's disease. *Can J Neurol Sci.* 1984;11:297–301.

Gaspar P, Gray F. Dementia in idiopathic Parkinson's disease. *Acta Neuropathol.* 1984;64:43–52.

Girotti F, Carella F, Pia Grassi M, et al. Motor and cognitive performances of parkinsonian patients in the on and off phases of the disease. *J Neurol Neurosurg Psychiatry.* 1986;49:657–660.

Girotti F, Soliveri P, Carella F, et al. Role of motor performance in cognitive processes of parkinsonian patients. *Neurology.* 1988a;38:537–540.

Girotti F, Soliveri P, Carella F, et al. Dementia and cognitive impairment in Parkinson's disease. *J Neurol Neurosurg Psychiatry.* 1988b;51:1498–1502.

Globus M, Mildworf B, Melamed E. Cerebral blood flow and cognitive impairment in Parkinson's disease. *Neurology.* 1985;35:1135–1139.

Goldenberg G, Wimmer A, Auff E, Schnaberth G. Impairment of motor planning in patients with Parkinson's disease: evidence from ideomotor apraxia testing. *J Neurol Neurosurg Psychiatry.* 1986;49:1266–1272.

Hietanen M, Teravainen H. The effect of age of disease onset on neuropsychological performance in Parkinson's disease. *J Neurol Neurosurg Psychiatry.* 1988;51:244–249.

Hovestadt A, De Jong GJ, Meerwaldt JD. Spatial disorientation in Parkinson's disease: no effect of levodopa substitution therapy. *Neurology.* 1988;38:1802–1803.

Hovestadt A, de Jong GJ, Meerwaldt JD. Spatial disorientation as an early symptom of Parkinson's disease. *Neurology.* 1987;37:485–487.

Huber SJ, Shuttleworth EC, Friedenberg DL. Neuropsychological differences between the dementias of Alzheimer's and Parkinson's diseases. *Arch Neurol.* 1989c;46:1287–1291.

Huber SJ, Shuttleworth EC, Paulson GW. Dementia in Parkinson's disease. *Arch Neurol.* 1986b;43:987–990.

Huber SJ, Shuttleworth EC, Christy JA, Rice RR. A brief scale for the dementia of Parkinson's disease. *J Neuropsychiatry Clin Neurosci.* 1990;2:183–188.

Huber SJ, Friedenberg DL, Shuttleworth EC, et al. Neuropsychological impairments associated with severity of Parkinson's disease. *J Neuropsychiatry Clin Neurosci.* 1989a;1:154–158.

Huber SJ, Friedenberg DL, Shuttleworth EC, et al. Neuropsychological similarities in lateralized parkinsonism. *Cortex.* 1989b;25:461–470.

Huber SJ, Shuttleworth EC, Paulson GW, et al. Cortical vs subcortical dementia: neuropsychological differences. *Arch Neurol.* 1986a;43:392–394.

Jaffe MJ, Bruno G, Campbell G, et al. Ganzfeld electroretinographic findings in Parkinsonism: untreated patients and the effect of levodopa intravenous infusion. *J Neurol Neurosurg Psychiatry.* 1987;50:847–852.

Kupersmith MJ, Shakin E, Siegel IM, Lieberman A. Visual system abnormalities in patients with Parkinson's disease. *Arch Neurol.* 1982;39:284–286.

Levin BE. Spatial cognition in Parkinson disease. *Alzheimer Dise Assoc Disord.* 1990;4:161–170.

Levin BE, Llabre MM, Weiner WJ. Cognitive impairments associated with early Parkinson's disease. *Neurology.* 1989;39:557–561.

Levin BE, Llabre MM, Ansley J, et al. Do parkinsonians exhibit visuospatial deficits? In: Streifler MB, Korczyn ADS, Melamed E, Yardin MBH, eds. *Advances in Neurology. Parkinson's Disease: Anatomy, Pathology, and Therapy,* vol 53. New York: Raven Press; 1990:311–315.

Lezak MD. *Neuropsychological Assessment.* New York: Oxford University Press; 1976.

Meier MJ, Martin WE. Intellectual changes associated with levodopa therapy. *JAMA.* 1970;213:465–466.

Mestre D, Blin O, Serratrice G, Pailhouse J. Spatiotemporal contrast sensitivity differs in normal aging and Parkinson's disease. *Neurology.* 1990;40:1710–1714.

Mohr E, Litvan I, Williams J, et al. Selective deficits in Alzheimer and Parkinsonian dementia: visuospatial function. *Can J Neurol Sci.* 1990;17:292–297.

Morris RG, Downes JJ, Sahakian BJ, et al. Planning and spatial working memory in Parkinson's disease. *J Neurol Neurosurg Psychiatry.* 1988;51:757–766.

Mortimer JA, Pirozzolo FJ, Hansch EC, Webster DD. Relationship of motor symptoms to intellectual deficits in Parkinson's disease. *Neurology.* 1982;32:133–137.

Ogden JA, Growdon JH, Corkin S. Deficits on visuospatial tests involving forward planning in high-functioning parkinsonians. *Neuropsychiatry Neuropsychol Behav Neurol.* 1990;3:125–139.

Oyebode JR, Barker WA, Blessed G, et al. Cognitive functioning in Parkinson's disease: in relation to prevalence of dementia and psychiatric diagnosis. *Br J Psychiatry.* 1986;149:720–725.

Piccirilli M, Piccinin L, Agostini L. Characteristic clinical aspects of Parkinson patients with intellectual impairment. *Eur Neurol.* 1984;23:44–50.

Pillon B, Dubois B, Bonnet A-M, et al. Cognitive slowing in Parkinson's disease fails to respond to levodopa treatment: the 15-objects test. *Neurology.* 1989;39:762–768.

Pirozzolo FJ, Hansch EC, Mortimer JA, et al. Dementia in Parkinson disease: a neuropsychological analysis. *Brain Cogn.* 1982;1:71–83.

Proctor F, Riklan M, Cooper IS, Teuber H-L. Judgment of visual and postural vertical by parkinsonian patients. *Neurology.* 1964;14:287–293.

Ransmayr G, Schmidhuber-Eiler B, Karamat E, et al. Visuoperception and visuospatial and visuorotational performance in Parkinson's disease. *J Neurol.* 1987;235:99–101.

Reitan RM, Boll TJ. Intellectual and cognitive functions in Parkinson's disease. *J Consult Clin Psychol.* 1971;37:364–369.

Riklan M, Diller L. Visual motor performance before and after chemosurgery of the basal ganglia in parkinsonism. *J Nerv Ment Dis.* 1961;132:307–314.

Riklan M, Zahn TP, Diller L. Human figure drawings before and after chemosurgery of the basal ganglia in parkinsonism. *J Nerv Ment Dis.* 1962;135:500–506.

Spicer KB, Roberts RJ, LeWitt PA. Neuropsychological performance in lateralized parkinsonism. *Arch Neurol.* 1988;45:429–432.

Starkstein S, Leigurda R, Gershank O, Berthier M. Neuropsychological disturbances in hemiparkinson's disease. *Neurology.* 1987;37:1762–1764.

Stern Y, Mayeux R, Rosen J. Contribution of perceptual motor dysfunction to construction and tracing disturbances in Parkinson's disease. *J Neurol Neurosurg Psychiatry.* 1984;47:983–989.

Stern Y, Mayeux R, Hermann A, Rosen J. Prism adaptation in Parkinson's disease. *J Neurol Neurosurg Psychiatry.* 1988;51:1584–1587.

Stern Y, Mayeux R, Rosen J, Ilson J. Perceptual motor dysfunction in Parkinson's disease: a deficit in sequential and predictive voluntary movement. *J Neurol Neurosurg Psychiatry.* 1983;46:145–151.

Taylor AE, Saint-Cyr JA, Lang AE. Frontal lobe dysfunction in Parkinson's disease: the cortical focus of neostriatal outflow. *Brain.* 1986;109:845–883.

Villardita C, Smirni P, Zappala G. Visual neglect in Parkinson's disease. *Arch Neurol.* 1983;40:737–739.

Villardita C. Smirni P, Le Pira F, et al. Mental deterioration, visuoperceptive disabilities and constructional praxis in Parkinson's disease. *Acta Neurol Scand.* 1982;66:112–120.

White OB, Saint-Cyr JA, Tomlinson RD, Sharpe JA. Ocular motor deficits in Parkinson's disease. III. Coordination of eye and head movements. *Brain.* 1988;111:115–129.

Wright MJ, Burns RJ, Gefen GM, Gefen LB. Covert orientation of visual attention in Parkinson's disease: an impairment in the maintenance of attention. *Neuropsychologia.* 1990;28:151–159.

Yamada T, Izuyuinn M, Schulzer M, Hirayama K. Covert orienting attention in Parkinson's disease. *J Neurol Neurosurg Psychiatry.* 1990;53:593–596.

6

Executive Function

ANN E. TAYLOR AND JEAN A. SAINT-CYR

When we consider the executive functions of the brain, we are speaking of the final stage of information processing in which external sensory input and interoceptive signals are integrated to determine a course of action. Anatomically, the posterior cortical areas (temporal, occipital, and parietal lobes) are largely concerned with the reception and initial analysis of auditory, visual, and tactile input. This information is received, identified, and mapped onto past experience for *goodness of fit*. If such input is in register with past experience and therefore easily understood, little effortful processing is required to select an appropriate response. In this case, strategic planning and goal monitoring, two of the higher order executive functions, are minimally challenged.

Demands on the planning and monitoring operations of the brain, however, change markedly when the environment presents a novel problem. Under these circumstances, familiar routines no longer suffice. According to Luria (1980), the creation of complex as opposed to routine behavioral programs involves the selection of salient sensory input, the planning and sequencing of motor output, and the constant updating of performance against original purpose. Descriptively, Lezak (1983) refers to such comprehensive and sophisticated mental activities as "the executive functions" of the brain. These include, but are not limited to, focused and sustained attention, fluency and flexibility of thought in the generation of solutions to novel problems, and the planning and regulating of adaptive goal-directed activity. Anatomically, there is mounting experimental and clinical evidence that the executive functions are the domain of the prefrontal cortical region, the final staging area of information processing before action (Glosser and Goodglass, 1990).

If one wishes to study the executive branch of behavior, clarification of the major subroutines supporting purposeful activity is critical. Whereas the principles governing the functions of the temporal, occipital, and sensorimotor zones are "reasonably well-known" (Luria, 1980), the nature of the supraordinate functions mediated by the frontal lobes and the principles that guide their activity are less well understood. Indeed, until the middle of this century, the frontal lobes were considered to be silent zones within the cerebral cortex, having no clearly defined purpose. Thanks to Milner and Petrides (1984), Goldman-Rakic (1987), Fuster (1980), Stuss and Benson (1986), and others, this situation is beginning to change.

Before considering the various routines that comprise executive function, their relevance to Parkinson's disease (PD) must be identified. PD mainly affects the physiological integrity of the basal ganglia, a complex neural network lying just below the cortex and intimately connected with it. If one follows the anatomical organization of the basal ganglia and its afferent and efferent pathways, as described by Alexander and colleagues (1986), it is apparent that widespread cortical input is processed in this region. Eventually, via sequential relay mechanisms, the product of processing within the multiple, segregated, and partially closed corticobasal ganglia loops is returned to subregions within the frontal lobes (Fig. 6–1).

Put simply, sensorimotor information, arriving from the sensorimotor cortex, undergoes transformation in the putamen, one of the major subdivisions of the neo-striatal portion of the basal ganglia. Output is relayed eventually to the supplementary motor area on the mesial surface of the frontal lobes. In contrast, nonmotor information, arriving from association areas within the cortical regions, is transformed within the caudate nucleus for eventual return to the prefrontal cortex. Accordingly, considerable information necessary to the formation of behavioral action plans is pro-cessed within the area of the brain most affected by PD and incorporated into the exec-utive decisions that determine response–selection. For this reason, a number of researchers have questioned to what extent PD may disrupt the abilities to plan and to regulate behavior.

Understandably, the programming and execution of motor activity have received considerable attention in this disorder. More recently, attention has turned to the non-motor area, which, for lack of a better term, has been labeled *complex* (i.e., nonmotor in nature) (DeLong et al, 1983). The term *cognitive* (replacing *complex*) generally refers to all the conscious processes involved in thought. However, it is possible that some nonmotor activity may occur at a subcognitive level, that is, independent of con-scious direction. In our view, subcognitive processes, particularly those engaged in the establishment of new behavioral routines, may rely heavily on the integrity of the basal

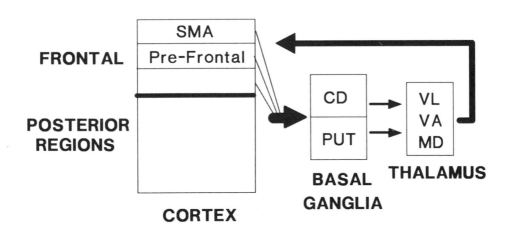

SMA - supplementary motor area   VL - ventralis lateralis
CD - caudate nucleus   VA - ventralis anterior
PUT - putamen   MD - medialis dorsalis

Figure 6–1. Corticobasal ganglia partially closed feedback system.

ganglia (Taylor et al, 1990a). In this case, adaptation to novel environmental contingencies would pose a problem for patients with basal ganglia disease. The failure would be executive in nature as opposed to more purely sensory or motor.

HISTORICAL PERSPECTIVES

Until Nauta's discovery (1964) of massive links between the prefrontal cortex and the basal ganglia, little thought was given to the possibility of more than motor consequences in PD. Indeed, James Parkinson declared that "the senses and the intellect remain uninjured." However, Proctor and colleagues, in 1964, began to compare the behavior of PD patients and patients with damage to the frontal lobes on a variety of cognitive tests. The deficits in both groups were highly similar. Follow-up studies in subhuman primates (where ablation could produce lesions within either the frontal lobes or their basal ganglia projection sites) supported this observation. Interestingly, wherever impairment on a specific cognitive test followed lesion within the dorsolateral or orbital frontal cortex, a comparable deficit emerged following lesion of the specific basal ganglia region to which these areas of the frontal lobes project (Johnson et al, 1968; Divac, 1972). Rosvold (1972), impressed with the consistency of such observations, hypothesized that the prefrontal cortex and the basal ganglia function together in a serial cortical-to-subcortical-to-spinal cord sequence. In his view, disruption at either the cortical or subcortical level would interfere with behavior originating in the frontal lobes, relayed (as he presumed) through the basal ganglia to the effector system. Given the experimental paradigms popular in those days, the behaviors perceived to be at risk in basal ganglia disease were short-term memory (delayed response tasks) and impulse control (go, no/go tasks).

As mentioned, however, more recent research has shown that, far from acting in a serial manner, the frontal cortex and the basal ganglia participate in a partially closed feedback loop system, where the majority of information processed within the basal ganglia is returned exclusively to the frontal area. Given that the frontal cortex is also in receipt of a vast amount of information arriving from other cortical and subcortical sources, it no longer seems reasonable to suppose that dysfunction within the basal ganglia should produce deficits equivalent to those associated with frontal cortical damage, nor that deficits originating in basal ganglia disease should be as extensive. In disorders largely confined to the basal ganglia, such as PD, the cortex remains intact, able to profit from multiple inputs crucial to its executive responsibilities. Thus, for PD patients, the real issue becomes detection of those specific executive routines that may be at risk as a result of basal ganglia dysfunction.

PROCESS ANALYSIS

Initially, the search for specific Parkinson-related deficits employed clinical tools with known sensitivity to frontal lobe integrity. The main technique used in many studies was the Wisconsin Card Sort Test (WCST), a task that requires both the formation of spontaneously developed strategies to solve novel problems and the switching of these strategies in response to fluctuating task demands (Lezak, 1983). Milner (1964) had demonstrated that performance on the WCST is reliably impaired in patients with damage to the dorsolateral frontal region.

This deceptively simple task involves the discovery, through trial and error, of which of three possible sorting principles (color, shape, or number) is correct at any point in time. An internal (unknown to the subject) set of rules governs correct sorting, changing arbitrarily after every sequence of 10 consecutively correct responses. In order to succeed, one must first formulate a plan (choose one of the contingencies), then switch plans after each correct run. Patients with damage to the dorsolateral frontal cortex preferentially perseverate on old, formerly successful strategies. The mental routine implicated in this deficit is flexibility of thought, an executive function lost when one cannot abandon a currently unsuccessful plan in favor of a more adaptive strategy.

Several investigations have confirmed that patients with PD have difficulty with the WCST (Bowen et al, 1976; Lees and Smith, 1983; Taylor et al, 1986), and interest is now focused on the form in which such failures occur. Whereas previously it was sufficient to compare deficits in frontal lobe and basal ganglia dysfunction, current research asks whether or not patients with cortical vs subcortical disease fail for similar or different reasons. Detection of a deficit can no longer be considered an end point in research. Today, among cognitive and neuropsychologists, detection is the beginning of process analysis, an exercise that explores the nature as well as the extent of behavioral impairments.

Unfortunately, the WCST, like many human experimental paradigms, is highly complex, simultaneously calling on a number of executive abilities (e.g., strategy development, flexible switching of plans, working memory, response monitoring). As such, it can lead to more than one type of error. Loss of flexible thinking is not the only route to impaired performance. For example, schizophrenic patients have great difficulty with the initial stage of category formation, that is, generating a workable hypothesis (Goldberg and Weinberger, 1988). In this case, thought appears too flexible.

Different forms of the WCST test have been used with PD patients, making direct comparisons between studies somewhat difficult. Nevertheless, if one considers the error pattern in two studies using the same version of the test in comparable groups of patients (Bowen et al, 1976; Taylor et al, 1986), a striking similarity emerges. In these two studies, PD patients had difficulty maintaining a stable strategy over the required sequence of 10 consecutive correct responses. In this case, the failure appeared to involve an inability to lock onto an adaptive plan. Choosing between a range of equally possible options became confusing. PD patients were able to form workable hypotheses but tended to abandon them prematurely, even when successful. Although Bowen and associates (1976) considered the problem to lie in short-term memory, that is, in the inability to remember which plan is correct at any moment, it is equally possible that PD patients fail to appreciate the full salience of a response outcome. Under these circumstances, facilitation through experience would suffer. Appreciation of the consequences of behavior, particularly in novel situations, is yet another executive ability necessary for success on this popular but highly complex multidimensional task. Given the numerous possible breakdown points in performing the WCST (and many other clinical tests), process analysis becomes difficult.

One strategy is to simplify task demands and thereby gain control over the mental routines involved. Flowers and Robertson (1985) employed a test of concept formation that involved only two possible solutions. This was presented to PD patients with the instruction to select either solution on the first set and then to switch to the other strategy once 10 correct trials had been completed. Errors were corrected at the time of commission to avoid confusion. This odd-man-out paradigm, in which the item that does not belong to a related group must be identified, did not provoke difficulty during plan selection. PD patients were quite capable of choosing size or shape as the initial rule. However, difficulty occurred when the rule had to be switched, confusion arising over which of the two alternatives was in play at the moment. Once again, it was apparent that in a novel situation, PD patients had difficulty maintaining a clear separation between the available options.

The importance of novelty in provoking a failure of executive functions in PD cannot be overemphasized. However, are all executive abilities affected in this disorder? If not, can specific task conditions be identified that are necessary for impaired performance? Finally, are executive abilities selectively implicated, or are functions predominantly dependent on regions other than the frontal lobes involved as well?

Several years ago, we conducted an exhaustive assessment of cognition in a clinically representative group of nondemented PD patients (Taylor et al, 1986). Ultimately, it could be seen that patients performed the majority of tasks in a normal manner. No deficit emerged on any test that presented material in an organized form or that depended on recourse to the stored lexicon of conventional knowledge or that provided explicit guidelines against which to check progress. This even applied to several tests sensitive to frontal lobe integrity for which there is documented evidence of impairment when this area is damaged. On this basis, it appeared that dysfunction within the basal ganglia is not the mirror image of disruption at the cortical level of the frontocaudate loop, in that the consequences are more restricted.

The task conditions that proved problematic for PD patients appeared consistent. They were not modality specific. Performance on any task, verbal, visual, or motoric, that required the patients to generate a solution to a novel problem without the help of external guidance or access to the stored knowledge base was impaired. This observation, although not explanatory, provided a clearer view of the circumstances under which the basal ganglia are important to the organization and direction of behavior.

METHODOLOGICAL ISSUES

Unfortunately, little specificity about the role of a neural system, such as the basal ganglia, can be gleaned from tests that employ a wide variety of mental operations during execution. After the observation that PD patients have difficulty solving problems when they must generate and monitor their own strategies and must alternate between strategies according to task conditions, interest shifted to parceling the relevant demands on the executive system. This effort has led to the adoption of much simpler experimental paradigms where a single cognitive domain can be studied in isolation. Accordingly, a number of investigators are turning to reaction time techniques that focus on one critical variable within the family of executive functions. At present, the control of selective attention is undergoing considerable study.

The manner in which one allocates attentional resources when confronted by a novel situation is critical to subsequent performance. The amount of information to which one can attend at any moment is limited and must be selected, with varying degrees of efficiency, from a vast array of input. Although we often are unaware of the details of this selective process, without it, subjective experience could not remain unified.

An early model of selective attention (Norman and Bobrow, 1975) conceived of an information processing system capable of varying its input according to stimulus conditions. In the active (effortful) mode, changes in the selection of what is attended to are driven by information stored in memory. In this case, the cue for allocating attention is internal. In the passive mode, which is less effortful, changes in the allocation of attention are driven by external (environmental) cues, no memory being required. Using a very simple reaction time test where subjects had to respond if they saw the letter T in a group of other letters, the model predicted that the externally driven condition (where T was always in the same place) would be easiest, followed by the memory-driven condition (where the location of T was presented on the first of two positions-to-be-learned). In addition, it was predicted that performance would be poorest in the uncued condition (where T appeared in random positions).

PD patients and healthy elderly control subjects were indistinguishable on this test (Cossa et al, 1989). In both cases, performance under directed attention, whether internally or externally driven, was superior to that in the uncued (random) condition. PD patients were considered to "maintain their ability to take advantage of cueing and show unimpaired skill in allocating attentional resources." On this basis, it was concluded that the basal ganglia are not involved in selective attention.

These results and the conclusions drawn from them raise a very serious issue concerning methodology. Is one task, no matter how well conceived and tightly controlled, sufficient to cover a complex domain, such as the allocation and selection of attention? Given the simplicity of the cognitive demands of the Norman and Bobrow (1975) paradigm, is it possible that the complexity of the decisions-to-be-made slipped below the threshold necessary to provoke problems in PD? Dedication to a particular theory and its accompanying experimental measures may hamper the advance of knowledge in a manner equal but opposite to the use of highly complex clinical tests where no parcellation of the subroutines at risk is possible.

A second reaction time paradigm has been used extensively to study the processes that comprise attention. In the Posner paradigm (Posner and Presti, 1987a), attention is divided into two compartments, one an automatic (preattentive) mechanism, the other an effortful focal processor. By alerting subjects with a cue indicating the direction in which an impending stimulus will appear, one can measure gains relative to noncued trials. If the directional cue is *valid* (80 percent of the trials), it presents an advantage. However, if the directional cue is *invalid* (i.e., the impending stimulus will appear in the direction opposite to that indicated by the cue), the advantage of the automatic orienting mechanism is lost. Attention covertly focused in the wrong direction must then be disengaged and rerouted to an alternate location.

Posner and associates (1987b) have demonstrated that reaction time to invalid, as opposed to valid, cues is considerably longer. They hypothesize that the greater expectation of a valid cue (80 percent of the trials) during this task predisposes the system to covertly orient to the impending target before presentation. If one expects something to happen in a certain location, attention automatically shifts to that site in advance of the event.

Several experiments suggest that the basal ganglia are important to the automatic process of covert (preattentional) orienting mechanisms. In the first of two experiments, Clark and co-workers (1989) demonstrated that suppression of either dopamine or norepinephrine transmission in healthy subjects facilitated disengagement from invalid cues. Although reaction time to valid cues remained unchanged, reaction time to invalid cues improved. Although some might argue that faster disengagement from an invalid cue improves attentional processing, it is equally likely that the weaker link between attention and its ultimate object under catecholamine suppression represents a loss in attentional vigilance.

In a second step, these authors (Wright et al, 1990) submitted PD patients to the Posner paradigm. Once again, although valid cueing significantly improved reaction time, there was a reduced effect of invalid cueing among patients. The more rapid disengagement of attention in the invalid condition by the PD group was interpreted to reflect instability in the process of attentional maintenance. The authors comment that tasks involving more substantial attentional demands than those represented by Norman and Bobrow's paradigm cast doubt on conclusions regarding intact attentional resources in PD. In their opinion, impairment in the maintenance of oriented attention may underlie some of the cognitive deficits reported in this disorder.

When a large group of PD patients was subdivided according to severity, the entire Posner effect disappeared in the older, more disabled subjects (Yamada et al, 1990), and in contrast to the Wright and colleagues' study (1990), even the advantage of valid cueing was lost. Yamada and associates speculated that the ability to shift attention covertly to an expected response location may be lost as the disease advances. These results imply that with progression, older, more disabled patients may rely increasingly on explicit, overt cues in order to focus attention, particularly during nonfamiliar tasks, such as those posed by reaction time experiments.

Task conditions, as well as disease factors, can influence the performance of PD patients on tests of attentional control. Brown and Marsden (1988) presented a more difficult reaction time test of internal (subject-directed) vs external (stimulus-bound) cueing than any mentioned previously. In this case, the words *red* and *green* appeared on a video screen printed in disgruent colors. On some trials, the word alone was read; on other trials, the color in which the word was printed had to be named. When patients were cued by a continual visual instruction announcing which task condition was in operation at the moment, PD patients had no difficulty. However, when patients had to cue themselves by constantly remembering which attribute was in use on a block of trials, performance was significantly poorer than that of the control group. The authors, using Norman and Shallice's model (1980) of an executive Supervisory Attentional System (SAS), believed to allocate its limited resources according to need, interpreted these results as a failure in working memory. *Working memory* in this model is the routine that supports *on line* recall of the operative details of any task during execution.

The proposed SAS has a limited capacity. Accordingly, it is only used when task demands are novel or when no external or preprogrammed information is available to facilitate decisions. Given the importance of the frontal lobe system to the direction and control of attention (Luria, 1980), the SAS would be vulnerable to dysfunction within this system, further reducing the limited reserves under its control. According to Brown and Marsden (1988), in PD, the SAS either suffers a depletion of resources or fails to allocate them efficiently. Thus, provided that the attentional demands of a task do not exceed what remains (externally cued condition), no deficit emerges. However, if the attentional demands do exceed the processing resources of the SAS (internally cued condition), deficits will be observed.

Results of carefully controlled laboratory experiments that attempt to parcellate the mental routines underlying the clinically observed weaknesses in executive ability in PD strongly indicate that one of the crucial determinants of cognitive impairment is disruption of focused attention. This may occur at an automatic level if covert attention is involved or at a conscious level if working memory is an important ingredient of the task. Deficits of attention may vary according to disease severity as well as to the nature of the task demands.

CURRENT THEORIES

Is a deficit in attention sufficient to account for all the executive impairments in Parkinson's disease? How do the basal ganglia contribute to this deficit, largely thought to be under the control of the frontal cortical system? What role do the basal ganglia play in the focus and sustaining of attention? If some light can be shed on these issues, one can predict with greater precision the conditions under which PD patients might have difficulty in real life situations.

In the motor executive domain, Robertson and Flowers (1990) have tested the ability of PD patients to learn complex programs and to alternate between them on a spontaneous (internally cued) basis. Patients had no difficulty learning, remembering, and generating several different five-step button-pushing sequences. However, when instructed to alternate between two sequences within the same block of trials in response to a neutral warning light, significantly more errors were made by patients than by control subjects. Since several investigators (Taylor et al, 1986; Brown and Marsden, 1988), have suggested that PD patients need an explicit external cue to initiate the correct response, a second experiment provided signal lights indicating the required path before actual performance. The error rate in the patient group dropped significantly. In these experiments, maintenance of the correct motor set was observed to require "continual stimulation or arousal" from an explicit external source.

Having demonstrated that patients could remember the motor sequences involved in their tasks, Robertson and Flowers (1990) concluded that the observed problem in alternating motor sets could not be explained by an inability to learn or to execute a new routine. In their opinion, the PD-related deficit lay at a higher (i.e., nonmotor) level involving the selection and maintenance of one plan of action when that plan is in direct competition with equally appropriate alternatives.

Motor control theorists have suggested that motor programs are not directly stored in memory in terms of all the pertinent details necessary to run each one (Schmidt, 1976). This would be unwieldy and wasteful of storage capacity. Instead, the schema or algorithm of the motor program that contains the abstract rules governing execution may be stored and later summoned to suit current requirements. If PD patients can execute a motor program only under external guidance, the problem may lie not with the algorithm itself but with internal control mechanisms, such as selection among the available algorithms appropriate to the task. A high level impairment at the level of algorithm selection (which includes inhibition of unwanted alternatives) would apply equally to nonmotor (cognitive) and motor-based executive deficits.

The selection and suppression of all the possible algorithms that might pertain in a situation would greatly slow performance if conducted on a conscious basis. If one had to consider all the options before initiating an action, one would, like PD patients, become motorically akinetic or cognitively inefficient, especially when confronted by a novel situation. Parsimony dictates that to some extent, high-order *set* selection is performed at a subcognitive level. Given the signposts provided by PD, the basal ganglia become a likely candidate.

We have proposed (Saint-Cyr et al, 1991) that the basal ganglia are important to the gradual establishment of limits on all the available response options one is offered when confronted with a new learning situation. Given the rich connections between the frontal cortex and the basal ganglia, the algorithm of new learning (whether motor or nonmotor) might follow a pattern as represented in Figure 6–2.

The crucial step in this schema is the activity that occurs once a favorable outcome is reached. Success/failure on tasks known to be sensitive to frontal lobe integrity appears to be recorded at a cortical level by postresponse neurons designed to register the specific nature of the consequences (Thorpe et al, 1983). Again, parsimony dictates that since a favorable outcome facilitates adaptive learning, it would undergo further neuronal initializing at the end point to protect its interests. Unfavorable outcomes would not receive this boost, thereby accruing less attention within the circuitry.

In our view, the basal ganglia participate in learning by further recognizing favorable response outcomes and promoting neural activity patterns that foster adaptive solutions. In this regard, Rolls and colleagues (1984) have identified a group of neurons within the caudate nucleus that respond selectively and uniquely to stimuli associated with task-specific meaning. These units are so selective that they do not fire if the same stimulus is encountered outside the test experience, where it carries no associated reward message.

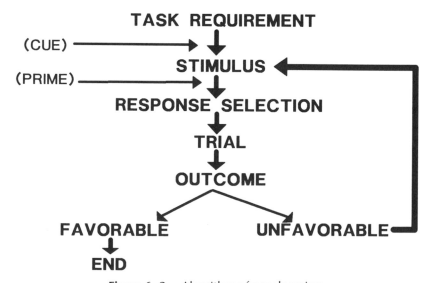

Figure 6–2. Algorithm of new learning.

At a subcortical level, neuronally based priority for the pathway that carries the most appropriate, task-specific message could shape the frontal cortex to favor one particular action plan over the alternatives. Such a mechanism would free the cortex to monitor progress and to perform other conscious cognitive routines necessary for efficient problem solving. In other words, we propose that the basal ganglia may automatically enhance a correct solution path, giving preference to appropriate response algorithms while inhibiting competing options. Practice would hone behavior that carries this advantage. Loss of such an advantage would force the cortex to be responsible for discriminating between each response–outcome, for reaffirming the links between stimulus and successful response, and for continually and actively defining and refining the theater of its operations. In combination, these activities would stretch attentional resources to and, perhaps, beyond their limit. In this case, either a cue before stimulus onset (to announce the rule-in-operation) or a prime before action (to prompt the favored response) (Fig. 6–2) would offset the loss. It is under these latter circumstances that PD patients retain their executive abilities (Lee and Brown, 1991).

SUMMARY

The executive abilities of the brain, which appear to be largely under the control of the frontal lobe system, are responsible for the planning and regulation of behavior. At no time are they more important than when one is confronted by a new situation, unable to rely on past experience (stored knowledge) or explicit guidelines (external cues). Given the intimate relationship between the basal ganglia and the frontal cortex, where the outflow of the former is exclusively directed to the latter, it is not surprising that PD patients may suffer some disruption of an executive nature.

As disrupted activity within the basal ganglia is the primary consequence of PD, the frontal cortex can continue to benefit from the input of all other regions. In this manner, the vast amount of knowledge stored throughout the brain can be used to plan and to regulate behavior operating under familiar algorithms.

However, work farmed out to the basal ganglia begins to suffer when this area undergoes a loss of dopamine regulation. Even familiar motor algorithms, such as walking, undergo change once the disease reaches clinical proportions. Given the greater preservation of dopamine within the caudate as opposed to the putamen in PD (Hornykiewicz, 1966), nonmotor (cognitive) algorithms remain better protected. Indeed, in the early stage of the disease, one must challenge the cognitive executive domain with highly demanding and novel tasks in order to see a failure of executive function (Taylor et al, 1990b). When the problem-to-be-solved requires the subject to plan and to execute a strategy using only internal resources to guide behavior, PD patients experience difficulty.

In PD, reliance on an external guidance system becomes crucial to efficient performance. This strongly suggests to us, and to other investigators (Robertson and Flowers, 1990; Sullivan et al, 1989), that the basal ganglia serve as an internal navigational system slowly placing useful limits on the options that lead to success. In all probability, this system is subcognitive in nature, relying on practice rather than on memory to set the context in which the frontal lobes problem solve most efficiently. This advantage is lost in PD placing all the demands of a novel situation under conscious control. Under these circumstances a limited SAS, responsible for mental or motor set maintenance, would be exhausted prematurely. In consequence, the ability to track a behavioral sequence by stringing together a task-appropriate algorithm would suffer. This is the executive ability at highest risk in PD.

ACKNOWLEDGMENTS

The authors wish to thank the Canadian Parkinson's Disease Foundation for their continued support of this work. Thanks are also due to Ms. Indrani Singh for her help with the illustrations.

REFERENCES

Alexander G, DeLong M, Strick P. Parallel organization of functionally segregated circuits linking basal ganglia and cortex. In: Cowan WM, ed. *Annual Review of Neuroscience.* Washington: Society for Neuroscience; 1986;9:357–81.

Bowen FP, Kamienny RS, Burns MM, Yahr MD. Parkinsonism: the effects of levodopa treatment on concept formation. *Neurology.* 1976;25:701–04.

Brown RG, Marsden CD. Internal versus external cues and the control of attention in Parkinson's disease. *Brain.* 1988;111:23–45.

Clark CR, Geffen GM, Geffen LB. Catecholamines and the covert orientation of attention in humans. *Neuropsychologia.* 1989;27:131–39.

Cossa FM, Della Sala S, Spinnler H. Selective visual attention in Alzheimer's and Parkinson's patients: memory and data-driven control. *Neuropsychologia.* 1989;27:887–92.

DeLong M, Georgopoulos A, Crutcher M. Cortico-basal ganglia relations and the coding of motor performance. *Exp Br Res.* 1983;7(suppl):30–40.

Divac I. Neostriatum and functions of prefrontal cortex. *Acta Neurobiol Exp Warsz.* 1972;32:461–477.

Flowers KA, Roberston C. The effect of Parkinson's disease on the ability to maintain a mental set. *J Neurol Neurosurg Psychiatry.* 1985;48:517–29.

Fuster JM. *The Prefrontal Cortex.* New York: Raven Press; 1980.

Glosser G, Goodglass H. Disorders in executive control functions among aphasic and other brain-damaged patients. *J Clin Exp Neuropsychol.* 1990;12:4:485–501.

Goldberg TE, Weinberger DR. Probing pre-frontal function in schizophrenia with neuropsychological paradigms. *Schizophr Bull.* 1988;14:179–83.

Goldman-Rakic PS. Circuitry of the primate prefrontal cortex and regulation of behaviour by representational knowledge. In: Plum F, Mountcastle V, eds. *Higher Cortical Function: Handbook of Physiology.* Washington DC: American Physiology Society; 1987;5:373–417.

Hornykiewicz O. Dopamine (3-hydroxytramine) and brain function. *Pharmacol Rev.* 1966;8:925–64.

Johnson T, Rosvold HE, Mishkin M. Projections from behaviorally-defined sectors of the prefrontal cortex to the basal ganglia, septum, and diencephalon of the monkey. *Exp Neurol.* 1968;21:20–34.

Lee C, Brown R. Use of advance information in Parkinson's disease. *Mov Disord.* 1991;(in press).

Lees AJ, Smith E. Cognitive deficits in the early stages of Parkinson's disease. *Brain.* 1983;106:257–70.

Lezak M. *Neuropsychological Assessment,* 2nd ed. New York: Oxford University Press; 1983.

Luria A. *Higher Cortical Functions in Man.* New York: Basic Books; 1980.

Milner B. Some effects of frontal lobectomy in man. In: Warren JM, Akert K, eds. *Frontal Granular Cortex and Behaviour.* New York: McGraw-Hill; 1964:313–34.

Milner B, Petrides M. Behavioral effects of frontal lobe lesions in man. *Trends Neurosci.* 1984;77:403–07.

Nauta WJH. Some efferent projections of the prefrontal cortex in the monkey. In: Warren J, Akert K, eds. *Frontal Granular Cortex and Behaviour.* New York: McGraw-Hill; 1964;379–409.

Norman DA, Bobrow DG. On data-limited and resource-limited processes. *Cognit Psychol.* 1975;7:44–67.

Norman DA, Shallice T. Attention to action: willed and automatic control of behavior. *University of California CHIP Report 99.* 1980.

Posner MI, Presti DE. Selective attention and cognitive control. *Trends Neurosci.* 1987a;10:13–17.

Posner MI, Inhoff AW, Friedrich FJ. Isolating attentional systems: a cognitive-anatomical analysis. *Psychobiology.* 1987b;15:107–21.

Procter F, Ricklan M, Cooper I, Teuber H-L. Judgment of visual and postural vertical by Parkinsonian patients. *Neurology.* 1964;14:273–87.

Robertson C, Flowers KA. Motor set in Parkinson's disease. *J Neurol Neurosurg Psychiatry.* 1990;59:583–92.

Rolls ET, Thorpe SJ, Boytim M, Peretti P. Responses of striatal neurons in the behaving monkey. Effects of iontophoretically applied dopamine on normal responsiveness. *Neuroscience.* 1984;12:1201–12.

Rosvold HE. The frontal lobe system: cortical-subcortical interrelationships. *Acta Neurobiol Exp.* 1972;32:439–60.

Saint-Cyr JA, Taylor AE. The mobilization of procedural learning: the "key signature of the basal ganglia." In Squire LR and Butters N, eds. *The Neuropsychology of Memory,* 2nd ed., New York: Guilford Press, 1992.

Schmidt RA. The schema as a solution to some persistent problems in motor learning theory. In: Stelmach GE, ed. *Motor Control: Issues and Trends.* New York: Academic Press; 1976.

Stuss DT, Benson DF. *The Frontal Lobes.* New York: Raven Press; 1986.

Sullivan EV, Sagar HJ, Gabrieli JDE, et al. Different cognitive profiles on standard behavioural tests in Parkinson's disease and Alzheimer's disease. *J Clin Exp Neuropsychol.* 1989;11:6:799–820.

Taylor AE, Saint-Cyr JA, Lang AE. Frontal lobe dysfunction in Parkinson's disease: the cortical focus of neostriatal outflow. *Brain.* 1986;109:279–92.

Taylor AE, Saint-Cyr JA, Lang AE. Sub-cognitive processing in the frontocaudate "complex loop". *Alzheimer's Dis Assoc Disord.* 1990a;4:150–160.

Taylor AE, Saint-Cyr JA, Lang AE. Memory and learning in early Parkinson's disease: evidence for a "frontal lobe syndrome". *Brain Cogn.* 1990b;13:211–32.

Thorpe SJ, Rolls ET, Maddison S. The orbitofrontal cortex: neuronal activity in the behaving monkey. *Exp Brain Res.* 1983;49:93–115.

Wright MJ, Burns GM, Geffen GM, Geffen LB. Covert orientation of visual attention in Parkinson's disease: an impairment in the maintenance of attention. *Neuropsychologia.* 1990;28:151–59.

Yamada T, Izyuuinn M, Schulzer M, Hirayama K. Covert orientation in Parkinson's disease. *J Neurol Neurosurg Psychiatry.* 1990;53:593–96.

7

Bradyphrenia in Parkinson's Disease

DANIEL ROGERS

The term *bradyphrenia* was coined by the French neurologist, Naville, in 1922 to describe a new psychiatric syndrome produced by the epidemic of encephalitis lethargica sweeping across Europe (Rogers, 1986). Bradyphrenia means slowing of mental function, but the syndrome was wider than this. It included impairment of attention, interest, initiative, and the capacity for sustained effort and work. There was lethargy of thought, movement, and affect. Cognitive functioning was slowed, but intelligence was spared except for a slight impairment of memory. An expressionless face was typical. Naville described bradyphrenia as loss of psychic tone. Those severely affected became uncommunicative and did nothing without constant prompting. In its extreme form, there could be complete loss of psychomotor activity. Naville speculated about a special psychomotor system whose physiology awaited elucidation.

A similar syndrome had been noted previously (Ball, 1882).

> An invisible weight seems to crush the intellect and slow down perception, movement and ideas. . . . The present case is obviously one of paralysis agitans with dementia, but one cannot help, on observing these symptoms, but think of certain cases of melancholic stupor, such as one sees in our mental asylums.

The author, France's first professor of psychiatry, is here describing bradyphrenia in Parkinson's disease (PD). Interestingly, he compares it to the psychomotor retardation of depressive illness. The overlap between PD and depressive illness has only recently been taken up again as a focus of interest. A hundred years ago, when Ball was writing, neurology and psychiatry were close together. Shortly afterward, psychiatry went its own way, interested in the mind but not the brain. Neurology left psychiatric disorders to the psychiatrists. Even the epidemic of encephalitis lethargica, which produced the whole spectrum of known psychiatric disorders, was not enough to bring them together again. This has only happened in the last 25 years.

RELATIONSHIP TO MOTOR IMPAIRMENT

Naville included motor features in his syndrome of bradyphrenia. Peripheral execution of movement could be slow, and there could be a delay between the impulse for movement and the start of its execution. What was especially slow, however, was the impulse for movement. At times, movements were performed correctly that at other times were completely impossible—kinesia paradoxica. Bradyphrenia could be associated with marked, generalized parkinsonism, but often there was no rigidity or tremor. It was not distinguished from akinesia. This slowly became accepted as a major motor component of the parkinsonian syndrome after the epidemic encephalitis. Up to then, akinesia, like bradyphrenia, had been considered a psychiatric syndrome. When akinesia became fully established in the 1960s, bradyphrenia became regarded as its mental corollary and was renamed by some *psychic akinesia.* The concept of motor akinesia is still evolving.

Contradictory findings among experimental studies of motor and cognitive slowing in PD have been present from the outset. Naville (1922) used a series of tests in which the motor element remained the same but the intellectual difficulty varied. Parkinsonian patients, both postencephalitic and not, had slowing of intellectual function compared with normal controls, and there was a relationship between this intellectual slowing and motor slowing. Worster-Drought and Hardcastle (1924) compared the performance of 19 postencephalitic patients, 17 of whom had some form of parkinsonian syndrome, and normal controls on a psychomotor reaction time task using an electrical apparatus. They found that in most of the patients, the psychomotor reaction time was prolonged, usually by about 50 percent, but that the cerebration time component of the total reaction time was not.

Different theoretical views on what is motor and what is mental may explain some of the contradictory conclusions of these and subsequent studies. Brumlik and Boshes (1966) compared the motor reaction times of 30 PD patients and 30 comparable normal subjects and found that about 75 percent of the PD patients showed slowness of limb movement. In over 50 percent, a peripheral factor was operating, but in all patients with delayed onset of movement, there was also a central factor. Evarts and colleagues (1981) carried out extensive assessments of reaction times and movement times in 29 patients with PD and 44 control subjects. They found that both reaction times and movement times tended to be longer in the PD patients but that there was no reliable correlation between delays in reaction time and delays in movement time. They believed that reaction time could be delayed due to central motor disorder, independent of bradykinesia. Angel and colleagues (1970) used a step function tracking task in which, on 50 percent of trials, the directional relationship between control and display was reversed, causing subjects to make numerous false moves. The duration of both false and correct responses was significantly longer in 8 PD patients compared to 8 controls. They thought that the PD patients had difficulty in sending motor commands from the highest level to the upper motor neurons.

Another reason for the different findings among experimental studies is that slowing of response, whatever its cause, is a feature of some, but not all patients with PD. Talland (1963) compared the reaction times of 25 PD patients and 25 matched normal controls and found that they were not significantly different. The reaction times of the most severely affected patients, however, were significantly longer than those of the controls and patients with mild or moderate disability. Garron and colleagues (1972) administered four cognitive tests with a computer-controlled teletype writer to 47 PD patients and an equal number of individually matched controls. A subgroup of the patients had significantly slower response times than the controls and the rest of the patients. Wilson and colleagues (1980) used a memory scanning test to minimize the motor requirement of a cognitive test. They compared 20 PD patients and 16 normal controls, matched for age and education, and found that the scanning speed of elements held in short-term memory was increased, but only in a subgroup of elderly PD patients.

The apparent conflict in the conclusions of different studies continues. Mortimer and colleagues (1982) compared the performance of 60 patients with idiopathic PD and matched normal controls on an extensive neuropsychological test battery. They found that performance of the PD patients was significantly poorer on 18 of the 23 individual tests. Poorer neuropsychological performance was always associated with increased bradykinesia. They suggested that cognitive impairment in PD might result from the same subcortical lesions causing the motor symptoms. Hansch and colleagues (1982) measured the auditory event-related potentials of 20 PD patients and found significantly increased latencies of the cognitive P300 component of these evoked potentials in the patients compared with normal controls. In addition, they found a significant and age-independent negative correlation in the PD patients between latency of the P300 component and their score on a digit–symbol substitution test. They believed that both of these abnormalities, the electrical and the neuropsychological, were reflections of a common disrupted aspect of cognitive function best described as bradyphrenia.

On the other hand, Rafal and colleagues (1984) carried out a series of tests on 10 patients with PD, including rate of memory scanning, orienting of attention in the visual fields, and time required to prepare a manual movement. The patients served as their own controls at different stages of treatment with L-dopa, including on and off states. The investigators found that overall reaction times were increased when patients were in the untreated state, but without a concomitant slowing of the purely cognitive components, and concluded that slowing of thought did not necessarily accompany slowing of movement in PD patients. Girotti and colleagues (1986) tested 21 PD patients on L-dopa treatment during on and off phases. Movement time was significantly lengthened in the off phase and mood worsened, but no variation in five tests of cognitive performance, including a speed test, was observed. The same authors (1988) tested 67 PD patients and 44 age- and education-matched controls for cognitive function and motor performance using reaction times and movement times. The performance of the PD patients was impaired significantly on visuoperceptual and perceptual motor tests but not when these test scores were adjusted for reaction and movement times. The authors believed that motor dysfunction played the major role in apparent cognitive impairment in PD.

Studies that examined the relationship between motor slowing and bradyphrenia have produced mixed results. This variability may be attributed to different theoretical views on what is motor and what is mental. Further, slowed responses are seen in some but not all patients with PD, and this may vary as a function of disease severity, age, or degree of overall cognitive impairment.

RELATIONSHIP TO DEPRESSIVE SYMPTOMS

Naville thought that the concept of bradyphrenia had implications for the relationship of motor and mental phenomena in a wide range of disorders, including depressive illness. Depression was another possible sequel of epidemic encephalitis. Steck (1931) distinguished different postencephalitic depressive syndromes, contrasting neurasthenia-like states that could lead to bradyphrenia and melancholic states with tearfulness, ideas of guilt and suicide, and hypochondriasis. Interestingly, he described bradyphrenia as a global impairment of mental activity, like dementia but without those symptoms normally ascribed to cortical function. Little further interest in the relationship of PD and depression was shown until the revival of a neuropsychiatric approach in the 1960s. A series of studies then found a higher prevalence of depression in PD patients than in matched control groups, which was independent of the degree of disability, the duration of the illness, and medication. The idea began to gain ground of an overlap between the physiological mechanisms underlying both PD and depression.

The development of treatment with dopamine agonists for PD, starting with levodopa in the 1960s, shed more light on this overlap. Ajuriaguerra (1971) studied 204 patients with PD and found depressive states in 70 percent. Like Steck, he divided these depressive states into two types. Sixy percent of his patients had simple depressive states characterized by some sadness but mainly by lack of drive and fatigability. A further 10 percent had more severe depressive symptoms or melancholia, with ideas of guilt, suicide, and hypochondriasis. All patients with simple depression had significant akinesia, and levodopa could produce a parallel improvement in motor and affective symptoms. In the second group with melancholia, levodopa produced a significant improvement in motor symptoms, with less effect on the depressive symptoms, requiring the addition of a tricyclic antidepressant. Several authors then examined the effect of levodopa on depressive illness and found that it had a therapeutic effect on depression with motor retardation, without being otherwise an effective antidepressant.

Van Praag and colleagues (1975) studied central dopamine metabolism in various disorders, including depression and PD, by means of the probenicid technique to measure dopamine metabolites in the cerebrospinal fluid (CSF). They concluded that decreased dopamine metabolism was associated with hypomotility rather than being specific for any particular disease or syndrome and that this decreased dopamine turnover was related to the cause of the hypomotility rather than simply being its consequence. Banki (1977) performed another CSF study of depressive illness and showed that dopamine turnover, as measured by homovanillic acid concentration, was reduced in depressed patients with retardation but not in those without. Anderson and colleagues (1980) carried out a placebo-controlled trial of the effect of treating depression in 19 PD patients already being treated with levodopa. The tricyclic had a significant clinical effect on their depressive symptoms, but motor retardation and inhibition of thought were not improved to the same degree as other depressive symptoms, with the implication that this was because of the pretreatment with levodopa.

The implication of all these studies was that there was probably a close relationship among akinesia, bradyphrenia, and the psychomotor retardation of depressive illness, with impairment of dopamine function as a common pathological factor.

Several studies have looked at the relationship of affective and cognitive impairment in PD. Brown and colleagues (1984) performed on two occasions a neuropsychological assessment of 16 patients with PD in both their on and off phases and control subjects matched for age and education. Subjects were asked to assess their affect and arousal on each occasion. In the on phase, the PD patients showed a significant impairment of accuracy, though not of total response time, on the cognitive task and of their affect–arousal score when compared with the normal controls. In their off phases, there was a further significant deterioration of accuracy on the cognitive task and their affect–arousal score, and there was a significant correlation in the cognitive score, the degree of motor impairment, and the impairment of affect–arousal. When a regression analysis was carried out, only the impairment of affect–arousal made a significant contribution to the cognitive impairment when considered independently, the correlation with motor impairment being mediated through the impairment of affect–arousal.

Starkstein and colleagues (1989) examined 78 patients with PD for the presence of depression using the Present State Examination and Hamilton Rating Scale and neuropsychological deficits using the Mini-Mental State Exam and an extensive neuropsychological battery. Severity of depression was found to be the single most important factor associated with severity of the cognitive impairment. Fifteen patients had major depression and 19 had minor depression according to DSM III criteria. The 15 with major depression were compared to 15 nondepressed PD patients, matched for age, education, and a wide variety of illness variables. The PD patients with major depression were significantly more impaired cognitively. This involved all aspects of neuropsychological function but was most prominent on tests of frontal lobe function. The authors believed that PD patients with major depression have more frontal lobe dysfunction than nondepressed PD patients.

Mayberg and colleagues (1990) measured regional cerebral glucose metabolism using positron emission tomography (PET) to compare 5 depressed PD patients with 4 nondepressed PD patients and 6 age-comparable normal subjects. Relative metabolic activity in the caudate and orbital inferior region of the frontal lobe was significantly lower in the depressed patients than in both the other two groups. In addition, there was a significant inverse correlation between relative glucose metabolism in the orbital inferior frontal lobe and depression scores. This and the findings of Starkstein and colleagues (1989) support the hypothesis that depression in PD is associated with frontal lobe dysfunction. Recent studies in patients with primary affective disorders also have described hypometabolism in the frontal lobe and caudate.

COMPARISON WITH OTHER NEUROLOGICAL ILLNESSES

In 1974, Albert and colleagues put forward the concept of *subcortical dementia* to characterize the cognitive disorder of progressive supranuclear palsy. Twenty-six of 42 cases of this disorder reported in the literature and 4 of their 5 cases had slowness of thought processes as a prominent clinical feature. Tests for various cognitive functions, including verbal abilities, perceptual–motor skills, and memory, would be performed adequately but only if the patients were given more than the normal amount of time. The slowing of cognitive and motor function shown by these patients, if severe, could produce a state approaching akinetic mutism. A similar syndrome was found in a variety of neurological illnesses, such as PD and Huntington's disease, in which prominent pathological changes were found in subcortical nuclei or frontal lobes. They called the slowing of thought processes, impaired ability to manipulate acquired knowledge, and forgetfulness, in the absence of the aphasia, agnosia, and apraxia of cortical dementia, such as Alzheimer's disease, *subcortical dementia.*

Albert did not compare his new syndrome to the previously described syndrome of bradyphrenia, but the two had many features in common. Both terms provided a needed conceptual advance in the understanding of two different components of cognitive ability—capability and access to that capability.

The association of bradyphrenia and depression was not confined to PD. All 5 of the patients with supranuclear palsy described by Albert and colleagues (1974) and 24 of the 42 PD patients they reported, had personality or mood changes, which they divided into two groups, the larger group including indifference, apathy, and depression. Mayeux and colleagues (1983), comparing patients with Parkinson's, Huntington's, and Alzheimer's diseases, showed that depression, absent in patients with Alzheimer's, was present in half the patients with Huntington's disease and correlated with their intellectual decline, again characterized as principally *subcortical dementia.*

RECENT STUDIES

Several recent studies have used the same principle as Naville originally did in testing for bradyphrenia—using tests of differing cognitive difficulty but with the same motor response, and now using computerized testing. Rogers and colleagues (1987) used two tests, a choice reaction time test involving nine digits and a more difficult digit-symbol substitution test involving the same nine digits. Thirty patients with PD were tested before starting any dopaminergic treatment, and 12 were retested after starting such treatment. The results were compared with those of 30 age- and education-matched patients with primary depressive illness, with 12 retested after improvement, and 30 similarly matched normal controls, with 12 tested on two occasions. The difference between the response times for the two tests was used as a measure of cognitive processing time. This was significantly increased in PD patients, but only in those with significant depressive symptoms. It also was significantly increased in patients with primary depression, but only in those who had significant clinical motor disorder. On retesting, cognitive processing time was significantly improved in the 12 patients with primary depression, whose Hamilton rating had improved significantly, but not in the 12 PD patients whose mean Hamilton rating had not. Change in response time for the digit–symbol substitution test in individual PD patients, however, correlated with change in their Hamilton rating. This study suggested a strong association between cognitive slowing and depression in PD patients and a large overlap between bradyphrenia in PD and psychomotor retardation in primary depressive illness.

Dubois and colleagues (1988) used several tasks with different levels of cognitive complexity, but with the same motor response, to assess central processing time by comparing reaction times for the different tasks. They tested 10 patients with progressive supranuclear palsy, 33 patients with idiopathic PD on dopaminergic treatment, and 20 age- and education-matched normal controls. Reaction times for the simpler and more complex tasks were increased in both patient groups, and these response times were associated with a frontal score on neuropsychological testing in both groups. Central processing time, however, was only increased in the patients with progressive supranuclear palsy. Depression scores were higher in both patient groups compared with controls, but no attempt to correlate response times with depression scores was made. Based on these findings, the authors suggest that the slowing in processing time they found could result partly from "nonspecific factors," such as depression or a decreased level of attention, but did not attempt to explore this possibility further.

Pierrot-Deseilligny and colleagues (1989) showed significant increases in choice reaction times and P300 latency in 25 patients with progressive supranuclear palsy compared with 14 age-matched controls. There was a significant correlation in the patients between their reaction times, as well as P300 latency, and an index of general intellectual deterioration, though not a specific frontal impairment score. P300 latency looks to be a promising electrophysiological method of investigating cognitive impairment, especially bradyphrenia.

PUTATIVE NEUROBIOLOGY OF BRADYPHRENIA IN PARKINSON'S DISEASE

In 1970, Hicks and Birren, reviewing research on psychomotor slowing in aging, psychosis, and brain damage, suggested that the same brain mechanisms underlie the slowing in all three groups, involving a cortical–subcortical system that was diffuse in location but specific as to structures. Ajuriaguerra (1975), reviewing the literature on the possible cerebral localization of akinesia, concluded that it could be produced by lesions close to the medial neuraxis anywhere from the frontal poles to the pons, including the cingulate gyri, septum, medial temporal lobes, thalamus, hypothalamus, and midbrain.

Price and colleagues (1978) found a marked decrease in dopamine levels in certain parts of the limbic forebrain in a postmortem study of PD brains and suggested that this might be an important factor in the etiology of the affective disorder in PD. Javoy-Agid and Agid (1980) found lesions of the mesocorticolimbic dopaminergic projection system in the brains of patients with PD and suggested that these might play a role in both the motor akinesia and the cognitive disorder of PD. Agid and colleagues (1984) suggested that involvement of the mesocorticolimbic dopaminergic system in PD was the basis of bradyphrenia and depression, since these two symptoms were often closely associated. Lesions in a single projection system innervating several areas with different functions would explain this association and the features bradyphrenia and depression shared in common. Loss of dopaminergic innervation to the prefrontal cortex would explain the similarity of bradyphrenia to frontal lobe syndromes. Bradyphrenia should be reversed by treatment with dopa, whereas impairment of more posterior cortical cognitive functions involving the cholinergic innominatocortical system should not.

Mayeux and colleagues (1987) compared the performance on a continuous performance task (CPT), as well as on tests of general intellect, memory, and reaction time, of 15 PD patients, 15 age-matched controls, and 21 mildly impaired patients with probable Alzheimer's disease and measured metabolites of the major biogenic amines in the CSF. In 10 of the PD patients, cognitive performance and CSF measures were similar to controls. In the remaining 5, performance on tests of general intellect, memory, and reaction time was similar to that of the Alzheimer's disease patients, but performance on the CPT was significantly less accurate than in the Alzheimer's disease, control, or other PD subjects. The CSF concentration of the major CNS metabolite of norepinephrine (MHPG) was significantly correlated with reaction time and accuracy on the CPT in the PD patients, with the highest levels in those with the lowest accuracy on the CPT. The authors defined bradyphrenia as an impairment of attention and vigilance and measured it by the accuracy on the CPT rather than the speed of cognitive processing. There was no relation between reaction time or CPT accuracy and Hamilton depression rating in the PD patients.

Pillon and colleagues (1989a) used a visual discrimination task consisting of 15 superimposed images of objects to evaluate slowing of cognitive processing in 70 PD patients compared with 20 age- and education-matched controls. They tested the PD patients after withdrawal from L-dopa and again during the maximal clinical effect of L-dopa. There was a mean 58 percent increase in the time needed to identify 12 of the 15 objects in the test in the PD patients after withdrawal from L-dopa compared with controls. There was no improvement after restarting L-dopa, although the motor disability score improved by 54 percent. There was a significant correlation between their score on the 15 objects test and global neuropsychological performance as well as disability score, thought to reflect residual disability due to nondopaminergic lesions, but not their akinesia score or depression score, which were deliberately measured with the Montgomery and Asberg scale to exclude any psychomotor component of the mood disorder. The authors believed that their results indicated a cognitive slowing in PD probably due to dysfunction of nondopaminergic neuronal systems.

Pillon and colleagues (1989b) analyzed the neuropsychological performance of 120 patients with idiopathic PD. Cognitive impairment was poorly correlated with akinesia and rigidity, symptoms that respond well to L-dopa treatment, and was not correlated at all with that part of the motor score that could be improved by the drug. In contrast, strong correlations were found between all neuropsychological test scores and axial symptoms, such as gait disorder and dysarthria, that respond little if at all to L-dopa treatment. The neuropsychological test scores were strongly correlated with the motor score of patients estimated when clinical improvement was maximal under L-dopa treatment, assumed to represent residual nondopaminergic motor dysfunctions. This suggested that the cognitive impairment they were measuring resulted from dysfunction of nondopaminergic neuronal systems. The neuropsychological tests used, however, were chosen to involve minimal motor activity, and patients were allowed unlimited time to perform them. Cognitive slowing was not assessed.

The same group (Dubois et al, 1990) investigated the contribution of cholinergic innervation to cognitive function by comparing two matched groups of 20 PD patients, except that one group was being given anticholinergic therapy and the other was not. They argued that anticholinergic therapy would amplify any preexisting subclinical cholinergic deficiency. On neuropsychological testing, the only difference between the two groups was severe impairment on frontal lobe function tests in the group taking anticholinergics. The authors argue that cerebral cholinergic deficit may contribute to subcorticofrontal dementia. The same neuropsychological tests were used as in the first study, except that the 15-objects test was used as a measure of cognitive slowing. The score on this test was poorer in the group taking anticholinergics, but the difference just failed to achieve statistical significance.

Despite the probable involvement of other neurotransmitter systems, deficiency of the dopamine projection pathways from brainstem to frontolimbic cortex still remains the most attractive basis for bradyphrenia.

SUMMARY

Bradyphrenia, a syndrome characterized by slowing of cognitive processing, impairment of concentration, and apathy, was first described as a sequel of epidemic encephalitis, associated with postencephalitic PD. More recently, there has been renewed interest in its association with idiopathic PD and other disorders, especially progressive supranuclear palsy. Subcortical dementia can be seen as an equivalent term for the same disorder. Bradyphrenia remains a controversial finding in PD for several reasons. It is not found in all PD patients and it has not been found at all in some studies. Its relationship to motor impairment is clouded by differing views of what is motor and what is mental. What one investigator will call slowing of central processing, another will call cognitive slowing. The cerebral localization offered for both akinesia and bradyphrenia in PD has been remarkably similar. A sharp distinction between motor and mental symptoms may be more apparent than real. The relationship with depressive symptoms has been clouded by differing views of the nature of depression. In cerebral terms, there is a close association between bradyphrenia and depression in PD and a close relationship, if not identity, between bradyphrenia and the psychomotor retardation of depressive illness. Dysfunction of dopamine projection systems from brainstem to frontolimbic cortex has been implicated in both bradyphrenia and depression, but other neurotransmitter systems could well be involved.

REFERENCES

Agid Y, Ruberg M, Dubois B, Javoy-Agid F. Biochemical substrates of mental disturbances in Parkinson's disease. In: Hassler RG, Christ JF, eds. *Advances in Neurology,* vol. 40. New York: Raven Press; 1984:211–218.

Ajuriaguerra J de. Etude psychopathologique des Parkinsoniens. In: Ajuriaguerra J de, Gauthier G, eds. *Monoamines, Noyaux Gris Centraux et Syndrome de Parkinson.* Geneva: Georg; 1971:327–351.

Ajuriaguerra J de. The concept of akinesia. *Psychol Med.* 1975;5:129–137.

Albert ML, Feldman RG, Willis AL. The "subcortical dementia" of progressive supranuclear palsy. *J Neurol Neurosurg Psychiatry.* 1974;37:121–130.

Anderson J, Aabro E, Gulmann N, et al. Antidepressive treatment in Parkinson's disease. *Acta Neurologica.* 1980;62:210–219.

Angel RW, Alston W, Higgins JR. Control of movement in Parkinson's disease. *Brain.* 1970;93:1–14.

Ball B. De L'insanité dans la paralysie agitante. *Encephale.* 1882;2:22–32.

Banki CM. Correlation between cerebrospinal fluid amine metabolites and psychomotor activity in affective disorders. *J Neurochem.* 1977;28:255–257.

Brown RG, Marsden CD, Quinn N, Wyke MA. Alterations in cognitive performance and affect-arousal state during fluctuations in motor function in Parkinson's disease. *J Neurol Neurosurg Psychiatry.* 1984;47:454–465.

Brumlik J, Boshes B. The mechanism of bradykinesia in parkinsonism. *Neurology.* 1966;16:337–344.

Dubois B, Pillon B, Legault F, et al. Slowing of cognitive processing in progressive supranuclear palsy. *Arch Neurol.* 1988;45:1194–1199.

Dubois B, Pillon B, Lhermitte F, Agid Y. Cholinergic deficiency and frontal dysfunction in Parkinson's disease. *Ann Neurol.* 1990;28:117–121.

Evarts EV, Teravainen H, Calne DB. Reaction time in Parkinson's disease. *Brain.* 1981;104:167–186.

Garron DC, Klawans HL, Narins FJ. Intellectual functioning of persons with idiopathic parkinsonism. *J Nerv Ment Dis.* 1972;154:445–452.

Girotti F, Carella F, Grassi MP, et al. Motor and cognitive performances of parkinsonian patients in the on and off phases of the disease. *J Neurol Neurosurg Psychiatry.* 1986;49:657–660.

Girotti F, Solivari P, Carella F, et al. Role of motor performance in cognitive processes of parkinsonian patients. *Neurology.* 1988;38:537–540.

Hansch EC, Syndulko K, Cohen SN, et al. Cognition in Parkinson's disease: an event-related potential perspective. *Ann Neurol.* 1982;11:599–607.

Hicks LH, Birren JE. Aging, brain damage and psychomotor slowing. *Psychol Bull.* 1970;74:377–396.

Javoy-Agid F, Agid Y. Is the mesocortical dopaminergic system involved in Parkinson's disease? *Neurology.* 1980;30:1326–1330.

Mayberg HS, Starkstein SE, Sadzot B, et al. Selective hypometabolism in the inferior frontal lobe in depressed patients with Parkinson's disease. *Ann Neurol.* 1990;28:57–64.

Mayeux R, Stern Y, Rosen J, Benson DF. Is "subcortical dementia" a recognizable clinical entity? *Ann Neurol.* 1983;14:278–283.

Mayeux R, Stern Y, Sano M, et al. Clinical and biochemical correlates of bradyphrenia in Parkinson's disease. *Neurology.* 1987;37:1130–1134.

Mortimer JA, Pirozzolo FJ, Hansch EC, Webster DD. Relation of motor symptoms to intellectual deficits in Parkinson's disease. *Neurology.* 1982;32:133–137.

Naville F. Les complications et les sequelles mentales de l'encephalite epidemique. *Encephale.* 1922;17:369–75, 423–436.

Pierrot-Deseilligny C, Turell E, Penet C, et al. Increased wave P300 latency in progressive supranuclear palsy. *J Neurol Neurosurg Psychiatry.* 1989;52:656–658.

Pillon B, Dubois B, Bonnet A-M, et al. Cognitive slowing in Parkinson's disease fails to respond to levodopa treatment: the 15 objects test. *Neurology.* 1989a;39:762–768.

Pillon B, Dubois B, Cusimano G, et al. Does cognitive impairment in Parkinson's disease result from nondopaminergic lesions? *J Neurol Neurosurg Psychiatry.* 1989b;52:201–206.

Price KS, Farley IJ, Hornykiewicz O. Neurochemistry in Parkinson's disease: relation between striatal and limbic dopamine. In: Roberts PJ, Woodruff GN, Iverson LL, eds. *Advances in Biochemical Psychopharmacology,* vol. 19. New York: Raven Press; 1978:293–300.

Rafal RD, Posner MI, Walker JA, Friedrich FJ. Cognition and the basal ganglia: separating mental and motor components of performance in Parkinson's disease. *Brain.* 1984;107:1083–1094.

Rogers D. Bradyphrenia in parkinsonism: an historical review. *Psychol Med.* 1986;16:257–265.

Rogers D, Lees AJ, Smith E, et al. Bradyphrenia in Parkinson's disease and psychomotor retardation in depressive illness: an experimental study. *Brain.* 1987;110:761–776.

Starkstein SE, Preziosi TJ, Berthier ML, et al. Depression and cognitive impairment in Parkinson's disease. *Brain.* 1989;112:1141–1153.

Steck H. Les syndromes mentaux postencephalitiques. *Schweiz Arch Neurol Psychiatr.* 1931;27:137–173.

Talland GA. Manual skill in Parkinson's disease. *Geriatrics.* 1963;18:613–620.

van Praag HM, Korf J, Lakke JPWF, Schut T. Dopamine metabolism in depressions, psychoses, and Parkinson's disease: the problem of the specificity of biological variables in behaviour disorders. *Psychol Med.* 1975;5,138–146.

Wilson RS, Kaszniak AW, Klawans HL, Garron DC. High speed memory scanning in parkinsonism. *Cortex.* 1980;16:67–72.

Worster-Drought C, Hardcastle DN. A contribution to the psychopathology of residual encephalitis lethargica. *J Neurol Psychopathol.* 1924;5:146–150.

8

Clinical Correlates
of Cognitive Impairment
in Parkinson's Disease

BONNIE E. LEVIN, RACHEL TOMER,
AND GUSTAVO J. REY

There is an overall lack of consensus concerning the nature of neuropsychological dyfunction in Parkinson's disease (PD). Although some PD patients develop dementia, the prevalence is unknown. The pattern of change also is controversial. It is assumed that once the diagnosis is made, there will be a steady downhill progression of the disease. This may apply to the motor symptomatology, but the issue has not yet been resolved with regard to the cognitive changes. It is also unknown whether patients with visuospatial impairments have a pattern of cognitive decline that differs from the memory deficits or executive dysfunction of other patients.

Early PD studies generally were descriptive and relied on retrospective chart review or informal bedside testing to identify patients with cognitive impairments. This approach probably missed more subtle forms of cognitive decline and was biased toward identifying only the most severe forms of dementia. In addition, studies repeatedly have used measures that confound PD symptomatology with such task demands as motor speed and manual dexterity.

There has been a trend to study motor symptomatology apart from cognition, and vice versa. Almost without exception, individual parameters are examined without controlling for other clinical factors that interact with the cognitive variable under investigation. Furthermore, the clinical course and rate of decline in PD may be influenced by factors that are independent of the disease, such as age and premorbid cognitive and psychological status. In this chapter, the clinical correlates that have been shown to influence the cognitive changes in PD are reviewed.

AGE AND AGE OF ONSET

Clinical subtypes of PD may be influenced by age at disease onset (Gibb and Lees, 1988). Mjones (1949) reported that motor symptoms in early-onset PD are more severe than in patients with late-onset disease. Lesser and colleagues (1979) also found younger patients to be more severely affected than older patients. Younger patients have more severe fluctuations of response to treatment and are more likely to develop dyskinesia (Kostic et al, 1991).

Other studies, however, indicate that older patients have more rapid disease progression, a poorer response to L-dopa, and a greater likelihood of developing dementia (Lieberman, 1974). Marttila and Rinne (1976) and Celesia and Wanamaker (1972) found that dementia increased with advanced age. Garron and associates (1972) compared 47 PD patients with 47 age-matched control subjects on timed measures of vocabulary, letter permutation, digit span, and word classification. PD subjects were divided into two groups based on analysis of time scores. Fast subjects had comparable motor responses and intelligence to controls, whereas the slow group was significantly older and showed greater intellectual impairment. There were no differences between the two groups in disease duration. The authors interpreted these findings as indicating that neither age nor PD alone compromises intellectual function but that it is the interaction of these two factors that leads to cognitive impairment. Portin and Rinne (1986) also recognized the influence of age over disease duration in predicting cognitive deterioration in PD. Elizan et al (1986) found that PD patients who exhibited abnormal mental status changes were older at disease onset and were more severely disabled earlier in their disease course than younger PD patients with normal mentation.

These early studies may be criticized, since they failed to employ standardized neuropsychological test batteries on their patient samples and, with one exception (Elizan et al, 1986), did not specifically address the issue of age of onset. However, when Hietanen and Teravainen (1988) used a comprehensive cognitive battery and examined the effect of age of onset, they found similar results. Two percent of the early-onset (< 60 years) PD patients were demented compared with 13 percent of the late-onset (> 60 years) group, despite comparable disease duration. Furthermore, patients with late-onset PD were inferior to early-onset patients on all cognitive measures.

Dubois and co-workers (1990) studied a group of early (<45 years) and late-onset PD patients (>65 years) matched on disease duration with tests of intellectual and memory function. Compared with age-matched control subjects, early-onset subjects exhibited mild memory problems and cognitive slowing. However, late-onset patients exhibited more global cognitive dysfunction, including marked impairment on a frontal lobe task. Dubois and colleagues (1990) concluded that late-onset PD is compounded by aging effects for which the early-onset group is able to compensate.

An important but unresolved issue is whether juvenile PD, defined as idiopathic PD that begins before the age of 40, is a separate clinical entity from classic PD. There is evidence to support both views. Yokochi and associates (1984) found clinical, pharmacological, and neuropathological similarities between juvenile and later-onset idiopathic PD. Gershanik and colleagues (Gershanik and Leist, 1986; Gershanik and Nygaard, 1990), Lima and co-workers (1987), and Quinn and colleagues (1987) drew the same conclusion. However, Barbeau and colleagues (Barbeau and Poucher, 1982; Barbeau and Roy, 1984) and Roy and associates (1983) consider juvenile PD to be a distinct entity consisting of several subgroups, of which three are inherited. One remaining question is whether juvenile PD, or very early PD, differs from that acquired later than 40 years of age but still defined as early onset. Ludin and Ludin (1989) addressed this question and found a hereditary subgroup of juvenile PD patients, but there were no differences in their neuropsychological profile, motor impairment, response to treatment, or medication side effects compared to a group with disease onset after 50 years. This study suggests that the distinction between juvenile and early-onset PD may not be valid because younger-onset PD patients will score higher on all cognitive measures by virtue of their age.

Significant differences in depression scores have been reported between early and late PD onset. Mayeux and associates (1981) found that depressed PD patients were more likely to be younger than nondepressed patients and exhibited fewer cognitive impairments. Santamaria and colleagues (1986) noted a similar pattern. Hietanen and Teravainen (1988) did not report early vs late onset differences in depression scores, although both groups were depressed relative to age-matched controls.

Starkstein and colleagues (1989) proposed that PD-related depression associated with early disease onset may have a different etiological basis than PD depression of later onset. They found a significantly higher frequency of depression in the early-onset group compared to the late-onset group (>55 years). Depression was significantly related to disease duration and performance on a dementia screening examination in the early but not the late onset group. Depression was related to Activities of Daily Living impairment in the later-onset group only. PD patients with late onset also exhibit more tremor and rigidity than early-onset patients, despite a relatively shorter disease duration.

The independent effects of age and age of disease onset cannot be completely disentangled because they are confounded by each other. Late-onset PD patients are, by definition, older. Early-onset PD patients can be divided into younger and older age groups, but symptom duration then becomes confounded by age of onset. Questions about the relative contribution of age and age of onset can best be addressed by studying four separate groups: an early-onset PD group compared with an age-matched control group and a older-onset PD group with the same disease duration as the early group compared to older healthy control subjects.

Despite marked variability in how investigators define *young* and *older* onset, there is considerable evidence indicating that the patient's age at the time of disease onset is a powerful predictor of subsequent cognitive decline. Future studies of age-related depletion of neurotransmitter systems and their synthesizing enzymes are of special importance in understanding the complex interaction between proposed subclinical lesions associated with the normative aging process and the progression of PD cognitive symptomatology.

SYMPTOM DURATION

The effect of symptom duration on cognitive performance in PD is unclear. It was believed that patients with PD would experience a steady downward progession of psychosocial functioning and intellect (Diller and Riklan, 1956; Hoehn and Yahr, 1967). However, other investigators have been unable to confirm any relationship between symptom duration and intelligence test scores, memory, perception, and problem-solving skills (Talland, 1962; Garron et al, 1972; Loranger et al, 1972). Most of these studies are open to criticism, in part due to the restricted test batteries or use of measures that confound motor speed and manual dexterity with problem-solving abilities.

Matthews and Haaland (1979) studied the effect of symptom duration on a sample of PD patients divided into three duration groups: <2 years (group I), 3–5 years (group

II), 6–15 years (group III). Differences between PD patients and controls were most frequently observed on the timed motor tasks, although mild cognitive impairments were demonstrated also on select measures. However, there was no evidence of progressive cognitive decline across the three duration groups. Maximal decline occurred within the first 5 years of disease onset, with no significant deterioration in the later duration group (6–15 years).

Despite several studies demonstrating minimal or no effect of disease duration on PD cognitive performance, it would be premature to dismiss this variable as an unimportant disease parameter. The fact that PD is a chronic progressive illness implies that disease duration must, by definition, exert some influence on the mental status changes observed during the course of the illness. One explanation is related to the way this variable is examined. Usually, symptom duration is studied in isolation (i.e., as a main effect or a single predictor). It is possible that this variable selectively interacts with other critical variables to influence the course of cognitive decline.

Levin and colleagues (1991) studied visuospatial decline in PD as a function of disease duration. One hundred eighty-three patients were compared with 90 controls on six visuospatial measures. Patients were divided into three cross-sectioned duration groups: early (1–4 years), mid (5–10 years), and advanced (>10 years). In addition, subjects were further divided into demented (Folstein MMSE < 24) and nondemented groups. The results indicated that the relationship between symptom duration and visuospatial decline was complex and depended in part on whether dementia was present. In the early duration group, demented and nondemented PD patients both exhibited facial recognition difficulties relative to controls. However, in the mid-duration group, demented subjects also exhibited difficulties on a mental object assembly task, embedded figures, and visuospatial judgments. Demented subjects in the advanced duration group exhibited pervasive visuospatial impairments. These findings suggest that the effect of disease duration on cognitive dysfunction in PD is best understood in the context of how it interacts with other clinical variables.

Since all of these studies are cross-sectional in nature, the interpretation of these data is limited. The issue of disease duration cannot be definitively resolved without employing a longitudinal design that also takes into account the influence of age of onset.

MEDICATION EFFECTS

The major neuropathology of PD is biochemical, that is, degeneration of the dopamine-producing cells of the zona compacta of the substantia nigra as well as dopamine-producing cells in the adjacent ventral tegmental area (Bernheimer et al, 1973). Therefore, the cognitive changes associated with PD ideally should be studied in medication-naive patients. This approach has limited application, however, because most untreated patients are in the earliest stages of the disease. This group is not representative of PD patients with the full range of motor and cognitive symptomatology and is thus a restricted sample.

An alternative approach is to study patients on drug holiday, although there is considerable evidence indicating that pharmacological intervention with dopaminergic agents may produce permanent CNS changes. These alterations may obscure the true relationship between the biochemical and cognitive changes associated with PD.

It is possible that some cognitive changes resulting from dopamine deficiency may be influenced by exogeneous dopaminergic agents (Brozoski et al, 1979). Therefore, special attention must be given to the medication status of PD patients when attempting to clarify the role of dopamine deficiency in cognition.

One approach to studying the effect of medication uses the on/off phenomenon observed in some PD patients treated with L-dopa. These patients manifest marked fluctuations in motor functions, ranging from normal or near normal (on) to severe disability (off). Assuming that these fluctuations reflect variations in the functional dopamine levels, examination of cognitive performance during on and off states in the same patient may be helpful in elucidating the relationship between dopamine deficiency and specific cognitive functions. This within-subject design offers the advantage of controlling for other subject variables known to influence cognitive performance in PD patients (e.g., age of onset, dementia).

Mohr and associates (1987) studied verbal, visuospatial, and motor functions in eight PD patients during on/off states. The profound changes in motor status were accompanied by a complex pattern of change in cognitive function. Performance on verbal fluency, embedded figures, and verbal and nonverbal immediate memory did not differ during on and off periods. However, delayed verbal memory was significantly improved during on compared to off periods.

Delis and colleagues (1982) reported similar patterns of performance on memory tasks in one patient with idiopathic PD who was tested during on and off phases. However, their patient also showed subtle language differences, including increased latency to correct response on a word retrieval task when off, increased perseverations on verbal fluency, and, surprisingly, increased number of responses on the same fluency measure during off as compared with the on period.

Brown and associates (1984) examined changes in general reasoning abilities for verbal, numerical, and spatial material and subjective affect–arousal state in 16 PD patients during on and off periods. The cognitive performance of the PD group was inferior relative to age- and education-matched controls in the on state and showed further decline during the off periods. However, the cognitive changes were mild relative to the severe motor fluctuations and were present only in a subgroup of PD patients.

There is evidence indicating affective changes during on/off periods that may be independent of cognitive fluctuations. Brown and associates (1984) found that subjective ratings of affect and arousal accounted for cognitive changes during the off but not on periods. Girotti and colleagues (1986) reported mood changes without accompanying cognitive fluctuations during on/off variations in 21 PD patients. In a review examining mood and sensory changes associated with on/off in L-dopa-treated PD patients, Sandyk (1989) concluded that off periods are associated with exacerbations of depression, anxiety, and sensory symptoms, whereas on periods are accompanied by normalization of mood and attenuation in the severity of the sensory symptoms.

The dissociation among motor, cognitive, and mood responses to L-dopa may reflect differential involvement of various branches of the dopaminergic system in PD or differential response of the nigrostriatal, mesocortical, and mesolimbic systems to pharmacological intervention. Brown and associates (1984) argued that severe fluctuations in the striatal dopamine system are not always associated with similar fluctuations in the mesolimbic and mesocortical systems. Gotham and colleagues (1988) reached the same conclusion in their study of the effect of L-dopa treatment on cognitive function in PD. They found a dissociation in the pattern of response on several measures believed to be sensitive to disruption of the prefrontal cortex. Verbal fluency was impaired only when patients were unmedicated. When the same patients were medicated, associative learning and subject-ordered pointing were impaired. Performance on the card sorting task was impaired when patients were on and off L-dopa. Taken together, these results may indicate that there is functional specialization within the frontal lobes and that dopamine may differentially affect one or more of these systems.

MOTOR SYMPTOMATOLOGY

Historically, PD has been regarded as a movement disorder. Much work has gone into the effort to characterize the pathophysiology underlying the cardinal motor symptoms of tremor, rigidity, and bradykinesia. There is now a considerable body of evidence implicating deterioration in localized regions of the brain and in specific neurotransmitter pathways.

An important strategy for studying cognitive impairment in PD is to relate patterns of neuropsychological dysfunction with specific motor deficits. A strong correlation would imply that a common pathophysiological mechanism underlies both patterns of dysfunction. Studies attempting to apply this approach to each of the cardinal PD signs are reviewed here.

Tremor

Although various types of tremor may coexist, tremor-at-rest is considered to be the cardinal feature of PD. Tremor has been found to be largely independent of other motor symptoms of PD and, relative to the other clinical features, is the least consistently responsive to anti-parkinson medication (Zetusky et al, 1985; Findley, 1988).

A weak relationship generally has been reported between tremor and the cognitive deterioration associated with PD (Lieberman, 1974; Mayeux and Stern, 1983; Mortimer et al, 1982; Zetusky et al, 1985). Mortimer and associates (1982) investigated neuropsychological performance and motor symptoms in 60 patients with idiopathic PD. They found no relationship between tremor and deterioration in any of the assessed cognitive domains, including measures of expressive language, visual scanning, psychomotor speed, timed and untimed visuospatial skills, set shifting, and verbal and visual memory. Mayeux and Stern (1983) also found tremor to be unrelated to performance on measures of attention, orientation, language, and memory in medically stable PD patients.

One study that did find a relationship between tremor and cognitive deterioration was reported by Reid and associates (1989). They found an association between increased tremor severity and prolonged choice reaction time, and impaired verbal learning and visual memory. However, these authors also noted a relationship between bradykinesia and widespread cognitive impairment. In addition, nearly one third of their subjects were over 70 years of age (older age of onset). Taken together, these finding suggest that the significant correlation between tremor and cognitive impairment may have been a nonspecific finding that reflects their sample's increased disease severity.

Bradykinesia

In contrast to tremor, bradykinesia consistently has been related to intellectual and cognitive deterioration in PD. Garron and colleagues (1972) reported that intellectual deterioration was particularly prominent among patients with severe akinesia. Lieberman (1974) studied 131 idiopathic PD patients before initiation of pharmacological intervention and observed that bradykinesia and gait disturbance were common clinical features among demented patients. In a series of 444 PD patients, Marttila and Rinne (1976) reported that demented patients were more bradykinetic than nondemented patients.

Investigators also have found highly significant relationships between bradykinesia and specific cognitive impairments. Mayeux and Stern (1983) found that increased bradykinesia was associated with impaired constructional praxis and complex attentional processes. Mortimer and co-workers (1982) also obtained significant correlations between ratings of bradykinesia and decreased performance on measures of psychomotor speed, visuospatial skills, and nonverbal memory. Reid and associates (1989) found increased bradykinesia to be related to impairment in word fluency, verbal learning, visual memory, constructional praxis, and information processing speed and capacity.

Rigidity

Although an inverse relationship between rigidity and overall mental status has been reported, these findings are less consistent and do not appear to involve as many cognitive variables as bradykinesia. Marttila and Rinne (1976) reported increased rigidity among demented patients. Rigidity also has been associated with impaired performance on constructional praxis, calculations, attention, verbal fluency, and recall of remote information (Mayeux and Stern, 1983; Reid et al, 1989). However, Mortimer and associates (1982) failed to find a relationship between rigidity and neuropsychological performance.

Although the extent of rigidity is not directly related to the degree of bradykinesia, these motor signs frequently coexist, since they both reflect disruption of dopaminergic neurotransmission in the basal ganglia (Mayeux and Stern, 1983; Cote and Crutcher, 1985). However, unlike other clinical features of PD, rigidity has been reported to correlate with all motor signs and may thus represent a general manifestation of disease severity (Zetusky et al, 1985).

SUMMARY

Although there are only a limited number of studies addressing the relationship between motor symptomatology and mental status functioning in PD, a consistent pattern of results emerges from the existing literature. Patients with predominant tremor exhibit relatively preserved mentation, whereas bradykinesia and rigidity are associated with greater intellectual decline.

The heterogeneous constellation of motor symptoms may constitute distinct PD subgroups that show differential rates and patterns of neuropsychological decline. The characterization of PD motor subgroups and their associated neuropsychological profile will provide critical information about the relationship between nigrostriatal degeneration and dementia. A major limitation is that most studies have been either retrospective or cross-sectional in nature and have relied on correlational analyses to interrelate motor symptoms with cognitive performance.

Given the complex interrelationships among motor, cognitive, affective, and demographic variables (e.g., age, age of onset, disease duration, and severity), it is important to investigate the relative contribution of each of these factors longitudinally. Studying each parameter in isolation implies that it exerts an independent effect on neuropsychological decline, an assumption that cannot be supported.

REFERENCES

Barbeau A, Poucher E. New data on genetics of Parkinson's disease. *Can J Neurol Sci.* 1982;9:53–60.

Barbeau A, Roy M. Familial subsets in idiopathic Parkinson's disease. *Can J Neurol Sci.* 1984;11:144–150.

Bernheimer H, Birkmayer W, Hornykiewicz O, et al. Brain dopamine and the syndromes of Parkinson and Huntington. *J Neurol Sci.* 1973;20:415–455.

Brown RG, Marsden CD, Quinn N, Wyke MA. Alterations in cognitive performance and affect-arousal state during fluctuations in motor function in Parkinson's disease. *J Neurol Neurosurg Psychiatry.* 1984;50:1192–1196.

Brozoski TJ, Brown RM, Rosvold HE, Goldman PS. Cognitive deficits caused by regional depletion of dopamine in prefrontal cortex of rhesus monkey. *Science.* 1979;205:929–932.

Celesia GG, Wanamaker WM. Psychiatric disturbances in Parkinson's disease. *Dis Nerv Syst.* 1972;33:577–583.

Cote L, Crutcher MD. Motor functions of the basal ganglia and diseases of transmitter metabolism. In: Kandel ER, Schwartz JH, eds. *Principles of Neural Sciences.* New York: Elsevier Science Publishing Co.; 1985:523–535.

Delis DC, Direnfeld L, Alexander MP, Kaplan E. Cognitive fluctuation associated with "on-off" phenomenon in Parkinson's disease. *Neurology.* 1982;3:1049–1052.

Diller L, Riklan M. Psychosocial factors in Parkinson's disease. *J Am Geriatr Soc.* 1956;4:1291–1300.

Dubois B, Pillon B, Sternic N, et al. Age-induced cognitive disturbances in Parkinson's disease. *Neurology.* 1990;40:38–41.

Elizan TS, Sroka H, Maker H, et al. Dementia in idiopathic Parkinson's disease: Variable associated with its occurrence in 203 patients. *J Neural Transm.* 1986;65:285–302.

Findley LJ. Tremors: differential diagnosis and pharmacology. In: Jankovic J, Tolosa E, eds. *Parkinson's Disease and Movement Disorders.* Baltimore, MD: Urban and Schwartzenberg; 1988:243–261.

Garron DC, Klawans HL, Narin F. Intellectual functioning of persons with idiopathic parkinsonism. *J Nerv Ment Disord.* 1972;154:445–452.

Gershanik OS, Leist A. Juvenile onset Parkinson's disease. *Adv Neurol.* 1986;45:307–312.

Gershanik OS, Nygaard TG. Parkinson's disease beginning before age 40. In: Streitler MB, Korczyn AD, Melamed E, Youdim MBM, eds. *Parkinson's Disease: Anatomy, Pathology and Therapy.* New York: Raven Press; 1990:251–258.

Gibb WRG, Lees AJ. A comparison of clinical and pathological features of young and old-onset Parkinson's disease. *Neurology.* 1988;38:1402–1406.

Girotti F, Carella F, Grassi MP, et al. Motor and cognitive performance of parkinsonian patients in the on and off phases of the disease. *J Neurol Neurosurg Psychiatry.* 1986;49:657–660.

Gotham AM, Brown RG, Marsden CD. "Frontal" cognitive function in patients with Parkinson's disease "on" and "off" levodopa. *Brain.* 1988;111:299–321.

Hietanen M, Teravainen H. The effect of age of disease onset on neuropsychological performance in Parkinson's disease. *J Neurol Neurosurg Psychiatry.* 1988;51:244–249.

Hoehn MM, Yahr MD. Parkinsonism: onset, progression, and mortality. *Neurology.* 1967;17:427–442.

Kostic V, Przedborski S, Flaster E, Sternic N. Early development of levodopa-induced dyskinesis and response fluctuations in young-onset Parkinson's disease. *Neurology.* 1991;41:202–205.

Lesser RP, Fahn S, Snider SR, et al. Analysis of the clinical problems in parkinsonism and the complications of long term levodopa therapy. *Neurology.* 1979;29:1253–1260.

Levin BE, Llabre MM, Reisman S, et al. Visuospatial impairments in Parkinson's disease. *Neurology.* 1991;41:365–369.

Lieberman AN. Parkinson's disease: a clinical review. *Am J Med Sci.* 1974;267:66–80.

Lima B, Neves G, Nova M. Juvenile parkinsonism: clinical and metabolic characteristics. *J Neurol Neurosurg Psychiatry.* 1987;50:345–348.

Loranger AW, Goodell H, McDowell FH, et al. Intellectual impairment in Parkinson's syndrome. *Brain.* 1972;95:405–412.

Ludin SM, Ludin HP. Is Parkinson's disease of early onset a separate disease entity? *J Neurol.* 1989;236:203–207.

Marttila RJ, Rinne UK. Dementia in Parkinson's disease. *Acta Neurol Scand.* 1976;54:431–441.

Matthews CG, Haaland KY. The effect of symptom duration on cognitive and motor performance in parkinsonism. *Neurology.* 1979;29:951–956.

Mayeux R, Stern Y. Intellectual dysfunction and dementia in Parkinson's disease. *Adv Neurol.* 1983;38:211–227.

Mayeux R, Stern Y, Rosen J, Leventhal J. Depression, intellectual impairment, and Parkinson's disease. *Neurology.* 1981;31:645–650.

Mjones H. Paralysis agitans: a clinical and genetic study. *Acta Psychiatry Neurol.* 1949;54(suppl):1–195.

Mohr E, Fabbrini G, Ruggieri S, et al. Cognitive concomitants of dopamine system stimulation in Parkinsonian patients. *J Neurol Neurosurg Psychiatry.* 1987;50:1192–1196.

Mortimer JA, Pirozzolo FJ, Hansch EC, Webster DD. Relationship of motor symptoms to intellectual deficits in Parkinson's disease. *Neurology.* 1982;32:133–137.

Portin R, Rinne UK. Predictive factors for cognitive deterioration and dementia in Parkinson's disease. In: Yahr MD, Bergmann KJ, eds. *Advances in Neurology,* vol 45. New York: Raven Press; 1986;413–416.

Quinn N, Critchley P, Marsden CD. Young onset Parkinson's disease. *Mov Disord.* 1987;2:73–91.

Reid WG, Broe GA, Hely MA, et al. The neuropsychology of de novo patients with idiopathic Parkinson's disease: the effects of age of onset. *Int J Neurosci.* 1989;48:205–217.

Roy M, Boyer L, Barbeau A. A prospective study of 50 cases of familial Parkinson's disease. *Can J Neurol Sci.* 1983;10:37–42.

Sandyk R. Locus Coeruleus-pineal melatonin interactions and the pathogenesis of the "on-off" phenomenon associated with mood changes and sensory symptoms in Parkinson's disease. *Int J Neurosci.* 1989;49:95–101.

Santamaria J, Tolosa E, Valles A. Parkinson's disease with depression: a possible subgroup of idiopathic parkinsonism. *Neurology.* 1986;36:1130–1133.

Starkstein SE, Berthier ML, Bolduc MS, et al. Depression in patients with early versus late onset of Parkinson's disease. *Neurology.* 1989;39:1441–1445.

Talland GA. Cognitive functions in Parkinson's disease. *J Nerv Ment Dis.* 1962;135:196–205.

Yokochi M, Narabayashi H, Iizuka R, Nagatsu T. Juvenile parkinsonism—some clinical, pharmacological, and neuropathological aspects. In: *Parkinson-Specific Motor and Mental Disorders. Advances in Neurology.* 1984;40:407–413.

Zetusky WJ, Jankovic J, Pirozzolo FJ. The heterogeneity of Parkinson's disease; clinical and prognostic implications. *Neurology.* 1985;35:522–526.

9

Cognition and Hemiparkinsonism

SERGIO E. STARKSTEIN

Early in the course of illness, most patients with Parkinson's disease (PD) show motor symptoms lateralized to either the left or the right side of the body. In fact, the Hoehn and Yahr classification of illness defines stage I of the disease as the period in which patients show only unilateral symptoms (Hoehn and Yahr, 1967). Nonetheless, although many studies have examined the presence of cognitive deficits in PD, surprisingly little research has addressed the potential influence of side of symptoms on cognitive disturbance.

This chapter reviews the most important findings in the study of intellectual impairment in patients with unilateral PD. The influence of confounding factors, such as depression and brain atrophy, also are examined. Whereas some studies have compared patients with unilateral symptoms to patients with bilateral symptoms, this review focuses only on the comparisons of patients with left-sided or right-sided motor symptoms.

METHODOLOGICAL CONSIDERATIONS

The study of asymmetries in cognitive deficits among patients with unilateral PD involves several important assumptions. First, it is assumed that patients with left-sided motor symptoms (left hemiparkinsonism, LHP) have dysfunction of the right hemisphere and that patients with right-sided motor symptoms (right hemiparkinsonism, RHP) have dysfunction of the left hemisphere. There are several findings supporting this assumption. Nahmias and colleagues (1985) examined the striatal uptake of 6-fluorodopa using positron emission tomography (PET) in patients with hemiparkinsonism. They found that whereas RHP patients had a significantly lower levodopa uptake in the left striatum, patients with LHP had decreased uptake in the right striatum. Henriksen and Boas (1985) examined regional cerebral blood flow (CBF) in 18 patients with either RHP or LHP using emission computed tomography (CT) of inhaled xenon-133 (^{133}Xe). They found that 16 of the 18 patients had significantly lower CBF in subcortical areas (probably corresponding to the striatum) contralateral to the affected side. Similarly, Perlmutter and Raichle (1985) found a significantly reduced blood flow in the frontal lobe contralateral to the affected side.

The second assumption is that the left hemisphere specialization for verbal functions and the right hemisphere specialization for visuospatial functions that was demonstrated in patients with cortical lesions (Warrington et al, 1986) is true also for lesions in subcortical structures, such as the striatum. The evidence is not conclusive, but several studies support this assumption (Naeser, 1982; Damasio et al, 1982).

The third assumption is that the asymmetrical dysfunction of the nigrostriatal dopaminergic pathway (which underlies the presence of asymmetrical motor symptoms in patients with hemiparkinsonism) is paralleled by an asymmetrical dysfunction in the brain areas underlying the cognitive dysfunction in hemiparkinsonism (Huber et al, 1989).

Several other factors are important to consider in examining a specific lateralization of cognitive deficits in hemiparkinsonism.

Handedness

Since handedness is related to cognitive asymmetries (i.e., left hemisphere dominance for language is significantly less frequent among left-handers than right-handers), studies of cognitive deficits in hemiparkinsonism should include only right-handed patients.

Neuropsychological Evaluation

Studies of lateralized cognitive deficits in PD were carried out assuming that the tasks used to measure left and right hemisphere dysfunction are sensitive and specific to unilateral dysfunction. Although some tasks have been demonstrated to be specific to unilateral dysfunction (i.e., the WAIS) (Warrington et al, 1986), other tasks, such as the Wisconsin Card Sorting Test (WCST), may not be as side-specific.

Medications

Several studies have demonstrated that the anticholinergic drugs frequently used in PD may produce deficits in cognitive function (Koller, 1984). Thus, the type and dose of medications are important variables to consider.

Overall Cognitive Impairment

RHP and LHP groups should be comparable in the overall severity of cognitive impairment. Otherwise, between-group differences may result because the group with more severe global cognitive deterioration performs worse on a more demanding task, regardless of the association between that particular task and the side of brain dysfunction.

Depression

The presence of depression is a significant confounding factor. In a recent study, we found that patients with PD and major depression had significantly more cognitive deficits than a group of nondepressed PD patients matched for age, education, and duration of illness (Starkstein et al, 1989). In another study, we demonstrated a specific association between side of motor symptoms and depression. Patients with RHP showed significantly higher depression scores than patients with LHP (Starkstein et al, 1990). This finding is consistent with studies of patients with lateralized cortical lesions (Starkstein and Robinson, 1989). Thus, patients with major depression should be excluded from studies on cognition in hemiparkinsonism.

COGNITIVE DECLINE IN PATIENTS WITH HEMIPARKINSONISM

We now review the findings of several studies that examined the presence of cognitive deficits in patients with hemiparkinsonism.

Bentin and colleagues (1981) examined 5 patients with RHP and 4 patients with LHP using a neuropsychological battery that included five tests of right hemisphere functions and four tests of left hemisphere functions. The main finding was that scores on the left hemisphere tasks were better than scores on right hemisphere tasks in the LHP group (i.e., patients with right hemisphere dysfunction). On the other hand, 2 of the 3 patients with superior performances on right hemisphere tasks belonged to the RHP group (i.e., patients with left hemisphere dysfunction).

Thus, even though the sample was small and precluded a more detailed statistical analysis, these findings suggested a lateralized pattern of cognitive deficits associated with the side of brain dysfunction.

Direnfeld and co-workers (1984) examined 5 patients with LHP and 4 patients with RHP. Inclusion criteria were based on the history of greater side of involvement as well as findings on the neurological examination. There were no significant between-group differences in demographic variables, neurological findings, medications, or global cognitive deterioration (as measured with the Mini-Mental State Exam, MMSE) (Folstein et al, 1975). Although differences in depression scores did not reach significance, the RHP group had mean depression scores almost twice that in the LHP group.

Even though there were no significant between-group differences in memory, visuospatial, language, or mental control tasks, the LHP group scored consistently lower than the RHP group in all four cognitive domains and had significantly worse overall dementia scale scores.

Zetusky and Jankovic (1985) have criticized the study by Direnfeld and colleagues (1984) on the grounds that the sample was small, the selection criteria were not defined, and the degree of asymmetry was not stated. They suggested that the more severe cognitive decline in the LHP group was related to their more severe bradykinesia. They also presented their own data showing a lack of association between cognitive decline and side of motor symptoms. Problems with Zetusky and Jankovic's suggestions are that the association between bradykinesia and cognitive impairment has not been demonstrated consistently (Taylor et al, 1986), they did not specify how many of their patients had hemiparkinsonism, and their cognitive evaluation was quite crude [a mental status examination with scores ranging from 0 (normal mental status) to 4 (global dementia)].

Chouza and associates (1984) examined 24 patients with hemiparkinsonism (13 RHP and 11 LHP). Inclusion criteria were based on neurological findings, and 32 percent of the patients had axial rigidity. The neuropsychological battery examined verbal and visuospatial memory, intelligence, and praxis. The authors found that 69 percent of the RHP patients had apraxia and somewhat lower IQs (although scores were not provided). On the other hand, apraxia was present in only 18 percent of the LHP group, who also showed deficits in visuospatial memory.

Although the finding of lower IQs in the RHP group (most of the tasks were verbally biased) and visuospatial deficits in the LHP group are in agreement with other studies, the finding of apraxia is unexpected. Other studies did not find apraxia in the early stages of PD (Lees and Smith, 1983).

Taylor and associates (1986) examined 10 RHP and 10 LHP patients matched for age, IQ, sex, disease duration, and severity. Patients were included in the study only if they had unilateral symptoms or there was a clear early history of unilateral involvement. All patients were right-handed. The main findings of the study were that the RHP group showed significantly lower scores on the free-recall section of the Rey Auditory-Verbal Learning Test (RAVLT: a verbal memory task) and on a test of verbal fluency, compared with the LHP group. On the other hand, the LHP group was significantly slower and more variable than the RHP group in several tests of visuospatial function. These authors concluded that differences between RHP and LHP groups were in agreement with "traditional concepts of hemisphere specialization with respect to language-located versus visual scanning demands, and consistent with dysfunction of the right (visuospatial) versus left (verbal) complex loops." The existence of these cortical–subcortical loops was postulated by Alexander and colleagues (1986) and include segregated connections between basal ganglia and frontal cortical areas that are specialized in either motor or cognitive complex functions.

We carried out a study that took into account some of the methodological problems discussed (Starkstein et al, 1987). Eighteen patients who were ambulatory and right-handed and had a normal CT scan were examined. None had clinical evidence of dementia, a family history of left-handedness, or neurological disorders other than PD. The severity of motor symptoms was rated using the Columbia Rating Scale, and only patients with at least a 3:1 ratio between sides were included in the study. Finally, RHP and LHP patients were matched for sex, age, education, duration of illness, and levodopa dosage. Our final sample was not large (9 RHP and 9 LHP), but we used stringent selection criteria to control for potentially important confounding variables that might otherwise have influenced the results of the study.

The RHP group had a significantly lower verbal IQ and performed significantly worse on a verbal memory task (the RAVLT) compared with the LHP group. They also obtained a significantly lower number of categories on the WCST (a test usually associated with frontal lobe functions). On the other hand, the LHP group showed a significant, albeit mild, hemispatial neglect (crossing-out lines to the right of the midline), similar to the finding reported by Villardita and colleagues (1983). We could not find significant between-group differences on a test of visuospatial memory or on Performance IQ.

Spicer and co-workers (1988) examined 15 patients with hemiparkinsonism (8 LHP and 7 RHP) using as inclusion criteria a ratio of affected/nonaffected side of at least 2:1. There were no significant between-group differences in demographic variables, duration of illness, and medications, although LHP patients had slightly higher depression scores.

A discriminant function analysis based on three left hemisphere tasks correctly classified 13 of the 15 patients into either RHP or LHP groups. On the other hand, there were no significant between-group differences on right hemisphere tasks.

Huber and colleagues (1989) examined the presence of cognitive deficits associated with hemiparkinsonism in a study that included two sets of comparisons: the first only included patients with unilateral motor symptoms, and the second included patients with motor symptoms predominantly on one side. In the first study, both groups (13 RHP and 10 LHP) were comparable in age, education, and duration of illness. The neuropsychological battery consisted of the MMSE, the Standard Progressive Matrices (a measure of visuospatial abstract reasoning), verbal memory tasks, and tests of calculation, language, and word list generation. No significant between-group differences were found on any of these tests.

The second set of patients (14 RHP and 17 RHP) were examined using the same neuropsychological battery, and again, no significant between-group differences were found in any of the tests.

Finally, Blonder and co-workers (1989) examined 21 right-handed patients with hemiparkinsonism (14 RHP and 7 LHP). Both groups were comparable in age, education, and duration of illness. They used a neuropsychological battery that examined language, memory, attention, abstraction, mental flexibility, sensorimotor, and visuospatial functions. After a Z-score transformation of individual test scores, patients with RHP showed significantly more impairment on verbal tasks, whereas patients with LHP showed significantly greater impairment in spatial functions.

SUMMARY OF FINDINGS

There are only five studies that took into consideration most of the important variables that might influence the final results in the study of cognitive deficits in hemiparkinsonism. All five studies had an adequate sample size, only included right-handed patients, used neuropsychological tasks associated with unilateral hemisphere dysfunction, excluded demented patients, had comparable groups in terms of age, education, duration of illness, and medications, and used quantitative motor evaluations to include patients in either the RHP or LHP groups. Unfortunately, the five studies have few neuropsychological tasks in common, making it difficult to replicate findings.

Four of the five studies showed that left hemisphere-related functions were significantly worse among patients with RHP. Among patients with LHP, three of the five studies showed significant deficits on some right hemisphere-related tasks (e.g., visuospatial deficits and mild neglect). Findings in other domains are more contradictory. For example, whereas one of the studies (Starkstein et al, 1987) showed significantly more deficits on the WCST in patients with RHP, another study showed significantly more deficits in patients with LHP (Blonder et al, 1989).

In summary, there is enough evidence to suggest that patients with RHP have significant verbally-related deficits. However, the evidence for visuospatial deficits in patients with LHP is somewhat less clear.

NEURORADIOLOGICAL FINDINGS IN PATIENTS WITH HEMI-PD

Chouza and colleagues (1984) examined CT scans from 13 RHP and 11 LHP patients for the presence of brain atrophy. They rated the severity of atrophy in various cortical and subcortical structures as absent, slight, mild, moderate, or severe. They found unilateral atrophy in 8 patients, which was contralateral to the affected side in 6 of them. Eight other patients had bilateral but asymmetrical atrophic changes, which were contralateral to the side of clinical manifestations in all of them. Ten of the 13 patients (77 percent) with RHP had predominant atrophy contralateral to the side of symptoms, as compared with 4 of the 11 patients (22 percent) with LHP ($X^2 = 11.2, p < 0.001$). Thus, in their sample, asymmetrical brain atrophy was significantly more likely among patients with RHP. The authors did not mention whether the atrophy was cortical or subcortical, and an important methodological limitation of the study was that quantified measures of brain atrophy were not made.

We performed a CT scan study that included 12 RHP and 12 LHP patients (Starkstein et al, unpublished observations). The inclusion criteria were the same as in our previous study (all patients were right-handed, with a 3:1 ratio of affected side, normal CRS scores, none were demented, and none had a focal brain lesion or any other degenerative brain disorder in addition to PD). CT scans were carried out parallel to the orbitomeatal line, and 10-mm thick slices were obtained. Area measurements were carried out using a digitizing tablet attached to a microcomputer. The following regions of interest were measured (Starkstein et al, 1988).

Bifrontal Ratio (BFR)

The BFR was calculated as the distance between the tips of the frontal horns divided by the distance between the inner tables of the skull along the same line, multiplied by 100.

Bicaudate Ratio (BCR)

The BCR was calculated as the minimal distance between the caudate indentations of the frontal horns divided by the distance between the inner tables of the skull along the same line, multiplied by 100.

Frontal Fissure Ratio (FFR)

The FFR was calculated as the maximal width of the interhemispheric fissure at the frontal level divided by the transpineal coronal inner table diameter, multiplied by 100.

Four Cortical Sulci Ratio (FCSR)

The FSCR was calculated as the sum of the widths of the four widest sulci divided by the transpineal coronal inner table diameter, multiplied by 100.

Frontal Horns Area (FH)

The FH was calculated as the average of the left and right frontal horns of the lateral ventricles at the level of the foramen of Monro, divided by the area demarcated by the inner table at the same level, multiplied by 100.

Ventricular Brain Ratio (VBR)

The VBR was calculated as the area of the lateral ventricles at the level of the waist, divided by the area demarcated by the inner table at the same level, multiplied by 100.

The study showed two main findings (Table 9–1). First, patients with LHP had significantly more medial frontal atrophy as measured by the FFR ($F_{1,22} = 4.30$, $p < 0.05$). Second, a 2-way analysis of variance with repeated measures [*factor 1:* group (LHP vs RHP), *repeated measure:* side (left vs right FH)] showed no significant group effect (i.e., both groups had similar frontal horn areas) but a significant effect for the repeated measure ($F_{1,22} = 8.17$, $p < 0.01$), which was the result of a larger left frontal horn in both LHP and RHP groups.

Thus, Chouza's as well as our own study demonstrated that in patients with hemiparkinsonism, the left frontal horn is significantly larger than the right frontal horn regardless of the side of symptoms. Although the finding of a larger left frontal horn in patients with RHP was an expected finding, it is not clear why patients with LHP did not show contralateral frontal horn atrophy, and this puzzling finding needs further study.

MECHANISM OF LATERALIZED COGNITIVE DEFICITS IN HEMIPARKINSONISM

Although several studies have examined the presence of lateralized cognitive deficits in hemiparkinsonism, the mechanism of this phenomenon has never been studied.

Table 9–1. CT measurements of cortical and subcortical atrophy in patients with left hemiparkinsonism (LHP) and right hemiparkinsonism (RHP)

	LHP ($n = 12$)	RHP ($n = 12$)
Bifrontal ratio	32.8 (3.3)[a]	31.9 (3.1)
Bicaudate ratio	14.6 (2.2)	13.0 (3.2)
Frontal fissure ratio*	9.8 (3.5)	6.7 (3.8)
Four cortical sulci ratio	14.2 (6.2)	10.4 (3.3)
Frontal horn area**		
Left	14.3 (3.7)	12.9 (4.5)
Right	13.0 (2.9)	11.1 (5.5)
Ventricular brain ratio	10.7 (1.1)	10.3 (2.3)

[a]Data are presented as mean (SD).
*$p < 0.05$.
**$p < 0.01$.

The finding of basal ganglia and frontal cortical dysfunction contralateral to the side of motor symptoms in patients with hemiparkinsonism may play an important role in the production of lateralized cognitive deficits in these patients (Nahmias et al, 1985; Perlmutter and Raichle, 1985). Whether the unilateral metabolic dysfunction is secondary to (1) faulty nigrostriatal dopaminergic transmission, (2) dopaminergic deficits in the mesocorticolimbic pathway, (3) unilateral DA/cholinergic imbalances, (4) remote metabolic cortical deficits, or (5) a combination of these factors remains to be established.

Only one study examined the presence of significant differences in the concentration of biogenic amines in the CSF between patients with RHP or LHP. Direnfeld and colleagues (1984) found significantly lower values of homovanillic acid (HVA) (a metabolite of dopamine) and acetylcholinesterase (a marker of cholinergic terminals) in the LHP as compared to the RHP group. On the other hand, no significant differences were found in levels of MHPG (a metabolite of norepinephrine), serotonin, 5-HT (a metabolite of serotonin), and DOPAC (a metabolite of dopamine).

Although the differences in HVA and acetylcholinesterase were rather weak and may have been the result of the longer duration and more severe disease of the LHP group, Direnfeld and colleagues (1984) made the interesting suggestion that their findings may be the result of an asymmetry in biogenic amine pathways. In support, asymmetries in the concentration of biogenic amines in cortical as well as subcortical regions have been found in rodents, primates, and humans (Geschwind and Galaburda, 1985). Thus, the presence of significant differences in cognitive performance between patients with LHP and RHP may be the result of a lateralized dysfunction of asymmetrical biogenic amine pathways.

CONCLUSIONS

Several studies have demonstrated significant cognitive deficits in the early stages of PD (Lees and Smith, 1983), which are most prominent in tests of frontal lobe functions. Studies that included patients with main unilateral motor symptoms demonstrated a significant association between the presence of right side motor symptoms and verbally related cognitive deficits and a less powerful association between left side motor symptoms and deficits in some visuospatial tasks.

Contralateral brain atrophy has been demonstrated in patients with right side motor symptoms, and an interaction between asymmetrical brain atrophy and dysfunction of dopaminergic pathways may underlie the presence of lateralized cognitive deficits in this group of patients. Patients with left-sided symptoms did not show contralateral brain atrophy, which may explain why lateralized cognitive deficits are not as prominent in this group of patients.

Future studies may examine differences in the longitudinal evolution of LHP and RHP groups in terms of progression of motor symptoms, cognitive decline, and presence of depression. Whether asymmetries in the mesocorticolimbic dopaminergic system underlie the presence of lateralized cognitive changes and whether changes in nigrostriatal and mesocorticolimbic pathways run in parallel remain to be established.

ACKNOWLEDGMENTS

This work was supported by a National Alliance for Research in Schizophrenia and Depression Young Investigator Award and a grant from the Instituto Di Tella. I would like to thank my friend Jason Brandt, Ph.D., for both his useful suggestions to this chapter and his help and advice during all these years.

REFERENCES

Alexander GD, Strick P. Parallel organization of functionally segregated circuits linking basal ganglia and cortex. *Annu Rev Neurosci.* 1986;9:357–381.

Bentin S, Silverberg S, Gordon HW. Asymmetrical cognitive deterioration in demented and Parkinson patients. *Cortex.* 1981;17:533–544.

Blonder LX, Gur RE, Gur RC, et al. Neuropsychological functioning in hemiparkinsonism. *Brain Cogn.* 1989;9:244–257.

Chouza C, Romero S, Laguardia G, et al. *Hemi-Parkinsonism: Clinical, Neuropsychological and Tomographic Studies.* New York: Raven Press; 1984.

Damasio AR, Damasio H, Rizzo M. Aphasia with nonhemorrhagic lesion in the basal ganglia and internal capsule. *Arch Neurol.* 1982;39:15–20.

Direnfeld LK, Albert ML, Volicer L, et al. Parkinson's disease: the possible relationship of laterality to dementia and neurochemical findings. *Arch Neurol.* 1984;41:935–941.

Folstein MF, Folstein SE, McHugh PR. Mini-Mental state: a practical method for grading the cognitive state of patients for the clinician. *J Psychiatr Res.* 1975;12:189–198.

Geschwind N, Galaburda AM. Cerebral lateralization: biological mechanisms, associations, and pathology: I. A hypothesis and a program for research. *Arch Neurol.* 1985;42:428–462.

Henriksen L, Boas J. Regional cerebral blood flow in hemiparkinsonian patients. Emission computerized tomography of inhaled [133]xenon before and after levodopa. *Acta Neurol Scand.* 1985;71:257–266.

Hoehn MM, Yahr MD. Parkinsonism: onset, progression and mortality. *Neurology.* 1967;17:427–442.

Huber SJ, Freidenberg DL, Shuttleworth EC, et al. Neuropsychological similarities in lateralized parkinsonism. *Cortex.* 1989;25:461–470.

Koller WC. Disturbance of recent memory function in parkinsonian patients on anticholinergic therapy. *Cortex.* 1984;20:307–311.

Lees AJ, Smith E. Cognitive deficits in the early stages of Parkinson's disease. *Brain.* 1983;106:257–270.

Naeser MA. Language behavior in stroke patients. Cortical vs. subcortical lesion sites on CT. *Trends Neurosci.* 1982;5:53–59.

Nahmias C, Garnett ES, Firnau G, Lang A. Striatal dopamine distribution in parkinsonian patients during life. *J Neurol Sci.* 1985;69:223–230.

Perlmutter JS, Raichle ME. Regional blood flow in hemiparkinsonism. *Neurology.* 1985;35:1127–1134.

Spicer KB, Roberts RJ, LeWitt PA. Neuropsychological performance in lateralized parkinsonism. *Arch Neurol.* 1988;45:429–432.

Starkstein S, Leiguarda R, Gershanik O, Berthier M. Neuropsychological disturbances in hemiparkinson's disease. *Neurology.* 1987;37:1762–1764.

Starkstein SE, Preziosi TJ, Berthier ML, et al. Depression and cognitive impairment in Parkinson's disease. *Brain.* 1989;112:1141–1153.

Starkstein SE, Preziosi TJ, Bolduc PL, Robinson RG. Depression in Parkinson's disease. *J Nerv Ment Dis.* 1990;178:27–31.

Starkstein SE, Robinson RG. Affective disorders and cerebral vascular disease. *Br J Psychiatry.* 1989;154:170–182.

Starkstein SE, Robinson RG, Price TR. Comparison of patients with and without post-stroke major depression matched for size and location of lesion. *Arch Gen Psychiatry.* 1988;45:247–252.

Taylor AE, Saint-Cyr JA, Lang AE. Frontal lobe dysfunction in Parkinson's disease: the cortical focus of neostriatal outflow. *Brain.* 1986;109:845–883.

Villardita C, Smirni P, Zappala G. Visual neglect in Parkinson's disease. *Arch Neurol.* 1983;40:737–739.

Warrington EK, James M, Maciejewski C. The WAIS as a lateralizing and localizing diagnostic instrument: a study of 656 patients with unilateral cerebral lesions. *Neuropsychologia.* 1986;24:223–239.

Zetusky WJ, Jankovic J. Laterality and symptom association in Parkinson's disease. *Arch Neurol.* 1985;42:1132.

III
DEMENTIA

10

Prevalence of Dementia in Parkinson's Disease

ALI H. RAJPUT

The issue of dementia in Parkinson's disease (PD) remained underexplored until after 1967, when Cotzias and colleagues (1967) reported dramatic improvement in the motor manifestations of PD patients taking levodopa. Current knowledge of the prevalence of dementia in PD is based primarily on studies conducted during the past 25 years. The literature is nonetheless voluminous and also controversial and somewhat difficult to interpret.

Several considerations are relevant to the prognosis and care of patients. The presence of dementia has implications for both the response to drug therapy and the probability of survival.

DEFINITION

The most commonly used measure to determine the magnitude of a given disorder in the general population is the point prevalence rate. It is defined as the ratio of the afflicted individuals present in the population at any given time. It usually is evaluated in the entire population but could be limited to a defined segment of the population (e.g., those over age 40 years, nursing home patients).

This chapter is aimed not at the prevalence of dementia in the general population but at the prevalence of dementia among all PD patients in the population. It is the measure of coprevalence of these two disorders in the general population that concerns us.

The association of these two conditions may start as (1) PD predating dementia, (2) simultaneous emergence of the two, or (3) dementia preceding the motor manifestations of PD. The presence of PD is essential for the present consideration.

The Parkinson syndrome (PS) is a heterogeneous group of disorders (Rajput et al, 1984b; Zetusky et al, 1985; Jellinger, 1987; Koller, 1987), and in the majority of cases, the cause is unknown (Rajput et al, 1984b). The terms idiopathic Parkinson's disease (IPD) and Parkinson's disease (PD), however, often are reserved for those patients with marked substantia nigra neuronal loss and Lewy body inclusions in some of the remaining neurons (Duvoisin and Golbe, 1989). PD accounts for the majority of PS cases (Rajput et al, 1984b). Epidemiological studies, therefore, have concentrated on measuring the frequency of dementia in PD cases.

Table 10–1 lists some of the commonly cited studies that deal with the frequency

Table 10–1. Summary of some pertinent studies

Study	Source of sample cases	Criteria for diagnosis dementia (and other abnormalities)	Frequency of dementia and significance interpreted by author	Other related information
Martin et al, 1973	Clinic patients (candidates for levodopa)	Neurologist assessment of orientation, word definition and proverb interpretation. After 7 days off anticholinergics. No controls	81%. Higher than reported before	All patients were on anticholinergics but tested when 1 week off anticholinergics. Is that sufficient time for reversal of drug effects? Higher frequency in advanced PD cases
Rajput and Rozdilsky, 1975	Clinic patients	Progressive intellectual loss leading to functional handicap. No controls	28%	—
Marttila and Rinne, 1976	All prevalence cases of parkinsonism in southern region of Finland	Celesia and Wanamaker criteria (1972)	29% prevalence	Used various sources to screen for PD and then examined the suspected patients but classified into only postencephalitic and idiopathic. The most comprehensive survey of prevalence rate
Mindham et al, 1982	Clinic patients	Clinical evaluation—memory, arithmetic, sentence learning, digit retention, general knowledge tests. Retrospectively selected psychiatric patients matched for age and sex used as controls	Initial 20% in cases and 24% in controls; 3 years later 33% in cases and 27% in controls. During 3 years, the rate of new cases of dementia was 4 times higher in PD patients than in controls	Evaluated patients on two separate occasions 3 years apart; only 13% of the demented PD patients at initial assessment survived to be reevaluated. The higher mortality in demented than nondemented and in controls led to dementia in 33% of patients and 27% of controls at the end of 3 years

Study	Population	Methods	Results	Comments
Brown and Marsden, 1984	Review	—	15%–20% dementia. Compared to expected age-matched population, 10%–15% additional risk of dementia in PD	Discuss sources of bias and evaluation methodology
McCarthy et al, 1985	Untreated new mild cases	Reasoning, reading vocabulary, verbal and visual memory, and calculation. Decline from premorbid level or below 10th percentile of expected. No controls	23%	—
Lees, 1985	Severely disabled older clinic cases	DSM III criteria. No controls	15% dementia. Somewhat similar to that expected in general population aged >65 years	The demented patients have higher mortality. These patients had long survival, which indicates that they were less likely to have dementia
Taylor et al, 1985	Clinic cases	Memory, visuospatial, psychomotor, and executive function. No controls	8%	This study indicates difficulty with detailed psychometrics. 7% had drug-related confusion, and 8% could not be tested adequately
Rajput et al, 1987	All community cases identified by physician contact	"Dementia" diagnosis by a physician on two separate occasions during 13 years. Two controls for each case	Up to the time of onset of PD, 5.9% dementia. At 5 years after diagnosis, cumulative probability of dementia 3.8 times higher than in the control group	Before onset of PD, the risk of dementia similar to the general population, but the risk significantly increases after onset of PD
Mayeux et al, 1988	Clinic patients onset after age 40 years	DSM III based on recorded information. Compared with the Baltimore longitudinal study of general population	Overall 10.9%. In elderly PD patients, dementia frequency 3.75 times higher than expected in control population	If onset of PD after 70 years, dementia is far more common. Demented patients were older at first evaluation (74 vs 64 years), and they had later age onset (65 vs 59 years). Demented patients had poor response to drug therapy and more rapid progression of disability

Table 10–1. Summary of some pertinent studies (*Continued*)

Study	Source of sample cases	Criteria for diagnosis dementia (and other abnormalities)	Frequency of dementia and significance interpreted by author	Other related information
Hietanen and Teravainen, 1988	Clinic case of less than 10 year duration	DSM III criteria. Age- and sex-matched controls	In 2% when onset of PD before 60 and in 25% when onset after 60 years	Disability more rapidly progressive and drug response poorer in late age onset PD. Even early-onset patients had (subdementia) cognitive impairment
Levin et al, 1989	Clinic patients of less than 3 year duration. No dementia by DSM III criteria	Six parameters—language, judgment, and reasoning, visuospatial/construction skills, attention, memory, and set shift ability. Age-, sex- and education-matched controls	None had dementia, but patients had significant cognitive impairment compared to controls	Memory, flexibility of set, visuospatial/construction, judgment, and language impaired compared to controls even in early and mild PD cases
Huber et al, 1989	Clinic patients	Cummings and Benson criteria. Age- and sex-matched controls	34%	An additional 50% of patients had (subdementia) cognitive impairment. Only 16% were normal. Those with longer duration of PD had greater tendency to dementia
Gibb, 1989	Review		10%–20%	—
Mohr et al, 1990	Clinic cases with exceptional professional distinction and no dementia. Mild severity of PD	DSM III criteria Memory, executive function, visuospatial skills, ego inventory state, visual retention, mosaic comparison. Age-, sex-, and profession-matched controls	None had dementia. Memory and cognitive deficits consistent features of PD	These were a highly selective group of executives. The executive function was not impaired, but memory and cognitive function declined compared to controls. Authors believe that such intellectual function abnormalities are "consistent" features of PD

of dementia and cognitive function assessment in PD. Some of these studies were not aimed strictly at determining dementia in PD and, therefore, do not bear directly on the prevalence rate. For example, the studies by Mohr and associates (1990) and by Levin and colleagues (1989) were aimed primarily at identifying subtle cognitive function impairment in early and mild PD patients when compared with matched healthy subjects. The patients in these two studies did not have dementia by the criteria commonly used. Most of the other studies aimed at determining the frequency of dementia in PD or reviewed the pertinent literature.

The prevalence of dementia can be determined most accurately by study of an entire community or of a sample representative of the population that includes PD patients of similar profile to the general population. Where the sample PD patients are not representative of the community at large, the results on the prevalence rate of dementia would deviate from that in the general population.

Another consideration regarding epidemiological studies is the accuracy of the clinical diagnosis, which in this case means the diagnosis of both PD and dementia.

Each study is like a snapshot, and the observations made may be valid only under those given circumstances. The accuracy of the observations is dependent on the methodological tools used in the study.

SAMPLE POPULATION

Most of the reported studies were conducted on patients referred to physicians or neurological clinics. Such patients were selected for a variety of reasons, including convenience, economics, and the special interest of the consulting neurologist. Thus, there is an unavoidable case selection bias in such studies, which are, therefore, liable to yield prevalence rate estimations that may not be applicable to the general population.

The 1987 report by Rajput and colleagues includes all the PD patients identified from the medical records of an entire community. Even that cannot be regarded as an all-inclusive study, however, since some PD patients may not have seen a physician or may not have been identified as having PD. An attempt based on a survey of community physicians by Pollock and Hornabrook (1966) is incomplete for similar reasons. The study by Marttila and Rinne (1976), conducted in southwest Finland (population 402,988), that used initial screening and subsequent verification of PD and of dementia by a neurologist is a bona fide prevalence study of dementia in PD in the general population.

DIAGNOSTIC ACCURACY

The next major consideration in evaluating different reports is to assess the diagnostic criteria used. The validity of epidemiological studies to a large extent depends on the correct clinical diagnosis, accurate data collection, proper analysis, and careful interpretation of the findings. In order to identify the presence of dementia in PD, the population at risk should be identified correctly (i.e., the diagnosis of PD should be correct).

Parkinson syndrome is a clinical diagnosis, and PD is overdiagnosed in 35 percent

(Rozdilsky et al, 1990) of early cases. The distinction between PD and other variants of Parkinson syndrome in which dementia is a known clinical feature is essential. These variants include progressive supranuclear palsy, Jakob-Creutzfeldt disease, Alzheimer's disease producing a Parkinson syndrome, and dementia-like features due to antiparkinsonian drugs. Almost all complex forms of PD are identified correctly within 5 years after onset of Parkinson syndrome (Rozdilsky et al, 1990). Studies that are limited to early cases (McCarthy et al, 1985; Levin et al, 1989) would, therefore, include a large proportion of Parkinson syndrome patients who do not have PD. Such studies would, however, not be handicapped by the possibility of drug-induced confusion being mistaken for dementia. For the purpose of determining prevalence rates, all cases—early and advanced—must be included. Hence, some errors in the diagnosis of early PD are unavoidable.

Although the diagnosis of Parkinson syndrome in well-established cases is easy, similar manifestations may be produced by Alzheimer's disease, which characteristically manifests as dementia (Pearce, 1974; Molsa et al, 1984; Rajput et al, 1990b). Some manifestations of Parkinson syndrome (e.g., cogwheel rigidity, stooped posture) are reported significantly more frequently in Alzheimer's disease than in the comparable general population (Galasko et al, 1990). Some patients diagnosed as having PD and Alzheimer's disease may have only Alzheimer's disease, which produces all the manifestations of dementia and PD (Rajput et al, 1990a,b). Dementia and Parkinson syndrome may coexist in a variety of other pathological entities (Chapters 11 and 13).

Several different sets of criteria have been used by different investigators to diagnose dementia. Before these are considered, the practical problems in assessing these patients should be addressed. PD patients may be confused due to dementia or drugs or may be uncooperative for other reasons, thus preventing proper psychometric assessments. The problem with evaluating these cases adequately is evident in the report by Taylor and colleagues (1985), who noted that 8 percent of the patients could not be evaluated satisfactorily, and an additional 7 percent developed confusion on drugs and may or may not represent early dementia. Mindham and associates (1982) classified 3 patients as having dementia at initial evaluation but 3 years later discovered that the diagnosis of dementia was erroneous. These two examples illustrate that satisfactory assessment of dementia in PD is not always possible.

DEMENTIA DIAGNOSIS

The psychometric assessments used by different workers vary widely. Diagnosis of dementia may be based on only history and clinical evidence of progressive memory loss and cognitive function impairment, resulting in decline of functional capabilities (Rajput and Rozdilsky, 1975). In another study, diagnosis was based on the fact that on at least two different occasions such a diagnosis was made (Rajput et al, 1987). Detailed cognitive function testing aimed at identifying subtle differences between early PD patients and matched subjects (Levin et al, 1989; Mohr et al, 1990) represents the other extreme.

The most commonly used assessments for dementia are the DSM IIIR criteria (American Psychiatric Association, 1987), Mini-Mental State testing (Folstein et al, 1975), Celesia and Wannamaker Criteria (1972), and Cummings and Benson criteria

(1983). Several workers have used modifications of these tests. The two most commonly used sets of criteria are DSM IIIR (American Psychiatric Association, 1987) and Cummings and Benson guidelines (1983). These criteria are discussed in detail in Chapter 3.

The false positive diagnosis of dementia by the Mini-Mental State (MMS) (Folstein et al, 1975) has been reported in 39.4 percent (Brown and Marsden, 1984) to 85 percent of the elderly population when measured against the DSM IIIR criteria (Gagnon et al, 1990). Therefore, the MMS can be used as a screening test, which should be followed by detailed psychometric assessment to make the diagnosis of dementia.

Three major sets of criteria used in the literature are outlined.

   I. The DSM IIIR criteria (American Psychiatric Association, 1987)
      "A. Demonstrable evidence of impairment in short-term and long-term memory. Impairment in short-term memory (inability to learn new information) may be indicated by inability to remember 3 objects after 5 minutes. Long-term memory impairment (inability to remember information that was known in the past) may be indicated by inability to remember past personal information (e.g., past Presidents, well known dates).
      B. At least one of the following:
         (1) impairment in abstract thinking, as indicated by inability to find similarities and differences between related words, difficulty in defining words and concepts and other similar tasks.
         (2) impaired judgment, as indicated by inability to make reasonable plans to deal with interpersonal, family and job related problems and issues.
         (3) other disturbances of higher cortical functions, such as aphasia (disorder of language), apraxia (inability to carry out motor activities despite intact comprehension and motor function), agnosia (failure to recognize or identify objects despite intact sensory function) and 'constructional difficulty' (e.g., inability to copy three dimensional figures, assemble blocks, or arrange sticks in specific designs).
         (4) personality change, i.e., alteration or accentuation of premorbid traits.
      C. The disturbance in A and B significantly interferes with work or usual social activities or relationships with others.
      D. Not occurring exclusively during the course of delirium.
      E. Either (1) or (2):
         (1) there is evidence from the history, physical examination, or laboratory tests of a specific organic factor (or factors) judged to be etiologically related to the disturbance.
         (2) in the absence of such evidence, an etiologic organic factor can be presumed if the disturbance cannot be accounted for by any nonorganic mental disorder, e.g., Major Depression accounting for cognitive impairment."
      The criteria for severity of dementia are as follows:
      Mild: Although work or social activities are significantly impaired,

the capacity for independent living remains, with adequate personal hygiene and relatively intact judgment.

Moderate: Independent living is hazardous, and some degree of supervision is necessary.

Severe: Activities of daily living are so impaired that continual supervision is required, e.g., unable to maintain minimal personal hygiene, largely incoherent or mute.

II. Cummings and Benson (1983) regard dementia if the patient has ". . . an acquired persistent impairment of intellectual function with compromise in at least 3 of the following spheres of mental activity: language, memory, visuospatial skills, emotion or personality, and cognitive (abstraction, calculation, judgment, etc.)".

III. Celesia and Wanamaker (1972) have classified dementia on the basis of the following: ". . . an irreversible deterioration of intellectual processes," and subdivided this as to the severity of their symptoms. "Grade 1 indicates mild impairment. The patient has difficulty in abstract thinking, concept formation and difficulty in calculation. He is self centered and shows blunting of interests or mental inertia. Often he shows emotional lability, has difficulty in distinguishing similarities or differences in words, is unable to interpret simple proverbs, shows graphic perseveration and defects in reproduction of drawings. Grade 2 indicates moderate impairment. The patient has a general impairment of cognitive functions, impaired judgment and insight, impairment of recent and past memory without disturbance of orientation. Grade 3 indicates severe impairment. The patient's impaired cognitive functions, memory and judgment are associated with disturbance in orientation. The patient is confused".

The most widely used criteria for dementia are those recommended by the American Psychiatric Association in DSM IIIR (1987). These criteria have been considered unsuitable for the diagnosis of dementia in PD by some experts, however, since they take into consideration social and occupational competence. Functional impairment consequent to the intellectual decline is not always possible to delineate when the physical handicap coexists (Brown and Marsden, 1984; McCarthy et al, 1985). Overall social competence depends not only on the individual's physical and intellectual capabilities but also on the social structure, such as employment and family support. In the population at risk for both PD and dementia, men are often employed outside the home whereas women are homemakers. Performance accountability, therefore, is more rigorous for men than for women, and demented PD men are recognized earlier than demented PD women (Rajput et al, 1990b; Ferini-Strambi et al, 1990).

Parkinson's disease patients evaluated by Cummings and Benson criteria (1983) may not show clear demarcation from normal to abnormal. In the study by Huber and colleagues (1989), 50 percent of the patients had "mild to moderate intellectual disturbance" but could not be classified as demented by these criteria. With half the patients in the borderline category, these criteria present no significant advantage over the DSM IIIR guidelines. Similar weaknesses can be found in the criteria of Celesia and Wannamaker (1972).

It is evident that no one definition is entirely satisfactory for diagnosis of dementia in PD. However, for the sake of uniformity in scientific communications and the practice of neurology, there should be standard criteria that are used by most, if not all, workers in the field. A modification of the criteria in DSM IIIR (American Psychiatric Association, 1987) that would take into consideration the physical disability in PD should be devised to facilitate and harmonize future studies of dementia in PD.

PREVALENCE RATE OF DEMENTIA IN PARKINSON'S DISEASE

When the sample population, the case ascertainment, and the methodology are all taken into account, the most reliable prevalence data are those reported by Marttila and Rinne (1976). Their study included all the possible cases of PD in a large population in Finland. They noted a 29 percent prevalence rate of dementia in PD. This study could be criticized for including only two subgroups of Parkinson syndrome, postencephalitic and idiopathic. For practical purposes, however, further subclassification would have made little difference, since early cases of PD are indistinguishable from most other variants of Parkinson syndrome, and late cases (which they excluded from consideration) are self-evident.

In strict terms, the studies that address the issue of dementia (whatever the definition), except that by Marttila and Rinne (1976), deal with the frequency within the given context only. A meaningful comparison of the reported prevalence ratio, therefore, is not possible. The reported rates vary widely—from 8 percent (Taylor et al, 1985) to 81 percent (Martin et al, 1973). Surprisingly, several studies (Rajput and Rozdilsky, 1975; Mindham et al, 1982; Huber et al, 1989) have reported rates very close to the 29 percent prevalence rate noted by Marttila and Rinne (1976). The weight of the scientific evidence so far is on the side of the 29% prevalence rate (Marttila and Rinne, 1976; Cummings, 1988).

The study by Rajput and associates (1987) that considered the premorbid health profile for an average of 40 years before diagnosis of PD observed no difference in the frequency of dementia in the patients compared to age- and sex-matched controls. That the risk of dementia is higher in PD patients than in matched controls is evident in the two studies where sequential evaluations were done (Mindham et al, 1982; Rajput et al, 1987). Mindham and colleagues (1982) noted that during the 3 years after initial assessment, new cases of dementia emerged four times more often in PD patients than in controls. Rajput and associates (1987) found that at 5 years after the nondemented patients and controls were matched, the cumulative probability of the diagnosis of dementia was 3.8 times greater in PD patients than in the control population.

This remarkably higher risk of dementia would not be evident if the studies were repeated at a later date without consideration of all the patients who developed dementia during the interval and died. The mortality rate among demented PD patients is significantly higher than in nondemented patients (Mindham et al, 1982; Rajput et al, 1990b; Starkstein et al, 1990; Marder et al, 1990) and controls. Consequently, the nondemented PD patients who survived longer would be compared with the control population. This is well illustrated in the report by Mindham and associates (1982). At initial evaluation, they noted dementia in 20 percent of PD patients compared with 24 percent among the controls. Although new cases of dementia emerged four times more frequently in PD patients, among those who survived 3 years, the frequency of dementia was only 33 percent compared with 27 percent in the controls because of the higher mortality rate in demented PD patients (Mindham et al, 1982). The differential mortality in the demented and nondemented PD patients could also explain the low frequency (15 percent) of dementia in the advanced elderly PD patients reported by Lees (1985).

That advanced age and PD together increase the risk of dementia is evident in several studies. Demented patients in general are older at onset of PD than are nondemented patients (Mayeux et al, 1988; Hietanen and Teravainen, 1988; Huber et al, 1989; Ebmeier et al, 1990). Hietenan and Teravainen (1988) noted dementia in 25 percent of the patients who had onset of PD after age 60 years. By contrast, only 2 percent of their PD patients with onset before age 60 years had dementia. They also compared patients in duration of PD and concluded that the duration of symptomatology alone is not critical for dementia. Given the fact that advanced age and the presence of PD together increase the risk of dementia, we expect that if the early-onset PD patients survived long, they would be at an increased risk of dementia.

Based on a review of the literature, Brown and Marsden (1987) estimated that PD patients had a 10 percent to 15 percent greater risk of dementia than the general population. The sequential studies by Rajput and associates (1987) and by Mindham and colleagues (1982) 5 years and 3 years after matching the nondemented PD patients and controls indicate the cumulative probability of dementia to be four times greater in the PD patients than in the controls. The 10 percent to 15 percent additional risk of dementia in PD suggested by Brown and Marsden (1984) would, therefore, be an underestimate.

COGNITIVE DYSFUNCTION THAT IS INSUFFICIENT FOR DIAGNOSIS OF DEMENTIA

The diagnosis of dementia is based on certain minimal qualitative and quantitative abnormalities, as noted previously. There are several psychometric studies and clinical observations that indicate that cognitive impairment of a lesser severity than is required for the diagnosis of dementia is very common among PD patients (McCarthy et al, 1985; Hietanen and Teravainen, 1988; Huber et al, 1989; Levin et al, 1989; Mohr et al, 1990). Mohr and colleagues (1990) conducted a series of psychometric assessments in normally functioning mild PD cases and noted that "cognitive impairment may be a consistant feature" of PD. Huber and associates (1989), who used the Cummings and Benson criteria (1983), found dementia in 34 percent, but an additional 50 percent of their patients had cognitive impairment in one or more categories that were not sufficient for the diagnosis of dementia; that is, 84 percent of the PD patients had some cognitive function abnormalities. Levin and associates (1989) evaluated 41 newly diagnosed PD patients and matched controls with a battery of cognitive function tests. None of the patients had dementia as determined by the DSM IIIR criteria. They assessed the subjects in six categories and noted a significant decline in five— language, judgment, visuospatial, construction, logical memory, and flexibility— among the patients as compared with the controls. A corollary of these tests has been noted in the clinical setting by several experienced workers as "nonspecific" intellectual changes associated with PD (Lees, 1985; McCarthy et al, 1985; Brown and Marsden, 1987).

The significance of the mild cognitive impairment in PD is unknown. There are two main possibilities. It may indicate nonspecific abnormality as might be seen in other chronic progressive diseases of the central nervous system. So far, there is no study addressing this issue. The second possibility is that these patients eventually would evolve into dementia. The detailed psychometric studies in early PD have been reported only recently, and the future course in these cases remains to be documented. Based on the observation over several years of follow-up that PD patients have a four times higher cumulative probability of dementia than controls (Mindham et al, 1982; Rajput et al, 1987), it is possible that those with mild cognitive function impairment during the early course would later develop dementia. Mild cognitive dysfunction is noted in nearly every early PD patient (Mohr et al, 1990), yet not all PD patients develop dementia regardless of duration of PD (Rajput et al, 1984a; Lees, 1985; Rajput et al, 1987). Further studies are needed to identify those cognitive function abnormalities in the early PD patients that accurately predict eventual dementia.

As noted earlier, new cases of dementia emerge at a far higher rate in PD than in the general population, and the prognosis is less favorable in demented PD patients. Information on the prevalence rate alone is not of sufficient value in counseling early PD patients about the future possibility of dementia. More meaningful information would be the probability of dementia during the remaining life of the patient.

Based on the literature on dementia in PD we can conclude the following.

1. The risk of dementia before the onset of PD is similar to that of the general population (Rajput et al, 1987).
2. Some cognitive function impairment (which is not sufficient for diagnosis of dementia) is very common during the early stages of PD.
3. Dementia is more likely in those patients who have PD onset after age 60 years (Hietanen and Teravainen, 1988; Mayeux et al, 1988).
4. New cases of dementia among PD patients are far more common than they are in the general population of the same age and sex. This was observed during 3 year and 5 year follow-ups (Mindham et al, 1982; Rajput et al, 1987). Lifetime risk of dementia is, therefore, significantly higher in PD than in the general population, but the relative risk remains to be determined.
5. Response to drug treatment is poor in demented PD patients (Mayeux et al, 1988; Hietanen and Teravainen, 1988).
6. Progression of disability is more rapid, and the mortality rate is higher in demented than in nondemented PD patients (Mindham et al, 1982; Mayeux et al, 1988; Starkstein et al, 1990).
7. Most studies are based on clinic populations. Only one study (Marttila and Rinne, 1976) fits the epidemiological criteria of the prevalence rate of dementia in the PD population.
8. The reported frequency of dementia, varying from 8 percent (Taylor et al, 1985) to 81 percent (Martin et al, 1973) of PD, is not applicable to the general population. The prevalence rate of dementia in the general PD population is 29 percent (Marttila and Rinne, 1976).
9. Because population-based prospective studies are difficult, highly useful information could be obtained with serial follow-ups of PD patients and matched controls to determine the extent of the greater lifetime risk of dementia in PD.

10. There should be uniform criteria for the diagnosis of dementia in PD. Because of the widespread use of DSM IIIR criteria, the best choice is a modified version of these criteria that considers the physical disability related to PD.

REFERENCES

American Psychiatric Association. Organic mental syndromes and disorders. In: American Psychiatric Association, ed. *Diagnostic nd Statistical Manual of Mental Disorders,* 3rd ed rev. (*DSM IIIR*. Washington, DC: American Psychiatric Association; 1987;97–123.

Brown RG, Marsden CD. How common is dementia in Parkinson's disease? *Lancet.* 1984;2:1262–1265.

Brown RG, Marsden CD. Neuropsychology and cognitive function in Parkinson's disease: an overview. In: Marsden CD, Fahn S, eds. *Movement Disorders,* 2nd ed. 1987;99–123.

Celesia GG, Wanamaker WM. Psychiatric disturbances in Parkinson's disease. *Dis Nerv Syst.* 1972;9:577–583.

Cotzias GC, Van Woert MH, Schiffer LM. Aromatic amino acids and modification of parkinsonism. *N Engl J Med.* 1967;276:374–379.

Cummings JL. Intellectual impairment in Parkinson's disease: clinical, pathologic, and biochemical correlates. J Geriatr Psychiatry Neurol. 1988;1:24–36.

Cummings JL, Benson DF. Dementia: definition, prevalence, classification and approach to diagnosis. In: *Dementia: A Clinical Approach.* Boston: Butterworths; 1983:1–34.

Duvoisin R, Golbe L. Toward a definition of Parkinson's disease. *Neurology.* 1989;39:746.

Ebmeier KP, Calder SA, Crawford JR, et al. Clinical features predicting dementia in idiopathic Parkinson's disease: a follow-up study. *Neurology.* 1990;40:1222–1224.

Ferini-Strambi L, Smirne S, Garancini P, et al. Clinical and epidemiological aspects of Alzheimer's disease with presenile onset: a case study. *Neuroepidemiology.* 1990;9:39–49.

Folstein MF, Folstein SE, McHugh PR. "Mini-Mental State": a practical method for grading the mental state of patients for the clinician. *J Psychiatr Res.* 1975;12:189–198.

Gagnon M, Letenneur L, Dartigues JF, et al. Validity of the Mini-Mental State Examination as a screening instrument for the cognitive impairment and dementia in French elderly community residents. *Neuroepidemiology.* 1990;143–150.

Galasko D, Kwo-Yuen PF, Klauber MR, et al. Neurological findings in Alzheimer's disease and normal aging. *Arch Neurol.* 1990;47:625–627.

Gibb WRG. Dementia and Parkinson's disease. *Br J Psychiatry.* 1989;154:596–614.

Hietanen M, Teravainen H. The effect of age of disease onset on neuropsychological performance in Parkinson's disease. *J Neurol Neurosurg Psychiatry.* 1988;51:244–249.

Huber SJ, Shuttleworth EC, Christy JA, et al. Magnetic resonance imaging in dementia of Parkinson's disease. *J Neurol Neurosurg Psychiatry.* 1989;52:1221–1227.

Jellinger K. The pathology of parkinsonism. In: Marsden CD, Fahn S, eds. *Movement Disorder,* 2nd ed. London; Butterworths; 1987;124–165.

Koller WC. Classification of parkinsonism. In: Koller WC, ed. *Handbook of Parkinson's Disease.* New York: Marcel Dekker Inc., 1987:51–80.

Lees AJ. Parkinson's disease and dementia. *Lancet.* 1985;1:43–44.

Levin BE, Llabre MM, et al. Cognitive impairments associated with early Parkinson's disease. *Neurology.* 1989;39:557–561.

Marder K, Mirabello E, Chen J, et al. Death rates among demented and nondemented patients with Parkinson's disease. *Ann Neurol.* 1990;28:2,295. Abstract.

Martin WE, Loewenson RB, Raesch JA, et al. Parkinson's disease: clinical analysis of 100 patients. *Neurology.* 1973;23:783–790.

Marttila RJ, Rinne UK. Dementia in Parkinson's disease. *Acta Neurol Scand.* 1976;54:431–441.

Mayeux R. Stern Y, Rosenstein R, et al. An estimate of the prevalence of dementia in idiopathic Parkinson's disease. *Arch Neurol.* 1988;45:260–262.

McCarthy R, Gresty M, Findley LJ. Parkinson's disease and dementia. *Lancet.* 1985;1:407.

Mindham RHS, Ahmed SWA, Clough CG. A controlled study of dementia in Parkinson's disease. *J Neurol Neurosurg Psychiatry.* 1982;45:969–974.

Mohr E, Juncos J, Cox E, et al. Selective deficits in cognition and memory in high-functioning parkinsonian patients. *J Neurol Neurosurg Psychiatry.* 1990;53:603–606.

Molsa PK, Martilla RJ, Rinne UK. Extrapyramidal signs in Alzheimer's disease. *Neurology.* 1984;34:1114–1116.

Pearce J. The extrapyramidal disorder of Alzheimer's disease. *Eur Neurol.* 1974;12:94–103.

Pollock M, Hornabrook RW. The prevalence, natural history and dementia of Parkinson's disease. *Brain.* 1966;89:429–448.

Rajput AH, Rozdilsky B. Parkinsonism and dementia: effects of L-dopa. *Lancet.* 1975;1:1084.

Rajput AH, Rozdilsky B, Rajput A. Levodopa efficacy and pathological basis of Parkinson syndrome. *Clin Neuropharmacol.* 1990a;13:553–558.

Rajput AH, Rozdilsky B, Rajput A. Alzheimer's disease with idiopathic Parkinson's disease: clinical, pharmacological and pathological observations. *Neurology.* 1990b;40:339. (Abstract).

Rajput AH, Stern W, Laverty WH. Chronic low-dose therapy in Parkinson's disease: an argument for delaying levodopa therapy. *Neurology.* 1984a;34:991–996.

Rajput AH, Offord KP, Beard CM, et al. Epidemiology of Parkinsonism: incidence, classification, and mortality. *Ann Neurol.* 1984b;16:278–282.

Rajput AH, Offord KP, Beard CM, et al. A case study of smoking habits, dementia and other illnesses in idiopathic Parkinson's disease. *Neurology.* 1987;37:226–232.

Rozdilsky B, Rajput AH, Rajput A. Diagnostic accuracy in Lewy body parkinsonism. *Neurology.* 1990;40(suppl 1):169.

Starkstein SE, Bolduc PL, Mayberg HS, et al. Cognitive impairments and depression in Parkinson's disease: a follow-up study. *J Neurol Neurosurg Psychiatry.* 1990;53:597–602.

Taylor A, Saint-Cyr JA, Lang AE. Dementia prevalence in Parkinson's disease. *Lancet.* 1985;1:1037.

Zetusky WJ, Jankovic J, Pirozzolo FJ. The hetrogeneity of Parkinson's disease: clinical and prognosyic implications. *Neurology.* 1985;35:522–526.

11

The Dementia Syndromes of Parkinson's Disease: Cortical and Subcortical Features

G. WEBSTER ROSS, MICHAEL E. MAHLER, AND JEFFREY L. CUMMINGS

This chapter describes the frequency and clinical correlates of dementia in Parkinson's disease (PD). It compares the patterns of cognitive and behavioral changes characteristic of dementia in PD to the dementia of Alzheimer's disease (AD), the prototype of a cortical dementia syndrome. It also reviews the neuropathology and neurochemistry of PD as it relates to intellectual changes in PD patients. The limited overlap and many differences in the neuropsychological profiles and neuropathology of demented patients with PD and AD suggest that dementia in PD is caused by concomitant AD in a minority of patients. The neuropsychological and neurobiological heterogeneity of PD indicates that there are multiple types of dementia in this disease.

OVERVIEW

Types of Dementia

Dementia is defined as an acquired and persistent loss of intellect affecting at least three of the following areas: (1) memory, (2) language, (3) visuospatial function, (4) complex cognition (such as abstraction, calculation, and judgment), and (5) emotion, including mood and personality (Cummings and Benson, 1983). According to this definition, dementia is a clinical syndrome and not a single entity or the outcome of one specific etiology. Within the dementia syndrome, distinctive patterns of intellectual deficits are associated with different etiologies.

There are two major patterns of neuropsychological deficits in dementia syndromes, identified as the cortical and subcortical subtypes (Cummings, 1986). Although these are anatomical terms, they are used to describe clinical syndromes, not to specify pathological anatomy in precise detail. Despite controversy regarding the cortical–subcortical dichotomy (Cummings and Benson, 1984; Whitehouse, 1986), the distinction between the two patterns has become an increasingly accepted and useful model for understanding the integration of brain structure and physiology mediating human cognitive function (Cummings, 1990).

Cortical dementia encompasses the constellation of aphasia, amnesia, agnosia, and apraxia, whereas subcortical dementia comprises the symptoms of slowing of cognition, defective recall, poor concept formation, and mood changes (Cummings, 1990). The clinical characteristics of cortical and subcortical dementia are contrasted in Table 11–1.

In cortical dementia, language function is abnormal early in the course, whereas language function is preserved until advanced stages of subcortical dementia (Cummings et al, 1985, 1988). This contrasts with the dysarthric speech commonly found in subcortical dementia and normal articulation until late phases of cortical dementia.

Memory function is affected by both types of dementia but in different ways (Cummings, 1986, 1990). Although spontaneous recall is impaired in both disorders, the processes of encoding and storing information are selectively preserved in subcortical but not in cortical dementia (Cummings, 1990). Thus, patients with subcortical dementia are aided by cueing, embedding, and priming strategies that do not help the memory loss in cortical dementia. Conversely, procedural memory is relatively spared in cortical dementia and impaired in subcortical dementia.

Visuospatial skills, calculation, abstraction, and frontal system functions are differentially affected by cortical and subcortical dementias (Cummings, 1986, 1990). In cortical dementia, visuospatial deficits occur early and affect constructional tasks. In subcortical dementia, visuospatial function is mildly involved early in the course and

Table 11–1. Comparison of cortical and subcortical types of dementia

Feature	Cortical dementia	Subcortical dementia
Language	Aphasia	Relatively preserved
Memory functions		
Recall	Impaired	Impaired
Recognition cues	Ineffective	Effective
Encoding	Ineffective	Effective
Priming	Absent	Present
Procedural	Intact	Impaired
Visuoperception	Severe impairment	Mild impairment
Calculation	Anarithmetria	Relatively preserved
Executive/frontal systems functions	Proportionate to overall intellectual impairment	Affected greater than overall impairment
Speed of information processing	Normal	Slowed
Personality/mood	No insight, unconcerned; depression infrequent	Insight, apathetic; depression frequent
Motor functions		
Speech	Normal articulation until late	Dysarthria early
Motor speed	Normal until late	Slowed
Posture	Normal until late	Stooped, rigid
Gait	Normal until late	Abnormal
Coordination	Normal until late	Abnormal
Adventitious movements	Absent except for myoclonus late in course	Chorea, tremor, dystonia, tics

may preferentially affect tasks, such as map reading (Brouwers et al, 1984). Anarithmetria occurs often in cortical dementia, whereas the calculation difficulties in subcortical dementia often involve more complex numerical sequencing and mathematical problem solving. Concept formation and frontal systems tasks are deficient in both cortical and subcortical dementia. These functions are disproportionately involved in subcortical dementia.

The two types of dementia are associated with different types of mood and personality changes (Pillon et al, 1986). Patients with subcortical dementia are more inert, indifferent, and disinterested. Patients with cortical dementia lack insight and are unconcerned about their deficits but have normal energy levels and may actively engage in purposeless activities. Major depression and other mood disorders are more common in subcortical dementia than in cortical dementia (Cummings et al, 1987).

Finally, in subcortical dementia, there is a slowing of the speed of information processing, which is not seen in cortical dementia (Cummings, 1990). Motoric slowing and specific abnormalities of motor function are also prominent in subcortical but not cortical dementias.

To summarize, cortical dementias affect the instrumental neuropsychological functions of language, memory, knowledge manipulation, perceptual recognition, and praxis. These are discrete functions corresponding to precise cortical localizations and depending on specific corticocortical connections (Cummings, 1986). The subcortical dementias affect the fundamental neuropsychological functions of arousal, timing, and sequencing, motor programming, motivation, and mood (Cummings, 1986). These functions depend on thalamocortical, corticostriatal, and limbic–striatal projections (Nauta, 1982).

Frequency of Dementia in Parkinson's Disease

Neuropsychological impairment is common in patients with Parkinson's disease, but there is little agreement on how often these deficits comprise a dementia syndrome. Cummings (1988) reviewed 27 studies of intellectual compromise in PD spanning 66 years and found that the frequency of dementia ranged from 4 to 93 percent, with a composite frequency of 39.9 percent. A recent study (Ebmeier et al, 1990) reported that 23.6 percent of 106 patients with PD fulfilled the *Diagnostic and Statistical Manual of Mental Disorders* (DSM IIIR) (American Psychiatric Association, [APA] 1987) criteria for dementia based on results of clinical examination and two dementia rating scales.

The wide range of reported frequencies of dementia in PD is due to variations in the definition of dementia, patient selection, and sensitivity of instruments used to evaluate cognitive function. Cummings (1988) emphasized that a major factor accounting for differences in the reported frequency of dementia was the method of cognitive assessment. The lowest figures were reported from studies using nonstandardized clinical examinations, and the highest rates were from studies applying standardized neuropsychological testing. In addition, the subcortical dementia syndrome of PD with deficits in concentration, psychomotor speed, and executive function may be overlooked in studies using tools sensitive only to cortical deficits, such as aphasia, amnesia, and agnosia. Mayeux and associates (1988) used DSM III (APA, 1980) criteria for primary degenerative dementia and found that 10.9 percent of PD patients were demented, whereas Pirozzolo and colleagues (1982) used the presence of neuropsychological deficits to define impairment and found that 93 percent of PD patients had abnormal cognitive function.

Clinical Correlates of Dementia in Parkinson's Disease

Several clinical factors, including age, age at onset, duration of illness, degree of disability, and type of treatment, have been investigated seeking clinical features predictive of dementia in PD. One of the strongest correlates of PD dementia is age of onset, with older-onset patients having a higher risk for dementia than those whose disease begins before age 55 (Hietanen and Teravainen, 1988; Dubois et al, 1990; Mayeux et al, 1988). In his review of dementia and PD, for example, Gibb (1989) combined the results of several studies and found that of 123 patients with disease onset before 46 years, only 1 patient had dementia. Elizan and colleagues (1986) compared groups of demented and nondemented PD patients and found the average age of onset of PD to be 52.7 years in the cognitively intact group and 58.8 years in the demented group. There was no significant difference in the duration of illness between the two groups. In their study of a somewhat older cohort of PD patients, Ebmeier and associates (1990) found the median age of onset to be 70 years for those patients meeting DSM IIIR criteria for dementia and 62 years for nondemented patients. The mean duration of illness was 5 years for demented and 7 years for nondemented patients. These data show, as Gibb (1989) states, that age is an important factor in the development of dementia in PD independent of the underlying disease process. Age alone, however, cannot explain the higher prevalence of dementia in PD than in the general population. In addition, age cannot account for the common presence of mild cognitive impairment in younger PD patients (Dubois et al, 1990; Hietanen and Teravainen, 1988).

Gender was not a determinant in the development of dementia in PD in two studies investigating this relationship (Elizan et al, 1986; Ebmeier et al, 1990).

Disease severity influences dementia prevalence rates, and several studies have shown that intellectual decline correlated directly with disease severity in demented PD patients (Elizan et al, 1986; Piccirilli et al, 1984; Hietanen and Teravainen, 1984; Huber et al, 1989). Mortimer and colleagues (1982) observed that the severity of bradykinesia correlated with the severity of dementia, whereas tremor was not correlated with cognitive deficit. These findings led to the proposal that the same subcortical pathophysiological process underlying the bradykinetic symptoms of PD were responsible for the subcortical pattern of intellectual decline. Although the methodology used by Mortimer and colleagues (1982) has been criticized (Nausieda et al, 1983), others also have found a parallel decline in certain motor symptoms (bradykinesia, gait difficulty, speech impairment) and intellectual function (Piccirilli et al, 1984; Zetusky 1985). Ebmeier and associates (1990) calculated age-corrected odds ratios for several motor impairment variables and found bradykinesia, diminished armswing, weakness of speech, and overall disability as assessed by the Hoehn and Yahr scale to be significant predictors of dementia. Although Elizan and colleagues (1986) did not find a significant difference in the pattern of motor dysfunction between demented and nondemented PD groups when initially assessed, PD patients with dementia developed more pronounced akinesia, rigidity, and gait difficulty as the illness progressed.

Parkinson's disease patients with dementia are at increased risk for developing confusional states induced by dopaminergic agents (Girotti et al, 1988; Sudarsky et al, 1989). Early studies reporting intellectual improvement with levodopa therapy (Loranger et al, 1972; Cummings 1988) suggested that intellectual impairment is in part related to dopamine deficiency. Improvement, however, is not sustained, and mental status changes return to pretreatment levels in 2 to 5 years. Cognitive and mood fluctuations occur during on/off episodes, with patients having improved memory, reasoning, and mood during on periods and the opposite during off periods (Delis et al, 1982; Brown and Marsden, 1984; Freidenberg and Cummings, 1989).

NEUROPSYCHOLOGICAL CHARACTERISTICS OF DEMENTIA IN PARKINSON'S DISEASE

The following discussion focuses on the clinical characteristics found in patients who fulfill the definition of dementia given in the introduction to this chapter. However, Pirozzolo and colleagues (1982) observed that neuropsychological deficits affect 93 percent of PD patients and that impairment extends in a broad spectrum without a precise demarcation between demented and nondemented patients. Therefore, the conclusions of studies making distinctions between the presence and absence of dementia in the PD patient should be regarded as tentative.

Attention and Concentration in Dementia in Parkinson's Disease

Intact alertness and attention are necessary for normal performance in other cognitive domains. PD patients with dementia are impaired on tests of sustained attention compared to normal controls (Girotti et al, 1988). In addition, these patients are more susceptible than cognitively intact patients to delirium and psychosis, which are characterized by abnormal attention (Girotti et al, 1988; Sudarsky et al, 1989).

Language Function in Dementia in Parkinson's Disease

Cummings and associates (1988) demonstrated that language function was relatively intact in PD patients with dementia. Most of the patients had deficits in the motor aspects of speech (rate, loudness, pitch, articulation, and intelligibility) as well as grammatical complexity, speech melody, and writing mechanics. Six of 16 subjects made naming errors. Other studies also have documented generally preserved linguistic ability (Bayles and Tomoeda, 1983; Pirozzolo et al, 1982; Huber et al, 1986b). Freedman and associates (1984) compared demented and nondemented PD patients on the Boston Naming Test (Kaplan et al, 1978). Although the average score of the demented patients was below that of the nondemented patients, their scores still fell within the normal range. Beatty and colleagues (1989) found that naming was impaired in PD patients with low scores on the Mini-Mental State Exam (MMSE) (Folstein et al, 1975) compared to PD patients with normal MMSE scores. Huber and co-workers (1989) also found anomia in PD patients with more severe dementia.

Visuoperceptual Function in PD Dementia

Numerous studies have demonstrated diminished visuospatial function independent of motor disability in patients with idiopathic PD, although those who are demented have greater impairments. Girotti and associates (1988) found that demented PD patients perform more poorly than nondemented patients on the Block Design subtest of the Wechsler Adult Intelligence Scale (WAIS) (Wechsler, 1955) and on Benton's Visual Line Orientation Test (Benton et al, 1978). The discrepancy on block designs, a timed test requiring visuomotor abilities, may be partly accounted for by the greater motor impairment found in the demented PD patients. However, performance on the line orientation test is independent of motor function. Beatty and associates (1989) also showed the performance of demented PD patients to be impaired on the line orientation test compared to normal controls and cognitively intact PD patients. In contrast, Huber and associates (1986a) found the performance of PD demented and nondemented patients to be similarly impaired compared to normal control patients on a pattern completion test.

Agnosias have not been described in PD patients with dementia (Pirozzolo et al, 1982; Huber et al, 1986b; Girotti et al, 1988), suggesting that cortical changes are not present in most cases.

Memory Function in PD Dementia

The pattern of memory loss in PD is one of relatively preserved recognition while performance on spontaneous recall tasks is poor (Flowers et al, 1984; Beatty et al, 1989). This profile is evident in patients with and without overt dementia and is apparent in both verbal and nonverbal learning tasks (Heindel et al, 1989). Recall deficits are demonstrable on paired-associate learning and auditory verbal learning tasks (Beatty et al, 1989; Huber et al, 1986b; Pillon et al, 1986). PD dementia patients also have been shown to have a greater deficit in date memory and temporal sequencing of remote events compared to content memory (Sagar et al, 1988b). Freedman and colleagues (1984) compared retrograde memory of demented and nondemented PD patients with normal controls using the famous faces test and found that the PD patients with dementia scored significantly below the controls. Performance by nondemented PD patients fell between that of normal controls and PD patients with dementia but still did not differ significantly from control values. Furthermore, a temporal gradient was absent, a finding that is similar to remote memory deficits in advanced Alzheimer's disease and Huntington's disease (HD) but is different from the amnesia of Korsakoff's syndrome or early Alzheimer's disease.

Implicit memory differs from explicit memory in that the latter refers to the conscious recollection of deliberately learned material, whereas the former refers to the spontaneous acquisition of skills and conditioned responses. PD patients have greater decay of implicit than explicit memory skills. Heindel and co-workers (1989) found that PD patients with dementia were impaired on a pursuit-rotor motor learning task and a lexical priming task, both tests of implicit memory. Furthermore, deficits on the motor learning task worsened with increasing severity of dementia but not with increasing motor impairment.

The pattern of impaired spontaneous recall, abnormal procedural memory, absence of a temporal gradient in remote recall, and relative preservation of recognition memory in PD dementia is characteristic of subcortical dementias. Lexical priming abnormalities are present in some cases of both cortical (e.g., Alzheimer's disease) and subcortical disorders and do not differentiate the two syndromes.

Executive Function in Parkinson's Disease Dementia

Executive function refers to anticipation, goal selection, preplanning, monitoring, and use of feedback in the performance of complex tasks and is generally attributed to the frontal lobes (Stuss and Benson, 1986) and frontal–subcortical connections. It also involves the ability to maintain one activity when faced with alternatives, cognitive flexibility to change an activity when appropriate, and speed of information processing (Flowers and Robertson, 1985). These abilities often are impaired in patients with PD (Cools et al, 1984; Flowers and Robertson, 1985). Beatty and colleagues (1989) compared cognitively impaired and intellectually normal PD patients on the Wisconsin Card Sort Test. They found that even intact PD patients had a mild inability to maintain the correct sorting principle, and impaired PD patients had significantly poorer performance, with fewer categories achieved and more perseverative responses.

Freedman and Oscar-Berman (1986) administered delayed alternation and delayed response tasks to normal control subjects and PD patients with and without dementia. On the delayed alternation task, a reward alternated between two wells after each correct response. The delayed response task required the subject to retrieve the reward following delays of between 0 and 60 seconds after seeing it placed in the well. Demented PD patients were impaired only on the delayed response task.

PD patients with dementia also perform poorly on tests of verbal fluency, another measure of frontal-subcortical function (Cummings et al, 1988; Beatty et al, 1989).

Mood Changes in Dementia in Parkinson's Disease

The syndrome of subcortical dementia commonly includes disturbances of mood. Major depression occurs in 40 to 60 percent of patients with PD (Cummings, 1988), and in some it may be the presenting symptom (Mayeux et al, 1981). Several studies have shown depression to be even more common in demented PD patients (Huber et al, 1986b), and Mayeux and colleagues (1981) demonstrated a direct correlation between increasing depression and worsening dementia. Piccirilli and associates (1984), however, did not find increased depression in PD patients with dementia.

Comment

In nearly every study, the performance of PD patients with dementia exhibited a spectrum of deficits from mild to severe. For example, Cummings and colleagues (1988) found that demented PD patients, in general, exhibited verbal output features characteristic of subcortical dementia with impaired motor function (dysarthria, mechanical agraphia) and preserved linguistic function (e.g., naming, comprehension). A subgroup of PD patients with dementia, however, manifested language abnormalities, including anomia, more characteristic of cortical dysfunction and Alzheimer's disease. A similar variability of performance among PD patients with dementia was found by

El-Awar and associates (1987) when assessing visuospatial skills. These observations emphasize the heterogeneity of intellectual impairments exhibited in PD with dementia and support the concept of multiple dementia syndromes in PD associated with variable cellular and biochemical pathology.

COMPARISON OF DEMENTIA IN ALZHEIMER'S DISEASE AND PARKINSON'S DISEASE

Alzheimer's disease (AD) is the prototype of the cortical dementias (Cummings and Benson, 1983). As such, it is useful to compare the dementia of AD and PD to determine similarities and differences. To the extent that both diseases are a cortical dementia, the features of the dementia syndrome should be similar.

Comparison of Memory Function

In neuropsychological comparisons of AD and PD, verbal memory has been the most intensively studied memory function. On a wide variety of recent verbal memory tasks, AD patients perform less well than PD patients with dementia (Huber et al, 1986b; Mildworf et al, 1986; Pillon et al, 1986; El-Awar et al, 1987; Heindel et al, 1989). This is true even when patients from the two groups are matched for overall dementia severity. AD also affects recall of previously learned verbal information differently than PD. Sagar and colleagues (1988a) found that both AD patients and mildly demented PD patients had more difficulty recalling recent than remote events. In addition, PD patients showed a relatively selective deficit in date memory and temporal sequencing compared to content memory for remote events, whereas the AD patients were equally impaired on both (Sagar et al, 1988b).

Sahakian and associates (1988) studied spatial recognition, matching-to-sample, and delayed matching to compare visuospatial memory in AD and PD. AD patients and those with more severe PD were impaired on pattern recognition tasks, and patients with mild PD were not. On the matching-to-sample test, PD patients were more impaired than controls, and the AD patients had no significant difficulty. On the delayed matching test, the AD patients deteriorated markedly with longer delay intervals, whereas the PD patients were not affected by the delay.

Freedman and Oscar-Berman (1987) tested tactile memory in AD patients and PD patients matched for dementia severity and found that the PD patients were more impaired. Both groups had difficulty changing to a new target pattern, again demonstrating both similarities and differences in their performances.

The ability to learn novel motor skills also distinguished AD and PD (Heindel et al, 1989), with demented PD patients significantly more impaired than AD or control subjects on a pursuit-rotor task. Difficulty on this task did not correlate with the extrapyramidal motor symptoms of PD but was significantly related to dementia severity.

Comparison of Language Function

The characteristic language disturbances of AD might be present in the dementia of PD if the latter were caused by co-occurring AD. However, whereas aphasia is common in AD (Cummings and Benson, 1983), consistent with the cortical dementia pattern, the studies cited previously demonstrate little language dysfunction in PD patients with dementia. Alzheimer's disease patients have decreased information content of spontaneous speech, impaired word list generation (verbal fluency), and more severe anomia than PD patients matched for severity of dementia (Bayles and Tomoeda, 1983; Cummings et al, 1988). Cummings and colleagues (1988) found that demented PD patients performed better than AD patients on tests of auditory comprehension, naming, and verbal fluency. Demented PD patients had significantly greater dysarthria and mechanical agraphia, shorter phrase length, and simplified grammar.

Comparison of Executive Function

There are also contrasts between AD and PD in executive functions mediated by the frontal lobe and its subcortical connections. Using delayed alternation and delayed response tests, Freedman and Oscar-Berman (1986) showed that AD patients were impaired on both tests while demented PD patients were impaired only on the delayed response task. Freedman and Oscar-Berman (1987, 1989) also demonstrated that AD patients made significantly more perseverative errors during the reversal phase of tactile and visual learning tests.

Pillon and co-workers (1986) found that performance on the Wisconsin Card Sort Test distinguished PD patients with intellectual deterioration from controls but did not differentiate AD patients and control subjects. PD patients displayed more prehension behaviors than normal controls and AD patients. Huber and colleagues (1986b) demonstrated greater apraxia and more severe impairment on Trail-making tests in AD than PD patients with dementia. Both of these skills are mediated by frontal–subcortical connections.

In sum, both AD and PD affect executive functions, but with different patterns of impairment.

NEUROBIOLOGY OF DEMENTIA SYNDROMES OF PARKINSON'S DISEASE

The morphological and biochemical changes found in PD patients with dementia are variable and reflect the broad spectrum of clinical characteristics. Furthermore, neuropsychological and neuropathological studies suggest that there may be several types of dementia syndromes reflecting a variety of cellular and biochemical changes in PD (Cummings, 1988). Some of these neurobiological changes overlap with those seen in AD.

Dementia and Classic PD Neuropathology

The classic pathology of PD includes the loss of pigmented neurons and the presence of Lewy bodies in the substantia nigra, ventral tegmental area (VTA), and locus ceruleus (Barbeau, 1986). These changes lead to denervation of the dopaminergic nigrostriatal and VTA–mesocortical pathways and the noradrenergic pathways from the locus ceruleus to cortex (Wooten, 1987).

Total cell loss in the substantia nigra in PD is highly variable and has not been shown to correlate with the presence or severity of dementia (Gaspar and Gray, 1984). Reduced cell counts in the medial substantia nigra specifically and reduced dopamine levels in the VTA have been correlated with dementia in PD (Javoy-Agid, and Agid, 1983; Rinne et al, 1989). Dopaminergic projections to mesial cortical and limbic structures arise from both these areas. In addition, studies have shown that neuronal loss in the locus ceruleus (the primary source of cortical norepinephrine) is greater in PD patients with dementia than in those without dementia, suggesting that diminished norepinephrine availability contributes to cognitive impairment (Gaspar and Gray, 1984; Chui et al, 1986; Cash et al, 1987).

There is ample evidence showing that dementia may occur in PD with pathology restricted to the brainstem pigmented nuclei. Helig and colleagues (1985) reported five demented PD patients with extensive cell loss and Lewy bodies in the substantia nigra and locus ceruleus, but without neuritic plaques (NP) or neurofibrillary tangles (NFT) in the cerebral cortex and with normal cell counts in the nucleus basalis. Chui and colleagues (1986) described the clinical and pathological aspects of four patients with dementia and PD. Abundant AD changes were not present in the cortex in any, and one had no alterations in nucleus basalis.

Alzheimer Type Pathology in Parkinson's Disease

There is considerable controversy regarding the frequency of Alzheimer-type pathology in PD and its relationship to dementia symptoms. Alvord and colleagues (1974) suggested that AD-type changes are more common in PD than in control subjects. Hakim and Mathieson (1979) found NP, NFT, granulovacuolar degeneration, and cortical cell loss in the brains of most PD patients and attributed dementia in PD to coexistent AD. Boller and colleagues (1980) found NP and NFT at autopsy in the brains of 15 of 36 PD patients, including 12 of 16 with some degree of dementia and 3 of 13 with normal mental status. The cognitive status of 7 patients was unknown, and the occurrence of AD pathology in the brains of patients without dementia suggests that the histological criteria for the diagnosis of AD may not have been rigorous. Gaspar and Gray (1984) found AD pathology in almost all demented PD patients and half of nondemented PD patients.

In contrast, Perry and colleagues (1983) reported AD pathology in only 1 of 7 demented PD patients. When Ball (1984) reanalyzed the data of Hakim and Mathieson (1979), there was no difference in the abundance of AD changes between PD patients with and without dementia. Ball's (1984) quantitative index of NFT was not different in 4 demented PD patients, 2 nondemented PD patients, and several normal aged controls. Jellinger and Riederer (1984) found no difference in the amount of AD pathology in 180 PD patients (101 with dementia) and age-matched control subjects. Jellinger (1987) reported a relationship between age at death and AD pathology in the brains of PD patients, with a frequency in those over 70 twice that of those under 70 (33 percent vs 17 percent). Xuereb and colleagues (1989) reported the specific histological criteria for AD in only 2 of 38 patients (5.3 percent) with PD. Half of the patients with no cortical pathology had dementia. In one of the few studies of the prevalence of AD in relatively unselected PD patients, Heston (1980) found only 12 cases of PD with marked dementia, none with AD pathology, in a review of 2204 necropsies from Minnesota state hospitals.

Atrophy of the nucleus basalis, a consistent finding and the cause of the cortical cholinergic deficit in AD (Whitehouse et al, 1982), is variable in PD. Several investigators have reported more pathology in the nucleus basalis of demented PD patients than in those without dementia (Whitehouse et al, 1983; Mann and Yates, 1983; Gaspar and Gray, 1984). Tagliavini and colleagues (1984), however, reported cell loss of 30 to 68 percent in nucleus basalis in all PD patients studied, with no statistically significant difference between those with and without dementia. Rogers and co-workers (1985) studied four demented PD patients, but only two had marked cell loss in nucleus basalis and the others had normal cell counts. Sudarsky and associates (1989) also described four patients with marked dementia, classic PD pathology, and moderately severe cell loss and Lewy body formation in the nucleus basalis without AD-type pathology in the cortex.

From these studies emerge several tentative conclusions. First, in PD patients with dementia, neuronal loss in the nucleus basalis is usually more severe than in those without dementia. Second, some patients with dementia have intact basal nuclei. Atrophy of nucleus basalis is not required for dementia in PD. Third, nucleus basalis atrophy often occurs without AD type pathology in the cerebral cortex of patients with PD.

The reported frequency of AD-type changes in PD brains in most studies is increased over the general population. The frequency of these pathologic changes depends on the age of the population examined. The pathological diagnosis of AD depends on the criteria used for the required abundance of histopathological alterations, and the application of these standards has been variable. There have been too few studies of unselected populations to determine if the true prevalence of AD is increased among PD patients. Although severe dementia in PD often is associated with AD-type cortical pathology (Boller et al, 1980) or atrophy of the nucleus basalis (Whitehouse et al, 1983), dementia in PD can occur in the absence of both these features (Heston, 1980; Helig et al, 1985; Chui et al, 1986). Concurrent AD exacerbates dementia severity in PD, but is not necessary for the development of dementia in PD. Moreover, the frequency of AD-type pathology in PD is lower than the nearly universal changes in mental status documented in PD.

Neurotransmitters, Receptors, and Neuropeptides in Parkinson's Disease

Dopamine concentrations are reduced in the caudate and frontal cortex of PD patients with and without dementia (Agid et al, 1987; Rossor, 1987). Norepinephrine levels in locus ceruleus are normal in non-demented PD patients, but diminished in demented PD patients (Cash et al, 1987). Norepinephrine levels in the cortex were reduced in both conditions (Agid et al, 1987; Rossor, 1987). Serotonin levels also are reduced in the frontal cortex in PD (D'Amato et al, 1987).

Dubois and colleagues (1983) found that choline acetyltransferase (CAT), a marker for cholinergic function, was reduced in PD. This reduction was greatest in PD patients with dementia, all of whom also had AD pathology. The degree of dementia correlated with the abundance of NP and NFT but not with the degree of CAT deficiency. Perry and associates (1985) found that CAT was reduced in the cortex of PD patients with overt dementia to levels comparable to those found in AD even in the absence of AD cortical histopathology. Atrophy of the nucleus basalis correlated with CAT levels in the temporal cortex. Gaspar and Gray (1984) also noted significant reductions in cortical CAT in demented PD patients compared to those without dementia, with a nonsignificant trend relating nucleus basalis atrophy to cortical CAT concentrations. Some nondemented PD patients have cortical CAT levels as low as those with overt intellectual changes (Gaspar and Gray, 1984; Perry et al, 1985). Whitehouse and colleagues (1988) found that CAT was reduced in PD with or without AD pathology, although the reductions were more marked in those with AD pathology. These observations indicate a relationship between nucleus basalis atrophy and CAT deficiency and between AD pathology and CAT deficiency. CAT deficiency is usually, but not invariably, accompanied by dementia.

Muscarinic cholinergic receptors (M1 and M2 subtypes) are increased in demented but not in nondemented, PD patients. Nicotinic cholinergic receptors were significantly reduced in PD with AD pathology, and in PD with dementia without AD pathology (Perry et al, 1987; Whitehouse et al, 1988). Serotonin S1 receptors were diminished in demented PD patients but not in those without overt dementia. S2 receptors were normal in PD patients with and without dementia (Perry et al, 1984). D'Amato and colleagues (1987) found no alterations in adenosine, phencyclidine, beta-adrenergic, and calcium antagonist receptors in PD.

Not all studies of neuropeptides in PD report similar results (Beal and Martin, 1986; Constantinidis et al, 1988), and in many studies, the mental status of the PD patients is not fully documented. Therefore, the relationship between neuropeptide changes and dementia in PD remains obscure. Concentrations of substance P in the substantia nigra and globus pallidus are diminished approximately 30 percent in PD patients with dementia. Somatostatin levels are 30 to 50 percent reduced in the cortex of PD patients with dementia, but there is no change in somatostatin in PD patients without dementia (Epelbaum et al, 1988). Cortical neuropeptide Y levels are normal in PD, as are levels of vasopressin. Vasoactive intestinal peptide is normal in both demented and nondemented PD patients (Jegou et al, 1985). Cholecystokinin is normal in the cortex in PD, but approximately 40 percent reduced in the substantia nigra. In PD, neurotensin is decreased in the hippocampus, and methionine enkephalin is reduced 50 to 70 percent in subcortical structures. Adrenocorticotropic hormone (ACTH) is normal in PD. Corticotropin-releasing factor (CRF) is reduced 50 to 80 percent in PD with AD type pathology. In other cases of PD, CRF reductions are variable (Whitehouse et al, 1987).

In the cerebrospinal fluid of PD patients with dementia, there are reductions in angiotensin-converting enzyme, homovanillic acid, and other metabolites of dopamine, whereas beta-endorphin, acetylcholinesterase, and somatostatin levels are normal (Zubenko et al, 1985, 1986; Jolkkonen et al, 1986, 1987).

SUMMARY

Nearly all neuropsychological studies demonstrate a spectrum of severity of intellectual deterioration in PD patients. In many cognitive domains, particularly memory and language, different patterns of abnormalities are evident in PD and AD even when subjects are matched for the overall severity of cognitive impairment (Pillon et al, 1986; Freedman and Oscar-Berman, 1987; Cummings et al, 1988). Although some PD patients with dementia perform above the level of AD patients, a few exhibit intellectual impairment quantitatively and qualitatively similar to AD. These observations emphasize the heterogeneity of intellectual impairment in PD and support the concept of multiple dementia syndromes in PD.

These multiple dementia syndromes may be associated with variable morphological and biochemical pathologies. Ten to 60 percent of PD patients show AD type neuropathology, and these patients also may have the neurochemical changes found in AD. Although severe dementia in PD often is associated with AD-type pathology in the cortex (Boller et al, 1980) or nucleus basalis (Whitehouse et al, 1983), many PD patients with dementia do not have this pathology but only the neurobiological manifestations of classic PD (Heston, 1980; Helig et al, 1985; Chui et al, 1986). Neuropsychological, neuropathological, and neurochemical comparison studies of AD and PD with dementia indicate that the dementia of PD is distinct from AD in a majority of cases.

At least three subtypes of the dementia syndromes of PD may be hypothesized. First, the dopamine deficiency ubiquitous in PD patients results in a dementia syndrome with the features of subcortical dementia: memory loss, executive function deficits and slowing of information processing, and mood changes, with relative preservation of linguistic skills. Often these changes are relatively mild in degree, but the cognitive deterioration may be marked when pathological changes confined to the subcortical nuclei are severe (Chui et al, 1986; Helig et al, 1985). Second, a more marked dementia syndrome commonly is present when atrophy of the nucleus basalis adds a cholinergic deficit to the dopaminergic and noradrenergic deficiencies of PD (Sudarsky et al, 1989). Third, some PD patients with dementia also have AD-type pathology. These patients have severe dementia characterized by a mixture of cortical and subcortical features (Gaspar and Gray, 1984; Perry et al, 1983).

ACKNOWLEDGMENTS

The authors acknowledge the support of the Department of Veterans Affairs and the French Foundation for Alzheimer's Research. Dr. Mahler receives support from the National Institute on Aging, Academic Award AG00260.

REFERENCES

Agid Y, Ruberg M, Dubois B, Pillon B. Anatomoclinical and biochemical concepts of subcortical dementia. In: Stahl SM, Iverson SD, Goodman ED, eds. *Cognitive Neurochemistry.* New York: Oxford University Press; 1987:248–271.

Alvord EC Jr, Forno LS, Kusske JA, et al. The pathology of parkinsonism: a comparison of degenerations in cerebral cortex and brainstem. *Adv Neurol.* 1974;5:175–193.

American Psychiatric Association. *Diagnostic and Statistical Manual of Mental Disorders,* 3rd ed. Washington, DC: American Psychiatric Association; 1980.

American Psychiatric Association. *Diagnostic and Statistical Manual of Mental Disorders,* 3rd ed rev. Washington, DC: American Psychiatric Association; 1987.

Ball MJ. The morphological basis of dementia in Parkinson's disease. *Can J Neurol Sci.* 1984;11:180–184.

Barbeau A. Parkinson's disease: clinical features and etiopathology. In: Vinken PJ, Bruyn GW, Klawans HL, eds. *Handbook of Clinical Neurology.* vol 5(49): Extrapyramidal disorders. New York: Elsevier Science Publishers; 1986:87–152.

Bayles KA, Tomoeda CK. Confrontation naming impairment in dementia. *Brain Cogn.* 1983;19:98–114.

Beal MF, Martin JB. Neuropeptides in neurological disease. *Ann Neurol.* 1986;20:547–565.

Beatty WW, Staton RD, Weir WS, et al. Cognitive disturbances in Parkinson's disease. *J Geriatr Psychiatry Neurol.* 1989;2:22–33.

Benton AL, Vourney NR, Hamshark K de S. Visuospatial judgment: a clinical test. *Arch Neurol.* 1978;35:364–367.

Boller F, Mizutani R, Roessmann U, Gambetti P. Parkinson disease, dementia, and Alzheimer disease: clinicopathologic correlations. *Ann Neurol.* 1980;7:329–335.

Brouwers P, Cox C, Martin A, et al. Differential perceptual-spatial impairment in Huntington's and Alzheimer's disease. *Arch Neurol.* 1984;41:1073–1076.

Brown RG, Marsden CD, Quinn N, Wyke MA. Alterations in cognitive performance and affect-arousal state during fluctuation in motor function in Parkinson's disease. *J Neurol Neurosurg Psychiatry.* 1984;47:454–465.

Cash R, L'Heureux R, Raisman R, et al. Parkinson's disease and dementia: norepinephrine and dopamine in the locus ceruleus. *Neurology.* 1987;37:42–46.

Chui HC, Mortimer JA, Slager U, et al. Pathologic correlates of dementia in Parkinson's disease. *Arch Neurol.* 1986;43:991–995.

Constantinidis J, Bouras C, Vallet PG. Neuropeptides in Alzheimer's disease and Parkinson's disease. *Mt Sinai J Med.* 1988;55:102–115.

Cools AR, Van Der Bercken JHL, Horstink MWI, et al. Cognitive and motor shifting aptitude disorder in Parkinson's disease. *J Neurol Neurosurg Psychiatry.* 1984;43:443–453.

Cummings JL. Subcortical dementia: neuropsychology, neuropsychiatry, and pathophysiology. *Br J Psychiatry.* 1986;149:682–687.

Cummings JL. Intellectual impairment in Parkinson'a disease: clinical, pathologic, and biochemical correlates. *J Geriatr Psychiatry Neurol.* 1988;1:24–36.

Cummings JL. Introduction. In: Cummings JL, ed. *Subcortical Dementia.* New York: Oxford University Press; 1990:3–14.

Cummings JL, Benson DF. *Dementia. A Clinical Approach.* Boston: Butterworths; 1983.

Cummings JL, Benson DF. Subcortical dementia: review of an emerging concept. *Arch Neurol.* 1984;41:874–879.

Cummings JL, Benson DF, Hill MA, Read S. Aphasia in dementia of the Alzheimer type. *Neurology.* 1985;35:394–397.

Cummings JL, Darkins A, Mendez M, et al. Alzheimer's disease and Parkinson's disease: comparison of speech and language alterations. *Neurology.* 1988;38:680–684.

Cummings JL, Miller B, Hill MA, Neshkes R. Neuropsychiatric aspects of multi-infarct dementia and dementia of the Alzheimer type. *Arch Neurol.* 1987;44:389–393.

D'Amato RJ, Zweig RM, Whitehouse PJ, et al. Aminergic systems in Alzheimer's disease and Parkinson's disease. *Ann Neurol.* 1987;22:229–236.

Delis D, Direnfeld L, Alexander MP, Kaplan E. Cognitive fluctuations associated with on-off phenomenon in Parkinson's disease. *Neurology.* 1982;32:1049–1052.

Dubois B, Pillon B, Sternic N, et al. Age-induced cognitive disturbances in Parkinson's disease. *Neurology.* 1990;40:38–41.

Dubois B, Ruberg M, Javoy-Agid F, et al. A subcortical-cortical cholinergic system is affected in Parkinson's disease. *Brain Res.* 1983;288:213–221.

Ebmeier KP, Calder SA, Crawford JR, et al. Clinical features predicting dementia in idiopathic Parkinson's disease: a follow-up study. *Neurology.* 1990;40:1222–1224.

El-Awar, M, Becker JT, Hammond KM, et al. Learning deficit in Parkinson's disease: comparison with Alzheimer's disease and normal aging. *Arch Neurol.* 1987;44:180–184.

Elizan TS, Sroka H, Maker H, et al. Dementia in idiopathic Parkinson's disease. *J Neural Transm.* 1986;65:285–302.

Epelbaum J, Javoy-Agid F, Enjalbert A, et al. Somatostatin concentrations and binding sites in human frontal cortex are differentially affected in Parkinson's disease associated dementia and progressive supranuclear palsey. *J Neurol Sci.* 1988;87:167–74.

Flowers KA, Robertson C. The effect of Parkinson's disease on the ability to maintain a mental set. *J Neurol Neurosurg Psychiatry.* 1985;48:517–529.

Flowers KA, Pearce I, Pearce JMS. Recognition memory in Parkinson's disease. *J Neurol Neurosurg Psychiatry.* 1984;47:1174–1181.

Folstein MF, Folstein SE, McHugh PR,. Mini-mental state: a practical method for grading the mental state of patients for the clinician. *J Psychiatry Res.* 1975;12:189–198.

Freedman M, Oscar-Berman M. Selected delayed response deficits in Parkinson's and Alzheimer's disease. *Arch Neurol.* 1986;43:886–90.

Freedman M, Oscar-Berman M. Tactile discrimination learning deficits in Alzheimer's disease and Parkinson's disease. *Arch Neurol.* 1987;44:394–98.

Freedman M, Oscar-Berman M. Spatial and visual learning deficits in Alzheimer's disease and Parkinson's disease. *Brain Cogn.* 1989;11:114–126.

Freedman M, Rivoira P, Butters N, et al. Retrograde amnesia in Parkinson's disease. *Can J Neurol Sci.* 1984;11:297–301.

Freidenberg DL, Cummings JL. Parkinson's disease, depression, and the on-off phenomenon. *Psychosomatics.* 1989;30:94–99.

Gaspar P, Gray F. Dementia in idiopathic Parkinson's disease. *Acta Neuropathol.* 1984;64:43–52.

Gibb WRG. Dementia and Parkinson's disease. *Br J Psychiatry.* 1989;154:596–614.

Girotti F, Soliveri P, Carella F, et al. Dementia and cognitive impairment in Parkinson's disease. *J Neurol Neurosurg Psychiatry.* 1988;51:1498–1502.

Hakim AM, Mathieson G. Dementia in Parkinson disease: a neuropathologic study. *Neurology.* 1979;29:1209–1214.

Heindel WC, Salmon DP, Shults CW, et al. Neuropsychological evidence for multiple implicit memory systems: a comparison of Alzheimer's, Huntington's, and Parkinson's disease patients. *J Neurosci.* 1989;9:582–587.

Helig CW, Knopman DS, Mastri AR, Frey W. Dementia without Alzheimer pathology. *Neurology.* 1985;35:762–765.

Heston LL. Dementia associated with Parkinson's disease: a genetic study. *J Neurol Neurosurg Psychiatry.* 1980;43:846–848.

Hietanen M, Teravainen H. The effect of age of disease onset on neuropsychological performance in Parkinson's disease. *J Neurol Neurosurg Psychiatry.* 1988;51:244–249.

Huber SJ, Shuttleworth EC, Paulson GW. Dementia in Parkinson's disease. *Arch Neurol.* 1986a;43:987–990.

Huber SJ, Freidenberg DL, Shuttleworth EC, et al. Neuropsychological impairments associated with severity of Parkinson's disease. *J Neuropsychiatry.* 1989;1:154–158.

Huber SJ, Shuttleworth EC, Paulson GW, et al. Cortical vs subcortical dementia: neuropathological differences. *Arch Neurol.* 1986b;43:392–394.

Javoy-Agid F, Agid Y. Is the mesocortical dopaminergic system involved in Parkinson's disease? *Neurology.* 1980;30:1326–1330.

Jegou S, Javoy-Agid F, Delbende C, et al. Cortical vasoactive intestinal peptide in relation to dementia in Parkinson's disease. *J Neurol Neurosurg Psychiatry.* 1985;48:842-843.

Jellinger LK. Pathologic correlations of dementia in Parkinson's disease. *Arch Neurol.* 1987;44:690-691.

Jellinger LK, Riederer P. Dementia in Parkinson's disease and (pre) senile dementia of Alzheimer type: morphological aspects and changes in intracerebral MAO activity. *Adv Neurol.* 1984;40:199-210.

Jolkkonen J, Soininen H, Halonen T, et al. Somatostatin-like immunoreactivity in cerebrospinal fluid of patients with Parkinson's disease and its relation to dementia. *J Neurol Neurosurg Psychiatry.* 1986;49:1374-1377.

Jolkkonen J, Soininen H, Riekkinen PJ. Beta-endorphin-like immunoreactivity in cerebrospinal fluid of patients with Alzheimer's disease and Parkinson's disease. *J Neurol Sci.* 1987;77:153-159.

Kaplan EF, Goodglass H, Weintraub S. *The Boston Naming Test.* Boston: E. Kaplan and H Goodglass; 1978.

Loranger AW. Goodell H, McDowell F, Lee JE. Intellectual impairment in Parkinson's syndrome. *Brain.* 1972;95:405-412.

Mann DMA, Yates PO. Pathological basis for neurotransmitter changes in Parkinson's disease. *Neuropathol Appl Neurobiol.* 1983;9:3-19.

Mayeux R, Stern Y, Rosen J, Leventhal J. Depression, intellectual impairment, and Parkinson's disease. *Neurology.* 1981;31:645-650.

Mayeux R, Stern Y, Rosenstein R, et al. An estimate of the prevalence of dementia in idiopathic Parkinson's disease. *Arch Neurol.* 1988;45:260-262.

Mildworf B, Globus M, Melamed E. Patterns of cognitive impairment in patients with Alzheimer's disease and Parkinson's disease: are they different? In: Fisher A, Hamin I, Lachman C, eds. *Alzheimer's Disease and Parkinson's Disease. Strategies for Research and Development.* New York: Plenum Press; 1986:135-140.

Mortimer JA, Pirozzolo FJ, Hansch EC, Webster DD. Relationship of motor symptoms to intellectual deficits in Parkinson's disease. *Neurology.* 1982;32:133-137.

Nausieda PA, Bieliauskas L, Glantz RH. Relationship of motor symptoms to intellectual deficits in PD [Letter]. *Neurology.* 1983;33:1390.

Nauta WJH. Limbic innervation of the striatum. In: Friedhoff AJ, Chase TN, eds. *Advances in Neurology, vol 35. Gilles de la Tourette syndrome.* New York: Raven Press; 1982:41-47.

Perry EK, Curtis M, Dick DJ, et al. Cholinergic correlates of cognitive impairment in Parkinson's disease: comparison with Alzheimer's disease. *J Neurol Neurosurg Psychiatry.* 1985;48:413-421.

Perry EK, Perry RH, Candy JM, et al. Cortical serotonin-S2 receptor binding abnormalities in patients with Alzheimer's disease: comparisons with Parkinson's disease. *Neurosci Lett.* 1984;51:353-357.

Perry EK, Perry RH, Smith CJ, et al. Nicotinic receptor abnormalities in Alzheimer's and Parkinson's disease. *J Neurol Neurosurg Psychiatry.* 1987;50:806-809.

Perry RH, Tomlinson BE, Candy JM, et al. Cortical cholinergic deficit in mentally impaired parkinsonian patients. *Lancet.* 1983;2:789-790.

Piccirilli M, Piccinin GL, Agostini L. Characteristic clinical aspects of parkinson patients with intellectual impairment. *Eur Neurol.* 1984;23:44-50.

Pillon B, Dubois B, Lhermitte F, Agid Y. Heterogeneity of cognitive impairment in progressive supranuclear palsy, Parkinson's disease, and Alzheimer's disease. *Neurology.* 1986;36:1179-1185.

Pirozzolo FJ, Hansch EC, Mortimer JA, et al. Dementia in Parkinson's disease: a neuropsychological analysis. *Brain Cogn.* 1982;1:71-83.

Rinne JO, Rummukainen J, Paljarvi L, Rinne UK. Dementia in Parkinson's disease is related to neuronal loss in the medial substantia nigra. *Ann Neurol.* 1989;26:47–50.

Rogers JD, Brogan D, Mirra SS. The nucleus basalis of Meynert in neurological disease: a quantitative morphological study. *Ann Neurol.* 1985;17:163–170.

Rossor M. The neurochemistry of cortical dementias. In: Stahl SM, Iverson SD, Goodman EC, eds. *Cognitive Neurochemistry.* New York: Oxford University Press; 1987:233–247.

Sagar HJ, Cohen NJ, Sullivan EV, et al. Remote memory function in Alzheimer's disease and Parkinson's disease. *Brain.* 1988a;111:185–206.

Sagar HJ, Sullivan EV, Gabrielli JDE, et al. Temporal ordering and short-term memory deficits in Parkinson's disease. *Brain.* 1988b;111:525–539.

Sahakian BJ, Morris RG, Evenden JL, et al. A comparative study of visuospatial memory and learning in Alzheimer-type dementia and Parkinson's disease. *Brain.* 1988;111:695–718.

Stuss DT, Benson DF. *The Frontal Lobes.* New York: Raven Press; 1986.

Sudarsky L, Morris J, Romero J, Walshe TM,. Dementia in Parkinson's disease: the problem of clinicopathological correlation. *J Neuropsychiatry Clin Neurosci.* 1989;1:159–166.

Tagliavini F, Pilleri G, Bouras C, Constantinidis J. The nucleus basalis of Meynert in idiopathic Parkinson's disease. *Acta Neurol Scand.* 1984;69:20–28.

Wechsler D, *Wechsler Adult Intelligence Scale Manual.* New York: Psychological Corporation; 1955.

Whitehouse PJ. The concept of subcortical dementia: another look. *Ann Neurol.* 1986;19:1–6.

Whitehouse PJ, Hedreen JC, White CL III, Price DL. Basal forebrain neurons in the dementia of Parkinson's disease. *Ann Neurol.* 1983;13:243–248.

Whitehouse PJ, Martino AM, Marcus KA, et al. Reductions in acetylcholine and nicotine binding in several degenerative diseases. *Arch Neurol.* 1988;45:722–724.

Whitehouse PJ, Price DL, Struble RG, et al. Alzheimer's disease and senile dementia—loss of neurons in the basal forebrain. *Science.* 1982;215:1237–1239.

Whitehouse PJ, Vale WW, Zweig RM, et al. Reductions in corticotropin releasing factor-like immunoreactivity in cerebral cortex in Alzheimer's disease, Parkinson's disease, and progressive supranuclear palsy. Neurology. 1987;37:905–909.

Wooten GF. Neurochemistry. In: Koller WC, ed. *Handbook of Parkinson's Disease.* New York: Marcel Dekker, 1987:237–251.

Xuereb JH, Tomlinson BE, Perry RH, et al. Dementia in Parkinson's disease: pathologic considerations. In: Nappi G. Caraceni T, eds. *Parkinsonism: Diagnosis and Treatment.* New York: Laurel House Publishing Company; 1989:45–54.

Zetusky WJ, Jankovic J, Pirozzolo FJ. The heterogeneity of Parkinson's disease: clinical and prognostic implications. *Neurology.* 1985;35:522–526.

Zubenko GS, Volicer L, Direnfeld LK, et al. Cerebrospinal fluid levels of angiotensin-converting enzyme in Alzheimer's disease, Pakinson's disease, and progressive supranuclear palsy. *Brain Res.* 1985;328:215–221.

12

Neuroimaging Correlates of Dementia in Parkinson's Disease

STEVEN J. HUBER AND SANDER L. GLATT

Although the pathological anatomy underlying the movement disorder in Parkinson's disease (PD) is well understood, the structural correlates of cognitive symptoms remain controversial. In addition to the progressive loss of dopaminergic substantia nigra cells classically associated with motor symptoms, alterations beyond the extrapyramidal structures exist (Rinne, 1978). Pathology studies have attributed dementia in PD to cortical cell loss similar to that observed in Alzheimer's disease (Boller et al, 1980; Hakim and Mathieson, 1979), but these findings have not been confirmed by others (Ball, 1984; Xuereb et al, 1989). Some researchers have demonstrated that neuronal loss in subcortical nuclei rather than cortical change is related to dementia in PD (Chui et al, 1986; Helig et al, 1985). This inconsistency may be due to small sample sizes, the lack of objective assessment of premorbid cognitive status, and variable criteria for establishing autopsy diagnoses.

Recent developments in neuroimaging provide powerful tools for examining structural correlates of neurobehavioral disturbances. These techniques allow researchers to examine large samples of patients in close temporal proximity to neuropsychological evaluation. Neuroimaging studies have identified the presence of cerebral atrophy, ventricular enlargement, caudate atrophy, frontal atrophy, and periventricular white matter abnormalities in some PD patients. Neuroimaging modalities may provide an excellent opportunity to study the clinicopathological correlates of cognitive impairments in patients with PD.

The seminal article that set the stage for current neuroimaging studies of dementia in PD was published by Selby (1968). Pneumocencephalograms were obtained in 250 PD patients referred for thalamic surgery. Results indicated that the prevalence of cerebral atrophy was greater in PD patients than in age-appropriate controls. Ventricular enlargement was not associated with motor symptoms, but cortical atrophy was associated with many symptoms, including rigidity, gait disturbance, and akinesia. Conversely, intellectual impairment was more common in patients with ventricular enlargement than in those with cortical atrophy.

This chapter reviews recent research correlating neuropsychological findings in PD with anatomical and physiological data derived from computed tomography (CT), magnetic resonance imaging (MRI), single photon emission computed tomography (SPECT), and positron emission tomography (PET). Methodological issues are discussed in the initial section that are necessary to examine the relationship between neuroimaging findings and cognitive dysfunction in PD in a reliable and valid manner.

GENERAL METHODOLOGY

Neuroimaging procedures have become indispensable tools to study the brain and are used routinely as part of the dementia evaluation. Their value in detecting secondary causes of dementia, such as tumors or hydrocephalus, is undeniable, but their value for the diagnosis of primary dementia is less clear. Cerebral atrophy is the most commonly identified neuroimaging change in degenerative conditions, and it lacks diagnostic specificity. Atrophy is determined by measures of ventricular dilatation or cortical sulcal enlargement. Studies using atrophy as a possible neuroimaging correlate of dementia will serve to illustrate some general methodological issues regarding neuroimaging studies in disorders without gross pathology, such as PD.

In studies that examined normal elderly subjects and patients with Alzheimer's disease, some have found a significant relationship between the degree of cerebral atrophy and the severity of cognitive impairment (Fox et al, 1975; deLeon et al, 1980; Jacoby and Levy, 1980), but others have not (Kaszniak et al 1979; Hughes and Gado, 1981; Wilson et al, 1982). Even in the studies that found the average degree of atrophy to be greater in demented patients, there was substantial overlap with the control subjects.

Several important methodological issues have been identified that could be responsible for the inconsistencies observed among studies. These methodological issues are discussed briefly and are considered necessary to adequately evaluate research related to neuroimaging correlates of cognitive dysfunction in PD. Further, these methodological constraints are necessary to incorporate into future research if we are to advance our understanding of this relationship.

The first issue relates to the method of neuropsychological assessment. Many studies have relied solely on subjective impressions of cognitive status, and the use of such subjective approaches invariably leads to low interrater reliability. Other studies used a wide variety of objective neuropsychological procedures, and the use of different methods of assessment makes comparability of these studies difficult, if not impossible. The need to develop standardized methods of neuropsychological assessment and standardized criteria to define dementia in PD is discussed in Chapter 3.

The second issue concerns the effect of age alone on the development of cerebral abnormalities. The one invariant finding among previous neuroimaging studies is that many cerebral changes systematically increase with age. Neither ventricular enlargement nor cortical atrophy is seen in young healthy individuals (Barron et al, 1976). In normal people over the age of 65, however, there is a positive correlation between advancing age and both progressive enlargement of the ventricles and cortical atrophy (Barron et al, 1976; Gyldenstad, 1977; Kaszniak et al, 1979; Jacoby and Levy, 1980). This potentially confounding variable is demonstrated most clearly in studies that found age to be the most reliable predictor of atrophy (Ford and Winter, 1980; Wilson et al, 1982; Inzelberg et al, 1987). The use of appropriate age-matched controls is necessary to determine whether cerebral abnormalities beyond those expected by age alone are present in association with dementia.

The final issue concerns the effect of disease severity alone on the development of cerebral abnormalities. It has been demonstrated that both cortical atrophy and ventricular enlargement become more prevalent with advancing disease (Schneider et al, 1979; Portin et al, 1984; Inzelberg et al, 1987). Thus, in order to identify specific neuroimaging abnormalities associated with the presence of cognitive decline in PD, it is necessary to control for the potential confounding effects of both age and disease severity. This could be accomplished most directly by the use of controls that are similar with respect to age and disease severity. Statistical methods, such as partial correlational or covariance techniques, also may be used to control for these potentially confounding variables. Even when the effects of potentially confounding variables are controlled using these statistical procedures, interpretation must be made cautiously (Adams et al, 1985).

The next section reviews current research examining the relationship between neuroimaging findings and cognitive impairment in PD. For ease of communication in a literature fraught with inconsistencies, only articles that adhere to the basic methodological constraints discussed are reviewed. These include objective assessment of cognitive status and some attempt to control for the potentially confounding effects of both age and disease severity.

NEUROIMAGING IN PARKINSON'S DISEASE

Computed Tomography

Schneider and colleagues (1979) examined the relationship between cerebral abnormalities detected by computed tomography (CT) and both disease severity and intellectual disturbances in 173 PD patients. Initial results indicated that both cortical atrophy and ventricular enlargement correlated with disease severity. The relationship between these CT parameters and performance on neuropsychological tests varied depending on the type of function tested. Measures of psychomotor speed and reaction time correlated with the extent of both cortical atrophy and ventricular enlargement. Interpretation of these results is not clear, however, since the effect of disease severity was not adjusted for in the statistical analysis. More specifically, since CT abnormalities increase with disease and performance on tasks that require manual manipulation decreases with disease severity (Lichter et al, 1988), there is no clear evidence that disease severity alone was responsible for these findings. Conversely, performance on the measure of general intelligence (HAWIE Vocabulary Test) did not correlate with either cerebral atrophy or ventricular enlargement.

Sroka and associates (1981) examined 93 patients with PD and 72 normal controls. The CT scans were evaluated for cortical atrophy and ventricular enlargement. Initial results indicated that age was correlated significantly with both increasing ventricular enlargement and sulcal size in both the patient and control groups. Therefore, corrections were employed to control for this factor before statistical comparisons of the patient groups. Patients were divided into those with typical idiopathic PD and those with atypical PD defined by the presence of a rapid or unusual course of disease. Patients with atypical PD were found more frequently to have an organic mental syndrome (OMS). Regardless of disease type, the primary finding was that the presence of OMS was more closely correlated with ventricular enlargement than cortical atrophy.

Portin and colleagues (1984) examined 28 PD patients in whom cognitive impairment was defined as normal/mild or moderate/severe based on scores derived from the Wechsler Adult Intelligence Scale (WAIS). The relationship between neuropsychological status and CT abnormalities was adjusted for significant relationships with demographic and motor factors using analysis of covariance for group comparisons and partial correlations when performances on individual measures were considered. Results indicated that ventricular enlargement, but not cortical atrophy, was associated with impaired overall mental status. Cortical atrophy (enlargement of the sylvian cisterns) did, however, exhibit a side-specific relationship to the type of cognitive function. Atrophy in the left insular region correlated with performance on verbal tasks, and right insular atrophy correlated with performance on visuospatial tasks. Ventricular dilatation was relatively symmetrical, and no such relationships could be established.

Inzelberg and colleagues (1987) examined 132 patients using a brief mental status examination and divided the patients into those with normal status, mild/moderate dementia, and severe dementia. Results indicated that age was the most robust factor related to both sulcal width (cortical atrophy) and ventricular enlargement (central atrophy). For all further analyses, age was covaried to control for this effect. After age adjustment, cortical atrophy was associated with disease severity but not with dementia. Severity of dementia was associated significantly with ventricular enlargement and even more closely with caudate pathology. Korczyn and associates (1986) also found intercaudate distance and width of the third ventricle to be the only significant correlates of dementia severity in PD.

Lichter and associates (1988) examined 39 PD patients with and 38 age- and sex-matched controls using various CT measurements. Neuropsychological evaluation included procedures related to perceptual motor skills, reaction time, executive functions, mood, and global intellectual status. Results indicated that disease severity did not correlate with any of the CT measures. Performance on the Block Design task correlated with the vast majority of CT measures. In contrast, global intellectual function as measured by the Mini-Mental State Examination (Folstein et al, 1975) correlated only with width of the anterior interhemispheric fissure and bicaudate diameter.

In summary, these results suggest that cognitive dysfunction in PD is associated with the extent of subcortical and frontal cortical atrophy but not with any measures of generalized cerebral atrophy compared with age-matched controls.

Magnetic Resonance Imaging

Magnetic resonance imaging (MRI) is superior to CT for visualization of many cerebral abnormalities, including cortical atrophy and ventricular enlargement. The greatest difference between the techniques is the enhanced sensitivity of MRI to periventricular white matter abnormalities (Friedland et al, 1984; George et al, 1986; Growdon and Corkin, 1986; Johnson et al, 1987a). The enhanced sensitivity of MRI to these lesions may be important, since intellectual abnormalities have been associated with white matter changes (Filley et al, 1988; Frazekas et al, 1987; Johnson et al, 1987a).

In the study of Johnson and colleagues (1987a), MRI and CT were compared not only for sensitivity to brain abnormalities but also for their relationship to dementia severity. Patients with mixed etiology, including Alzheimer's disease, vascular disease, and PD were examined for dementia severity using the Blessed Dementia Scale (BDS) (Blessed et al, 1968). Results indicated that subcortical white matter abnormalities, enlargement of the basal and sylvian cisterns, and ventricular enlargement were more evident by MRI than by CT. The only MRI finding to correlate significantly with severity of dementia was periventricular white matter pathology, but the magnitude of this relationship was modest at best ($p < 0.03$). Further, since no controls were used, the diagnostic specificity of this finding is uncertain.

Growdon and Corkin (1986) examined two patients, one demented and one nondemented, to illustrate the potential power of MRI for examining structural correlates of dementia in PD. Presence or absence of dementia was determined by scores on the BDS (Blessed et al, 1968). Results indicated that there was no significant difference in the extent of cortical atrophy between patients, and midbrain structures appeared normal in both patients, but the demented patient had significantly greater ventricular enlargement compared with the nondemented patient.

Recent studies have suggested that it is now possible to examine the substantia nigra using MRI, the anatomical site classically associated with PD. This is of interest, since cognitive and motor features in PD tend to parallel one another (Mayeux et al, 1981; Mortimer et al, 1982; Huber et al, 1988). Thus, MRI may provide a more direct and a quantifiable measurement of this relationship compared with indirect clinical measures of disease severity. Despite the optimism associated with first article to identify a reduction in width of the pars compacta portion of the substantia in PD (Duguid et al, 1986), subsequent studies have noted several difficulties associated with this procedure (Braffman et al, 1988; Huber et al, 1990; Stern et al, 1989). All studies have found substantial overlap between patients and controls, there is an inconsistent relationship between disease severity and narrowing of the pars compacta, and reduction in width may be present only in patients with relatively advanced disease. Precise evaluation of the pars compacta using MRI is hampered by the fact that this structure cannot be measured directly but is identified as the transition in signal intensity among the cerebral peduncle, reticular substantia nigra, and the red nucleus.

We examined potential MRI correlates of dementia in PD (Huber et al, 1989a). Patients and age- and education-matched controls were examined using a neuropsychological battery that assessed memory, visuospatial skills, cognition, language, and depression. Three groups were studied: PD patients meeting criteria for dementia (Cummings and Benson, 1983), PD patients without dementia and matched for age and disease severity with the demented group, and normal controls. MRI measures included total surface area of the brain minus the area of the ventricles as a gross measure of brain atrophy, several measures of ventricular enlargement, intercaudate width, high signal white matter lesions, and width of the pars compacta portion of the substantia nigra. The last procedure is presented graphically in Figures 12–1 and 12–2 and described in detail elsewhere (Huber et al, 1990). Results indicated that none of the 13 MRI measures were significantly greater in the demented than the nondemented PD patients.

MRI findings in PD studies deserve further comment. First, although MRI is clearly more sensitive to the detection of white matter lesions than is CT (Johnson et

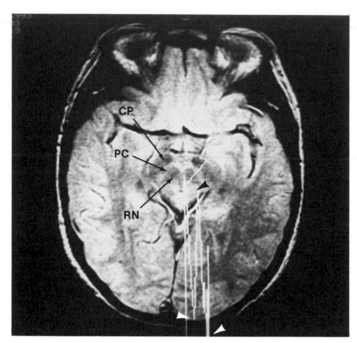

Figure 12–1. A spin-echo axial image (repetition time 3000 milliseconds, echo time 30 milliseconds) in which the high signal band of the pars compacta (PC) is outlined by the cerebral peduncle (CP) anteriorly and the red nucleus (RN) posteriorly. The center line used to construct the histographic plot of average signal intensities across these structures is shown at left. The actual plot of the relative pixel intensities is seen directly below. Arrowheads indicate the measurement points. (From Huber et al., Arch Neurol. 1990;47:735–737.)

al, 1987a), the significance of these abnormalities to dementia is unclear. Even though these abnormalities occur in patients with dementia (Frazekas et al, 1987; Johnson et al, 1987a), they are observed also in controls, and their diagnostic specificity is uncertain (Brandt-Zawadski et al, 1985; Zimmerman et al, 1986). Erkinjuntti and associates (1984) found high signal white matter abnormalities in patients with vascular dementia but not in those with primary dementia (i.e., Alzheimer's disease). Hunt and colleagues (1989) found that neuropsychological performance decreased and the severity of white matter lesions increased with advancing age in normal individuals. However, when the data were corrected for age, there was no correlation between neuropsychological performance and the extent of white matter abnormalities. Thus, these changes may be of limited clinical usefulness for identification of dementia in elderly patients. Finally, the pathological process underlying these high signal foci is uncertain and may not be associated uniformly with infarction or demyelination (Lotz et al, 1986; Rezeak et al, 1986; Johnson et al, 1987a).

The studies reviewed here that met the minimum methodological requirements are summarized in Table 12–1. Cortical atrophy was not sensitive to PD dementia in any study. In contrast, central atrophy (ventricular enlargement) and intercaudate width were consistently associated with intellectual impairment. This pattern suggests

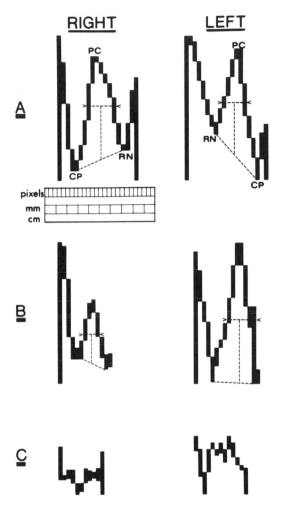

Figure 12–2. Representative histographic plots drawn to scale of a normal control (A), a patient with mild Parkinson's disease (B), and a patient with severe disease (C). The choice of measurement points for the cerebral peduncle (CP), pars compacta (PC), and red nucleus (RN) for contrast and for width measurements are shown in subject A. Patient B had predominantly unilateral symptoms contralateral to the narrowed side. The measurement points are not discernible for patient C. (From Huber et al., 1990.)

that dementia in PD may result primarily from subcortical pathology. These findings should be interpreted cautiously, however. To validate this trend, future studies must employ appropriate control subjects and standardized neuropsychological assessment. Each of the studies in Table 12–1 used different neuropsychological procedures.

EMISSION TOMOGRAPHY

CT and MRI visualize brain structure but provide no information about physiology. It would be useful to examine the physiological consequences of the structural changes

Table 12–1.   Representative studies that examined the relationship between neuroimaging abnormalities and intellectual impairments in Parkinson's Disease

Authors	Method of neuropsychological assessment	Central atrophy	Neuroimaging Measures		White matter lesions
			Cortical atrophy	Caudate width	
Sroka et al (1981)	chart reviews (DMA)	+[a]	−	NA[b]	NA
Portin et al (1984)	WAIS	+	−	NA	NA
Inzelberg et al (1987)	Short Mental Status	+	−	+	NA
Korczyn et al (1986)	Questionnaire	+	−	+	NA
Lichter et al (1988)	MMSE	+	−	+	NA
Growden and Corkin (1986)	BDS	+	−	NA	NA
Huber et al (1989a)	Cummings and Benson Criteria for Dementia	−	−	−	−

[a]+, positive relationship; −, negative relationship.
[b]NA, not analyzed.

identified in PD and interconnected neuronal pathways to answer important questions. How does a lesion in the substantia nigra affect striatal and cortical function? Are there functional deficits in brain regions that control cognition?

Positron emission tomography (PET) and single photon emission computed tomography (SPECT) construct an image of physiological parameters collected by noninvasive means. Emission tomography measures the regional cerebral distribution of selected radionuclides. These radionuclides may be bound to agents that are distributed in the brain in relation to blood flow, metabolism, or the presence of specific neurochemical receptors. An in vivo functional brain image "in the living patient" (Perlmutter, 1988) is derived from the tomographic measurements of regional radionuclide activity.

Cerebral Blood Flow

Studies measuring brain physiology in PD were first performed using xenon-133 inhalation technique. Lavy and colleagues (1979) measured regional blood flow in 60 PD patients and 51 age-matched controls. Mean regional cerebral flow (rCBF) was significantly reduced in PD, most prominently in the oldest subjects. This was not related to disease duration. Since deficits in cortical metabolism had been identified in Alzheimer's disease (Frackowiak et al, 1981), Globus and co-workers (1985) speculated that a deficit in rCBF in PD may occur specifically with cognitive dysfunction. However, they were unable to demonstrate a relationship between presence and severity of dementia in PD and reduced rCBF, suggesting differences between these dementia syndromes. Bes and colleagues (1983) used the xenon-133 inhalation method to demonstrate that rCBF was most prominently diminished in the frontal lobes of patients with PD compared with age-matched controls. Cognitive function was not evaluated. A more sensitive quantitative method, xenon contrast CT was used to measure rCBF in 14 PD patients, 3 of whom were noted to be demented (Tachibana et al, 1985). Cortical and subcortical flow was decreased significantly in patients compared with controls. This was most evident in the patients with dementia.

Positron Emission Tomography

It was hoped that the powerful technology of PET would unravel the pathophysiological basis of both motor and cognitive dysfunction in PD. PET quantitatively measures the regional distribution of positron emitting radiopharmaceuticals selected either for their ability to monitor cellular metabolism or to bind to a specific neurochemical receptor. Isotopes used in studies of PD include ^{15}O (e.g., $H_2^{15}O$) and ^{18}F [(^{18}F) fluorodeoxyglucose or (^{18}F) 6-fluorodopa], which label compounds that are inserted into cellular metabolism, or ^{11}C [(^{11}C)-N-methylspiperone or (^{11}C)raclopride], ligands of the dopaminergic receptor (Perlmutter, 1988). Unfortunately, studies of dopaminergic receptors with PET have not demonstrated a relationship with cognitive dysfunction in PD.

Presynaptic dopaminergic storage has been measured with $^{18}F_6$-fluorodopa, which is converted to fluorodopamine and stored in the striatum. Garnett and colleagues (1984) demonstrated marked differences in contralateral striatal dopaminergic storage in six patients with mild hemiparkinsonism. Leenders and associates (1986) studied seven patients with mild bilateral PD and five patients with more severe disease and levodopa-induced motor fluctuations. There were marked differences in striatal tracer uptake, with the greatest change in patients with on/off. The authors suggest that the severe deficit in striatal storage capacity for dopamine may underlie motor fluctuations. Cognitive status was not measured. Eidelberg and co-workers (1990) found a relationship between striatal uptake of fluorodopa, using $^{18}F_6$-fluorodopa, and bradykinesia but not with dementia.

Studies of cerebral and basal ganglia metabolism in PD have not yielded clear conclusions. A number of investigators have measured rCBF and oxygen (^{15}O) or glucose [(^{18}F)fluorodeoxyglucose] metabolism in patients with clinical hemiparkinsonism to allow for side to side comparisons. Perlmutter and Rachle (1985) measured rCBF with $H_2^{15}O$ in 11 nondemented patients with hemiparkinsonism before and after oral levodopa. They found that although there was no difference between sides in total hemispheric blood flow, there was a significant decrease in inferior frontal mesocortical flow in patients with PD compared with controls that did not improve with dopaminergic therapy. There was also a loss of coupling of pallidal blood flow between hemispheres in PD patients. They noted that patients with the mildest symptoms had an increase in pallidal blood flow that did not occur in those with more advanced disease. Martin and colleagues (1984) similarly noted contralateral pallidal hypermetabolism with (^{18}F)fluorodeoxyglucose in 4 PD patients with mild hemiparkinsonism. Wolfson and associates (1985) noted a similar increase in both blood and metabolism measured by $H_2^{15}O$ in the contralateral basal ganglia of 6 patients with PD and normal cognition. A corresponding decrease in both blood flow and metabolism was noted in the frontal lobe contralateral to the symptomatic limbs.

Perlmutter (1988) suggested that pallidal metabolism may be dependent on the stage of disease, increasing in early disease due to the recent loss of the inhibitory effect of dopamine. Decreased dopaminergic activity similarly may lead to decreased cortical blood flow, particularly in the frontal lobes with its prominent dopaminergic mesocortical input (Wolfson et al, 1985). The effect of exogenous levodopa may not be particularly advantageous. Leenders and colleagues (1985) demonstrated that dopaminergic stimulation acutely increased blood flow in cortex and basal ganglia without significantly affecting oxygen metabolism. The oxygen extraction ratio (OER) is a measure of the metabolic demand vs oxygen delivery. In Alzheimer's disease, OER is unchanged, reflecting the preservation of autogegulation in matching blood flow to metabolism (Frackowiak et al, 1981). This allows extrapolation about metabolic function from more readily available measures of rCBF. Although OER was unchanged in PD as compared with controls before dopaminergics, the acute use of dopaminergic agents resulted in an increase in blood flow but without a corresponding change in metabolic demand, decreasing OER (Leenders et al, 1985). They suggest that dopaminergics cause vasodilatation through dopaminergic receptors on the cortical vessels. This raises questions about the usefulness of SPECT and other measures of rCBF in PD, since changes may not reflect alterations in cerebral function.

The studies of cerebral metabolism in PD without overt dementia suggest that there is diminished global cortical activity, most prominently involving the frontal lobe (Brooks and Frackowiak, 1989; Perlmutter, 1988). This is consistent with the clinical description of the cognitive deficits in subcortical dementia. Subtle deficits in executive frontal lobe functions (Taylor et al, 1986) are present in functionally unimpaired PD patients. Patients with a subcortical dementia matched in severity to patients with Alzheimer's disease demonstrate less difficulty with memory, language, and orientation but more severe problems with speed of information processing and mood (Huber et al, 1989b), suggestive of frontal lobe dysfunction.

Only isolated reports deal with cerebral metabolism in PD patients with frank dementia. Kuhl and colleagues (1984) reported that cortical metabolism studied with (^{18}F)fluorodeoxyglucose was markedly decreased in nine PD patients as compared with controls. This change correlated with severity of dementia and bradykinesia. A severe deficit in parietal metabolism had developed in one patient with increasing dementia scanned twice over a 4 year interval. Focal deficits in posterior parietal function have been observed in patients with Alzheimer's disease (Frackowiak et al, 1981)

The pathological basis of dementia in PD has not been defined clearly. Severe dementia with characteristics suggestive of Alzheimer's disease may develop in patients with the motor manifestation of PD. Neuropathological studies have shown that cortical senile plaques and neurofibrillary tangles identical to those in Alzheimer's disease are found in some patients with clinical and neuropathological evidence of PD (Hakim and Mathieson, 1979; Boller et al, 1980). Others have noted that well-characterized subcortical dementia is not associated with cortical Alzheimer's disease pathology (Chui et al, 1986), and most patients with PD and dementia do not have Alzheimer's disease (Ball, 1984; Yoshimura, 1988). It seems likely that dementia in PD includes both patients with PD and Alzheimer's disease as well as a specific subcortical PD dementia syndrome (de La Monte et al, 1989)

PET has not been used effectively to study dementia in PD. A combined approach using both measures of dopamingergic activity and cerebral metabolism in clearly defined homogeneous PD populations may be required to identify the alterations in neuronal networks that underlie the PD dementia syndromes (Eidelberg et al, 1990)

Single Photon Emission Computed Tomography

SPECT, a more recently developed imaging modality, uses isotopes and imaging technology familiar to nuclear medicine physicians and has become widely available in clinical medicine. Qualitative images are obtained of the regional distribution of gamma-emitting radiopharmaceuticals selected for their ability to penetrate the blood–brain barrier, distribute in brain in proportion to blood flow, and be retained in a fixed regional distribution long enough to be imaged. Although SPECT at present yields only a qualitative image of the rCBF, the primary advantage over PET is its relatively modest expense, permitting large-scale studies. Radiopharmaceuticals that have been used clinically include (^{123}I)N-isopropyl iodoamphetamine (IMP) and (^{99m}Tc)hexamethylpropylene amine oxide (HMPAO). These agents are reliable indicators of cerebral blood flow (Kuhl et al, 1982; Neirinckx et al, 1987) and approximate perfusion images derived from PET (Nishizawa et al, 1989). Studies of basal ganglia activity with SPECT have not demonstrated clear abnormalities in PD (Nagel et al, 1991).

SPECT studies have replicated the identification of posterior parietal deficits in Alzheimer's disease (Jagust et al, 1987; Johnson et al, 1987b) previously noted using PET (Frackowiak et al, 1981). Smith and colleagues (1988) studied 16 PD patients with HMPAO, 9 of whom had evidence of dementia using the Mini-Mental State Examination (Folstein et al, 1975). Two of 7 nondemented and 6 of 9 demented patients had patchy cortical areas of diminished activity. The authors, experienced with SPECT in Alzheimer's disease, specifically noted that the scan appearance was not characteristic of Alzheimer's disease and that the severity of the cortical deficit was consistent with their cognitive status. Pizzolato and associates (1988) used HMPAO and semiquantitative methodology to study 36 PD patients. Nine were demented by Mini-Mental State criteria, and 6 had unilateral disease. Parietal cortical activity was significantly diminished bilaterally in PD. This deficit paralleled the severity of both motor disability and dementia.

SUMMARY

Emission tomography is a potentially powerful technique for evaluation of the underlying pathophysiology of both the motor and cognitive disorders identified in patients with PD. The results to date, however, have been disappointing. Studies suggest that there may be cortical deficits in blood flow and metabolism, particularly in the frontal lobe in functionally unimpaired PD patients and in the posterior parietal region in PD patients with overt dementia. Further work is required to understand the pathophysiology of the cerebral cortical metabolic deficits with PET, which would allow large-scale studies with SPECT for clinical correlations. Progress in this area is also dependent on more refined examination of cognitive status in patients with PD.

REFERENCES

Adams KM, Brown GG, Grant I. Analysis of covariance as a remedy for demographic mismatch of research subjects: Some sobering simulations. *J Clin Exp Neuropsychol.* 1985;7:445–462.

Albert M. Subcortical dementia in Alzeheimer's Disease. In: Katzman R, Terry RD, Bick KL, eds. *Senile Dementia and Related Disorders.* New York: Raven Press; 1978.

Ball MJ. The morphologic basis of dementia in Parkinson's disease. *Can J Neurol Sci.* 1984;11:180–184.

Barron SA, Jacobs L, Kinkel WR. Changes in size of normal lateral ventricles during aging determined by computerized tomography. *Neurology.* 1976;26:1011–1013.

Bes A, Guell A, Fabre N, et al. Cerebral blood flow studied by xenon-133 inhalation technique in parkinsonism: loss of hyperfrontal pattern. *J Cereb Blood Flow Metab.* 1983;3:33–37.

Blessed G, Tomlinson BE, Roth M. The association between quantitative measures of dementia of senils change in the cerebral grey matter of elderly subjects. *Br J Psychiatry.* 1968;114:797–811.

Boller F. Mizutani T, Roessmann U, Gambetti P. Parkinson's disease, dementia and Alzheimer's disease. Clincopathological correlations. *Ann Neurol.* 1980;7:329–335.

Braffman BH, Grossman RI, Goldberg HI, et al. MR imaging of Parkinson's disease using spin-echo and gradient echo sequences. *AJNR.* 1988;9:1093–1099.

Brandt-Zawadski M, Fein G, VanDyke C, et al. MR imaging of the aging brain: patchy white matter lesions and dementia. *AJNR.* 1985;6:675–682.

Brooks DJ, Frackowiak R. PET and movement disorders. *J Neurol Neurosurg Psychiatry.* 1989;Special Suppl:68–77.

Chui HC, Mortimer JA, Clager U, et al. Pathologic correlates of dementia in Parkinson's disease. *Arch Neurol.* 1986;43:991–995.

Cumming JL, Benson DF. *Dementia: A Clinical Approach.* Stoneham, Mass: Butterworth Publishers Inc; 1983.

de la Monte SM, Wells SE, Hedley-Whyte ET, Growdon JH. Neurological distinction between Parkinson's dementia and Parkinson's plus Alzheimer's disease. *Ann Neurol.* 1989;26:309–320.

deLeon MJ, Ferris SH, George AE, et al. Computed tomography evaluation of brain-behavior relationships in senile dementia of the Alzheimer's type. *Neurobiol Aging.* 1980;1:59–79.

Duguid JR, De La Paz R, DeGroot J. Magnetic resonance imaging of the midbrain in Parkinson's disease. Ann Neurol. 1986;20:744–747.

Eidelberg D, Moeller JR, Dhawan V, et al. The metabolic anatomy of Parkinson's disease: complementary [^{18}F] fluorodeoxyglucose and [^{18}F] fluorodopa positron emission tomographic studies. *Mov Disord.* 1990;5:203–213.

Erkinjuntti T, Sipponen JT, Livanainen M, et al. Cerebral NMR and CT imaging in dementia. *J Comput Assist Tomogr.* 1984;8:614–618.

Filley CM, Franklin GM, Heaton RK, Rosenberg NL. White matter dementia: clinical disorder and implications. *Neuropsychiatry Neuropsychol Behav Neurol.* 1988;1:239–254.

Folstein MF, Folstein SE, McHugh PR. Mini-Mental State: a practical guide for grading the mental state of patients for the clinician. *J Psychiatry Res.* 1975;12:189–198.

Ford CV, Winter J. Computerized axial tomograms and dementia in elderly patients. *J Gerontol.* 1980;36:164–169.

Fox JH, Topel JR, Huckman MS. Use of computerized tomography in senile dementia. *J Neurol Neurosurg Psychiatry.* 1975;38:948–953.

Frackowiak RSJ, Pozzilli C, Legg NJ, et al. Regional cerebral oxygen supply and utilization in dementia. *Brain.* 1981;104:753–778.

Frazekas F, Chawluk J, Alavi A, et al. MR abnormalities at 1.5 T in Alzheimer's dementia and normal aging. *AJNR.* 1987;8:421–426.

Friedland RP, Budlinger TF, Brant-Zawadski M, Jagust WJ. The diagnosis of Alzheimer's type dementia: a preliminary comparison of positron emission tomography and proton magnetic resonance. *JAMA.* 1984;252:2750–2752.

Garnett ES, Nahmias C. Firnau G. Central dopaminergic pathways in hemiparkinsonism examined by positron emission tomography. *Can J Neurol Sci.* 1984;11:174–179.

George AE, de Leon MJ, Kalnin A, et al. Leukoencephalopathy in normal and pathologic aging: 2. MRI of brain lucencies. *AJRN.* 1986;7:567–570.

Globus M, Mildworf B, Melamed E. Cerebral blood flow and cognitive impairment in Parkinson's disease. *Neurology.* 1985;35:1135–1139.

Growdon J, Corkin S. Cognitive impairments in Parkinson's disease. In: Yahr MD, Bergman KJ, eds. *Parkinson's Disease. Advancing in Neurology, vol 45.* New York: Raven Press; 1986:383–92.

Gyldenstad C. Measurements of the normal ventricular system and hemispheric sulci of 100 adults with computed tomography. *Neuroradiology.* 1977;14:201–204.

Hakim AM, Mathieson G. Dementia in Parkinson disease: a neuropathologic study. *Neurology.* 1979;29:1209–1214.

Helig CW, Knopman DS, Mastri AR, Frey W. Dementia without Alzheimer pathology. *Neurology.* 1985;35:762–765.

Huber SJ, Chakeres DW, Paulson GW, Khana R. Magnetic resonance imaging in Parkinson's disease. *Arch Neurol.* 1990;47:735–737.

Huber SJ, Paulson GW, Shuttleworth EC. Relationship of motor symptoms, intellectual impairment, and depression in Parkinson's disease. *J Neurol Neurosurg Psychiatry.* 1988;51:855–858.

Huber SJ, Shuttleworth ED, Christy JA, et al. Magnetic resonance imaging in dementia of Parkinson's disease. *J Neurol Neurosurg Psychiatry.* 1989a;52:1221–1227.

Huber SJ, Shuttleworth ED, Freidenberg DL. Neuropsychological differences between the dementias of Alzheimer's and Parkinson's diseases. *Arch Neurol.* 1989b;46:1287–1291.

Hughes CP, Gado M. Computed tomography and aging of the brain. *Neuroradiology.* 1981;23:391–396.

Hunt AL, Orrison WW, Yeo RA, et al. Clinical significance of MRI white matter lesions in the elderly. *Neurology.* 1989;39:1470–1474.

Inzelberg R, Treves T, Reider I, et al. Computed tomography brain changes in Parkinsonian dementia. *Neuroradiology.* 1987;29:535–539.

Jacoby RJ, Levy R. Computed tomography in the elderly. 2. Senile dementia: diagnosis and functional impairment. *Br J Psychiatry.* 1980;136:256–269.

Jagust WJ, Budinger TF, Reed BR. The diagnosis of dementia with single photon emission computed tomography. *Arch Neurol.* 1987;44:258–262.

Johnson K, Davis K, Buonhanno S, et al. Comparison of magnetic resonance and rotogen ray computed tomography in dementia. *Arch Neurol.* 1987;44:1075–1080.

Johnson KA, Mueller ST, Walshe TM, et al. Cerebral perfusion imaging in Alzheimer's disease. Use of single photon emission computed tomography and iofetamine hydrochloride I 123. *Arch Neurol.* 1987b;44:165–168.

Kaszniak AW, Garron DC, Fox JH, et al. Cerebral atrophy, EEG slowing, age, education and cognitive functioning in suspected dementia. *Neurology.* 1979;29:1273–1279.

Korczyn AD, Inzelberg R, Treves T, et al. Dementia of Parkinson's disease. In: Yahr MD, Bergmann J eds. Advances in Neurology (45). New York: Raven Press; 1986:399–403.

Kuhl DE, Barrio JR, Huang S-C, et al. Quantifying local cerebral blood flow by N-isopropyl-p-[^{123}I] Iodamphetamine (IMP) tomography. *J Nucl Med.* 1982;12:196–203.

Kuhl DE, Metter EJ, Riege WH. Patterns of local cerebral glucose utilization determined in Parkinson's disease by the [^{18}F] fluorodeoxyglucose method. *Ann Neurol.* 1984;15:419–424.

Lavy S, Melamed E, Cooper G, et al. Regional cerebral blood flow in patients with Parkinson's disease. *Arch Neurol.* 1979;36:344–348.

Leenders KL, Palmer AJ, Quinn N, et al. Brain dopamine metabolism in patients with Parkinson's disease measured with positron emission tomography. *J Neurol Neurosurg Psychiatry.* 1986;49:853–860.

Leenders KL, Wolfson L, Gibbs JM, et al. The effect of L-dopa on regional cerebral blood flow and oxygen metabolism in patients with Parkinson's disease. *Brain.* 1985;108:171–191.

Lichter DG, Corbett AJ, Fitzgibbon GM, et al. Cognitive and motor dysfunction in Parkinson's disease. *Arch Neurol.* 1988;45:854–860.

Lotz PR, Ballinger WE, Quisling RG. Subcortical ateriosclerotic encephalopathy: CT spectrum and pathologic correlation. *AJRN.* 1986;7:817–822.

Martin WRW, Beckman JH, Calne DB, et al. Cerebral glucose metabolism in Parkinson's disease. *Can J Neurol Sci.* 1984;11(suppl 1):169–173.

Mayeux R, Stern Y, Rosen J, Fahn S. Depression, intellectual impairment, and Parkinson's disease. *Neurology.* 1981;31:645–650.

Mortimer JA, Pirozzolo FJ, Hansche EC, Webster DD. Relationship of motor symptoms to intellectual deficits in Parkinson's disease. *Neurology.* 1982;32:133–137.

Nagel JS, Ichise M, Holman BL. The scintigraphic evaluation of Huntington's disease and other movement disorders using single photon emission computed tomography perfusion brain scans. *Semin Nucl Med.* 1991;21:11–23.

Neirinckx RD, Canning LR, Piper IM, et al. Technetium-99m d, 1-H-M-PAO: a new radiopharmaceutical for SPECT imaging of regional cerebral blood perfusion. *J Nucl Med.* 1987;28:191–202.

Nishizawa S, Tanada S, Yonekura Y, et al. Regional dynamics of N-Isopropyl-(^{123}I)p-iodoamphetamine in human brain. *J Nucl Med.* 1989;30:150–156.

Perlmutter JS. New insight into the pathophysiology of Parkinson's disease: the challenge of positron emission tomography. *TINS.* 1988;11:203–208.

Perlmutter JS, Raichle ME. Regional blood flow in hemiparkinsonism. *Neurology.* 1985;35:1127–1134.

Pizzolato G, Dam M, Borsato N, et al. [^{99m}Tc]-HM-PAO SPECT in Parkinson's disease. *J Cereb Blood Flow Metab.* 1988;8(Suppl 1):S101–S108.

Portin R, Raininko R, Rinne UK. Neuropsychological disturbances and cerebral atrophy determined by computerized tomography in Parkinson patients with long-term levadopa treatment. In: Hassler RG, Christ JF, eds. *Advances in Neurology.* New York: Raven Press;1984:219–227.

Rezek DL, Morris JC, Fulling KH, et al. Periventricular white matter lucencies in SDAT and healthy aging. *Neurology.* 1986;36(suppl 1):263.

Rinne UK. Recent advances in research on Parkinsonism. Acta Neurol Scand (Suppl). 1978;67:77–113.

Schneider E, Fischer P, Jacobi P, et al. The significance of cerebral atrophy for the symptomatology of Parkinson's disease. *J Neurol Sci.* 1979;42:187–197.

Selby G. Cerebral atrophy and parkinsonism. *J Neurol Sci.* 1968;6:517–559.

Smith FW, Besson JAO, Gemmell HG, Sharp PF. The use of technetium-99-M-HM-PAO in the assessment of patients with dementia and other neuropsychiatric conditions. *J Cereb Blood Flow Metab.* 1988;8:S116–S122.

Sroka H, Elizan T, Yahr M, et al. Organic mental syndrome and confusional states in Parkinson's disease: relationship to computerized tomographic signs of cerebral atrophy. *Arch Neurol.* 1981;38:339–342.

Stern MB, Braffman BH, Skolnick BE, et al. Magnetic resonance imaging in Parkinson's disease and parkinsonian syndromes. *Neurology.* 1989;39:1523–1526.

Tachibana H, Meyer JS, Kitagawa Y, et al. Xenon contrast CT-CBF measurements in parkinsonism and normal aging. *J Am Geriatr Soc.* 1985;33:413–421.

Taylor AE, Saint-Cyr JA, Lang AE. Frontal lobe dysfunction in Parkinson's disease. *Brain.* 1986;109:845–883.

Wilson RS, Fox JH, Huckman MS, et al. Computed tomography in dementia. *Neurology.* 1982;32:1054–1057.

Wolfson LI, Leenders KL, Brown LL, Jones T. Alterations of regional cerebral blood flow and oxygen metabolism in Parkinson's disease. *Neurology.* 1985;35:1399–1405.

Xuereb JH, Tomlinson BE, Perry RH, et al. Dementia in Parkinson's disease: pathologic considerations. In: Nappi G, Caraceni T, eds. *Parkinsonias: Diagnosis and Treatment.* New York: Laurel House Publishing Company; 1989:45–54.

Yoshimura M. Pathological basis for dementia in elderly patients with idiopathic Parkinson's disease. *Eur Neurol.* 1988;28(Suppl 10:29–35).

Zetusky WJ, Jancovic J, Pirozzolo RJ. The heterogeneity of Parkinson's disease: clinical and prognostic implications. *Neurology.* 1985;35:522–526.

Zimmerman RD, Fleming CA, Lee BCP, et al. Periventricular hyperintensity as seen by magnetic resonance: prevalence and significant. *AJNR.* 1986;7:13–20.

13

Pathological Correlates of Dementia in Parkinson's Disease

HELENA CHANG CHUI AND LYNN S. PERLMUTTER

Affective and cognitive as well as motor disturbances commonly are associated with idiopathic Parkinson's disease (PD) (Mortimer et al, 1985). The degree of cognitive impairment warranting the designation of dementia, however, is subject to interpretation and depends to a large measure on the methods of ascertainment. Methodological variability partially explains the wide range in the estimated prevalence of PD dementia–between 30 percent and 70 percent (for review see Mortimer et al, 1985; Cummings, 1988). The risk of developing dementia appears to increase with age (Yoshimura, 1988; Mayeux et al, 1990) but is not a simple function of disease duration. Some studies suggest that certain subgroups of patients, such as those more elderly (Lieberman et al, 1979; DuBois et al, 1990) or with less tremor (Lieberman, 1974; Mortimer et al, 1982; 1984; Zetusky et al, 1985), appear to be at greater risk for developing cognitive disturbances.

The typical dementia syndrome associated with PD has been termed "subcortical," being characterized by four cardinal features: memory impairment, deterioration of intellect, psychomotor retardation (bradyphrenia), and affective disturbance (Albert, 1978; Cummings and Benson, 1984). In addition, patients with PD commonly show impaired visuospatial skills (Villardita et al, 1982; Boller et al, 1984) and difficulty in shifting set (Cools et al, 1984; Flowers and Robertson, 1985; Taylor et al, 1986;). Language skills generally are spared, although a few patients appear to develop frank cortical symptoms such as aphasia and apraxia (Mortimer et al, 1985; Chui et al, 1986; Byrne et al, 1989). The factors that determine the pattern of cognitive deficits associated with PD remain unknown. Identification of their pathological substrates should facilitate the elucidation of pathogenetic mechanisms and the development of treatment strategies.

The typical brainstem pathologic changes associated with PD were described many years ago (Lewy, 1913), but substantial variability in the neuropathology has been recognized recently. Neocortical lesions, such as neurofibrillary tangles, senile plaques (Boller et al, 1980), and cortical Lewy bodies (Okazaki et al, 1961), may develop in a subset of PD patients. Further, variable patterns of subcortical pathology appear to influence both the motor and behavioral symptomatology for individual cases. The objectives of this chapter are twofold: first, to review the types of pathological changes associated with PD and, second, to discuss the relationship between these changes and dementia.

CORTICAL VS SUBCORTICAL BASIS FOR PD DEMENTIA

Several brain-behavioral principles are suggested by a review of the anatomical organization of the brain. Cortical and subcortical neurons, for example, have distinct patterns of interneuronal connectivity. On the one hand, cortical association neurons send and receive projections from multiple but highly specific targets (Mesulam, 1990) and seem well suited to provide the anatomical substrate for specific knowledge and skills. On the other hand, a subset of subcortical neurons project widely and diffusely to the cerebral mantle (Mesulam, 1990), a pattern of connectivity apparently better suited to the role of modulating cerebral cortical function. These neurons might, for example, set the tone or level of cortical excitability and thus the likelihood of informational transfer. Informational content itself, however, would be contained within the networks of cortical association neurons.

Comparisons of the brain-behavioral disturbances associated with the most prevalent dementing disorder, namely, Alzheimer's disease, (AD) and PD demonstrate the differences between cortical and subcortical dementias. Although there is some involvement of subcortical and brainstem neurons in AD, prominent pathological changes occur in limbic and neocortical association cortices (Kemper, 1984; Chui, 1989). The clinical hallmarks of AD include severe impairment of episodic memory, semantic knowledge, and basic language (aphasia), movement (apraxia), and recognition (agnosia) skills. In a subset of PD patients, pathological changes may occur in the cerebral cortex, but in most cases, this brain region is spared. Instead, pathological changes are confined largely to subcortical and brainstem nuclei. The typical behavioral disturbances associated with PD include depression, bradyphrenia, mental inefficiency, and difficulty shifting set (for reviews see Cummings, 1988; Chui, 1989). Aphasia, apraxia, and agnosia rarely are seen. Thus, the nature of behavioral disturbances associated with cortical vs subcortical pathology differs, supporting the notion that networks of cortical neurons contain specific informational content, whereas subcortical projection neurons modulate cortical tone.

CORTICAL BASIS FOR DEMENTIA IN PARKINSON'S DISEASE

In a subset of PD patients, the development of dementia may in fact result from pathological lesions in the cerebral cortex. Two scenarios appear most likely. First, some investigators have posited that the development of dementia in PD signifies the copresence of AD lesions in cerebral cortex (Hakim and Mathiesen, 1979; Boller et al, 1980). This finding might represent an increased susceptibility in PD to other neuronal cytoskeletal degenerations. On the other hand, the prevalence of AD increases with age (9 percent over age 65, 19 percent over age 85) (Davies et al, 1988), and the association of cortical lesions with PD may represent the chance co-occurrence of these two diseases. Second, a subset of PD patients with dementia may have a newly described clinicopathological entity known as diffuse Lewy body disease (DLBD). In DLBD, Lewy bodies (LB) are found in deep cortical neurons as well as in classic brainstem loci. The actual prevalence of this disease is, however, unclear. The pathological features of this syndrome have been defined only in the past decade (Kosaka et al, 1980), and few cases have been diagnosed antemortem (Crystal et al, 1990). Thus, in some PD patients, dementia may indeed result from cortical lesions.

Concomitant Alzheimer's Disease

The finding of hippocampal neurofibrillary tangles in many PD patients (Hakim and Mathiesen, 1979) prompted a systematic search for the simultaneous occurrence of AD in PD. The lack of universally accepted criteria for the diagnosis of AD has, however, resulted in widely disparate estimates of PD-concomitant AD. When cortical plaques or tangles are considered sufficient for the diagnosis of AD, the reported frequency of PD-concomitant AD ranged from 42 percent to 75 percent (Boller et al, 1980; Gaspar and Gray, 1984; Yoshimura, 1988). When both neocortical plaques and tangles are required for diagnosis (Tomlinson et al, 1970), however, the frequency of PD-concomitant AD was only 0 to 10 percent of all PD patients (Heston, 1980; Perry et al, 1983; Xuereb et al, 1990) and 12 percent of those who were demented (Xuereb et al, 1990). Thus, the reported prevalence of PD-concomitant AD varies from a high of 75 percent to approximately chance levels.

Accumulating evidence suggests that the senile plaque is not a specific marker for AD. Plaque densities do not always correlate well with mental status, and large numbers may be found in elderly individuals with normal mental status (Tomlinson et al, 1968; Crystal et al, 1988; Katzman et al, 1988). Indeed, one study reported that the use of plaque counts alone resulted in the misclassification of several nondemented PD patients as AD (Xuereb et al, 1990). Because plaques frequently occur without tangles in PD (Tagliavini et al, 1984; Nakano and Hirano, 1984; Yoshimura, 1988; Rinne et al, 1989a,b; Braak and Braak, 1990), the use of plaque-dependent criteria (Khachaturian, 1985) may lead to the overdiagnosis of AD in PD. Thus, both plaques and tangles, rather than plaques alone, should be used to determine the frequency of PD-concomitant AD.

Plaques with certain morphological characteristics may be more specifically related to dementia. Some plaques are comprised of both amyloid and degenerating neurites (Wisniewski and Terry, 1973), whereas others contain only amyloid proteins in various structural forms (Rozenmuller et al, 1989). Senile plaques in AD are characterized by prominent neuritic formations, whereas those associated with either normal aging or PD typically contain amyloid but not neurites (Dickson et al, 1990; Braak and Braak, 1990). Thus, the plaques most commonly associated with PD more closely resemble those associated with aging than with AD and may thus reflect an aging, rather than disease, process.

Diffuse Lewy Body Disease

Attention has focused on patients in whom Lewy bodies are not confined to brainstem neurons but are found widely dispersed throughout the cerebral cortex (Okazaki et al, 1961; Kosaka et al, 1976). This clinicopathological entity has been referred to by several designations, including (1) diffuse Lewy body disease (DLBD) (Kosaka et al,

1980), (2) senile dementia of the Lewy body type (Perry et al, 1990), and (3) Lewy body variant of AD (Hansen et al, 1990). Cortical LB are more subtle in appearance than their brainstem counterparts. At the light microscopic level, they are less eosinophilic, often irregular, and do not have well-defined halos (Yoshimura, 1988; Tiller-Borcich and Forno, 1988). Despite these morphological differences, cortical and brainstem LB are thought to arise from similar pathogenetic processes.

In DLBD, LB are observed within deep small cortical neurons of the temporal–frontal lobes and cingular–insular–entorhinal cortices, as well as in the more familiar brainstem nuclei (Dickson et al, 1987; Gibb et al, 1987; Byrne et al, 1987; Yoshimura, 1988; Burkhardt et al, 1988; Kosaka et al, 1988). In up to 76 percent of DLBD cases, concomitant Alzheimer's disease lesions (plaques more often than tangles) may be seen (Byrne et al, 1989; Perry et al, 1990; Kosaka, 1990). When specifically sought, cortical LB are not uncommon in PD. They have been reported in 7 percent of general autopsies (Byrne et al, 1989) and in 15 percent to 26 percent of those with dementia (Ditter and Mirra, 1987; Joachim et al, 1988; Byrne et al, 1989). Thus, it is possible that a substantial number of PD patients with dementia actually may have DLBD, with or without associated plaques and tangles.

The clinical syndrome of DLBD, first described retrospectively, has been reviewed recently (Kosaka, 1990). In over half of the cases, progressive dementia is the presenting symptom (Burkhardt et al, 1988; Gibb et al, 1989; Byrne et al, 1989; Kosaka, 1990; Crystal et al, 1990). Aphasia and apraxia, traditionally regarded as cortical symptoms, are common. Psychosis and depression also are seen frequently. Extrapyramidal signs (such as gait disturbance, rigidity, akinesia) develop eventually but may be mild or absent initially. In a recent review, AD was diagnosed clinically in approximately one third of the cases and PD in approximately one quarter (Kosaka, 1990). Thus, DLBD may represent a new disease entity previously misidentified as either AD or PD.

SUBCORTICAL BASIS FOR PD DEMENTIA

Subcortical and brainstem neurons are classically targeted in idiopathic PD. The nigral–striatal neurons of the substantia nigra, pars compacta (SNpc) are at particular risk and have received the most attention. Degeneration of these neurons results in classic motor symptomotology, such as akinesia and rigidity. Even the earliest pathological descriptions, however, recognized more widespread subcortical and brainstem involvement (see Jellinger, 1986, for a review). LB and neuronal loss also occurs in other dopaminergic nuclei of the ventral mesencephalic tegmentum, including the nucleus paranigralis. Pathological changes are prominent also in the hypothalamus, vagal dorsal motor nucleus, dorsal and median raphe, locus ceruleus (LC), and nucleus basalis (NB). In addition, milder degrees of neuronal loss are noted in numerous other sites. These changes result in a variety of nonmotor symptoms that also are associated with PD, such as autonomic dysfunction and affective and cognitive disturbance.

Of the many subcortical and brainstem nuclei affected by PD, those that project to the cerebral cortex are the most relevant to higher cortical functions. These include the nucleus paranigralis, dorsal and median raphe, LC, and NB. Most previous studies have focused on the relationship between single subcortical nuclei and mental status (Whitehouse et al, 1983; Rinne et al, 1989a,b; Chan-Palay and Asan, 1989). In PD, however, several of these anatomical loci usually are affected concomitantly. Thus, it is often difficult to discern the unique contribution of each nuclear lesion to behavior. In this section, we review each of these subcortical regions, its anatomical connectivity, relevant experimental lesion studies, and involvement in PD. The relationship between lesions in these various nuclei and affective–cognitive disturbance is examined.

Substantia Nigra and Related Dopaminergic Nuclei

Several subgroups of dopaminergic neurons have been identified in the midbrain (Fig. 13–1B,C). Based on their target regions, they have been divided into the mesostriatal and mesolimbic systems (Agid et al, 1984a; Graybiel et al, 1990). The mesostriatal system includes the SNpc (A9) and the perirubral–retrorubral nuclei (A8), which project to different compartments of the striatum (caudate-putamen). The mesolimbic system is comprised of the nucleus paranigralis (A10), which is located in the ventral mesencephalic tegmentum just medial to the SNpc. This system projects to limbic and paralimbic structures, such as septum, olfactory tubercle, nucleus accumbens, and amygdala, as well as to medial prefrontal, cingulate, entorhinal, and piriform cortices. By virtue of its anatomical connectivity, the mesolimbic loop appears to be most relevant for higher cortical function. However, a role for the mesostriatal pathway should not be dismissed prematurely.

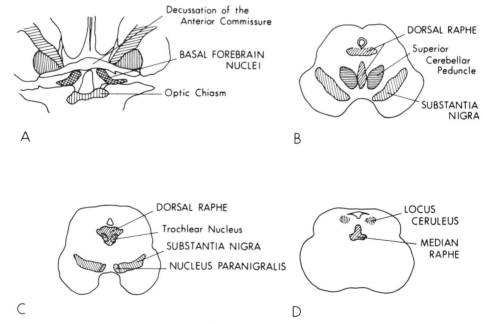

Figure 13–1. Subcortical and brainstem nuclei relevant to Parkinson's dementia. **A.** Basal forebrain nuclei, including the nucleus basalis (coronal section at the level of the decussation of the anterior commissure). **B.** Substantia nigra and dorsal raphe (caudal midbrain at the level of the superior cerebellar peduncle). **C.** Substantia nigra, nucleus paranigralis, and dorsal raphe (caudal midbrain at the level of the trochlear nucleus). **D.** Locus ceruleus and median raphe (rostral pons at the level of the aqueduct).

The mesostriatal system is most severely affected in PD, with a 50 percent to 85 percent loss of neurons reported (Jellinger, 1986). Rigidity and bradykinesia are thought to occur when the loss of striatal dopamine surpasses an 80 percent threshold (Hornykiewicz, 1982). Not surprisingly, loss of neurons in the ventral lateral SNpc has been correlated with severity of motor symptomatology (Rinne et al, 1989a,b). Recently, however, the existence of nonmotor striatal–thalamocortical circuits, which involve dorsolateral prefrontal, lateral orbitofrontal, and anterior cingulate cortices, have been described (Alexander et al, 1986). Although the functional role of these circuits is unknown, their anatomical connectivity suggests a possible contribution to visuospatial integration (Stern, 1983), spatial memory, the ability to switch behavioral set, and motivational state (Alexander et al, 1986). Thus, involvement of certain subsets of the mesostriatal pathway may be relevant to cognitive as well as motor impairments seen in PD.

Neuronal loss is seen also in the nucleus paranigralis, although degeneration generally is less extensive than in the SNpc (Javoy-Agid and Agid, 1980; Agid et al, 1984a,b; German et al, 1989; Goto et al, 1989; Graybiel et al, 1990). In animals, lesions of the nucleus paranigralis result in perseveration and disruption of delayed alternation (Galey et al, 1977; Simon et al, 1980). This may represent the animal correlate of impaired ability to shift set, which is commonly seen in PD. In humans, severe dementia has been associated with prominent degeneration of this pathway (Torack and Morris 1986, 1988), although other brainstem nuclei were involved in these cases as well. In PD, the severity of medial dopaminergic neuronal loss has been associated with the degree of cognitive impairment (Rinne et al, 1989a,b). Although specific behavioral correlations are lacking in human studies, these findings suggest that lesions of this system may underlie some of the cognitive impairments associated with PD.

Dorsal and Median Raphe

Two groups of brainstem serotonergic-synthesizing neurons have been identified that project to cerebral cortex: the mesencephalic dorsal raphe (nucleus supratrochlearis) and the pontine median raphe (nucleus centralis superioris) (Fig. 13–1B,C,D). In the rat, the dorsal and median raphe neurons project to similar overlapping target regions within the forebrain (Conrad et al, 1974; Azmita and Segal, 1978). However, the two projection systems have distinct morphological and anatomical characteristics. Dorsal raphe neurons give rise to slower-conducting nonmyelinated axons that branch profusely and do not appear to target particular neurons. Median raphe neurons, on the other hand, have faster-conducting myelinated axons that synapse on specific neurons (Korofsky and Molliver, 1987).

Some controversy has surrounded the involvement of the dorsal raphe in PD. Whereas one study reported a 42 percent loss of large dorsal raphe neurons (Jellinger, 1986), another reported relative sparing of this nucleus (Mann and Yates, 1983). Using specific markers, Halliday and colleagues (1990a) reported significant loss of catecholaminergic but not serotonergic neurons in the dorsal raphe. Thus taken together, the evidence suggests that the dorsal raphe is relatively spared in PD. On the other hand, a 60 percent loss of serotonergic neurons has been reported in the median raphe (Halliday et al, 1990a,b). Such neuronal loss could account for the 30 percent to 50 percent decrease in serotonin markers reported in PD cerebral cortex (D'Amato et al, 1987). It also would result in the selective loss of the faster-conducting myelinated serotonergic axons and might contribute to the slowing of mental processes associated with PD (Halliday et al, 1990a).

A major role has been postulated for serotonin in the regulation of mood (van Praag, 1982). In a study of 43 PD patients, those with major depression had the greatest reduction of a cerebrospinal fluid (CSF) metabolite of serotonin (Mayeux et al, 1984). Since these patients did not have lower levels of dopaminergic and noradrenergic metabolites, these findings suggest that specific alterations in serotonin metabolism may predispose PD patients to depression. Changes in these CSF metabolites most likely result from loss of serotonergic neurons, such as occurs in the median raphe. Thus, this alteration may contribute to the affective disturbance associated with PD.

Locus Ceruleus

The LC (Fig. 13–1D) gives rise to ascending noradrenergic projections that terminate on cerebral blood vessels and neurons in the cerebellum, hypothalamus, striatum, septum, hippocampus, and neocortex (Mann, 1983). In PD, destruction of the LC is a consistent feature (50 percent to 80 percent loss compared to age-matched controls) (Chui et al, 1986; Mann and Yates, 1983; Mann et al, 1983; Jellinger, 1986) and is observed throughout its rostral–caudal length (Chan-Palay and Asan, 1989).

The normal physiological role of the LC has been principally determined from animal studies. Stimulation of the LC results in reduced cerebral blood flow, increased brain vascular permeability (Raichle et al, 1975), and inhibition of spontaneous activity in its target neurons (Katayama et al, 1981). In animals, lesions of the LC are associated with several behavioral deficits. These include decrements in attention and response to reward, as well as in learning and memory consolidation (Mason and Iversen, 1978; Ogren et al, 1980). The behavioral alterations resulting from lesions of the human LC are less clear. PD patients with a history of depression have been said to show the greatest LC loss, but the status of the serotonergic raphe was not examined in these patients (Chan-Palay and Asan, 1989).

A complex relationship between norepinephrine and bradyphrenia has been reported (Mayeux et al, 1987). Bradyphrenia, or slowing of thought, is a frequent symptom of PD and subcortical dementia. Unlike bradykinesia, bradyphrenia is not responsive to levodopa (Rafal et al, 1984) but has been associated with increased CSF levels of a noradrenergic metabolite (Mayeux et al, 1987; Stern et al, 1984). It is unknown whether these patients did or did not exhibit cell loss in their LC, although our own experience has shown rather uniform involvement of the LC in PD (Fig. 13–2). A correlative study of the level of CSF noradrenergic metabolites and LC neuron counts is necessary to clarify the significance of this paradoxical finding.

Nucleus Basalis

Neurons in the basal forebrain (Fig. 13–1A) receive inputs rather selectively from limbic and paralimbic cortices (Mesulam and Mufson, 1984) but project widely to cere-

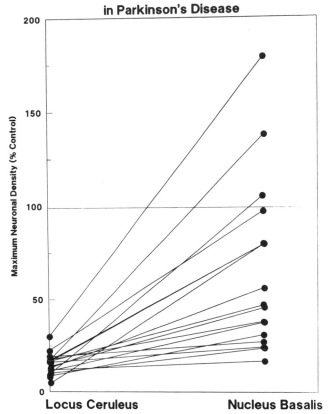

Figure 13–2. Maximum neuronal densities in the locus ceruleus and nucleus basalis in Parkinson's disease, expressed as a percentage of normal control values (*n* = 17 Parkinson's disease; *n* = 10 controls).

bral cortex (Mesulam et al, 1983). These neurons have been divided into several subgroups: (1) medial septal nucleus (Ch1), which projects to the hippocampus, (2) vertical nucleus of the diagonal band (Ch2), the major source of innervation to the hippocampus and hypothalamus, (3) horizontal nucleus of the diagonal band (Ch3), which projects to the olfactory bulb, and (4) nucleus basalis of Meynert (Ch4), which provides the primary source of extrinsic cholinergic input to neocortex (Johnston et al, 1979). Thus, the NB appears anatomically situated to control the major cholinergic innervation of the entire cerebral mantle in response to emotional stimuli.

Although a great deal is now known about the interconnections and neurochemistry of the basal forebrain, much remains to be learned about its role in behavior. In humans, acute cholinergic antagonism is associated with an impairment of recent memory (Drachman and Leavitt, 1974; Drachman, 1977). Physiological studies in animals have shown that NB neurons demonstrate tonic activity that changes with delivery of a reward (DeLong, 1972). In rodents, bilateral lesions of the NB acutely result in significant deficits in the acquisition of a spatial memory task (Murray and Fibiger, 1985; Bartus et al, 1985). Over several weeks, however, performance shows gradual and complete recovery (Bartus et al, 1985). These findings suggest that NB plays an important but complex role in mediating recent memory. Its pattern of afferent connections and electrophysiological characteristics suggests that this modulation may be related to the expectation or delivery of a reward.

The involvement of the NB in PD has long been recognized and was included in the original pathological descriptions of the disease (Lewy, 1913). Although neuronal loss appears to occur throughout the NB itself (Rogers et al, 1985), the diagonal band of Broca is relatively spared (Jellinger, 1986). A 30 percent to 80 percent loss of neurons has been reported in several series (for review, see Arendt et al, 1983; Candy et al, 1983; Whitehouse et al, 1983; Gaspar and Gray, 1984; Nakano and Hirano, 1984; Tagliavini et al, 1984; Ball et al, 1984; Rogers et al, 1985; Ezrin-Water and Resch, 1986). A greater degree of neuronal loss occurs in patients with dementia (Whitehouse et al, 1983; Gaspar and Gray, 1984; Jellinger, 1986; Yoshimura, 1988), with one series suggesting a 60 percent to 70 percent symptomatic threshold (Jellinger, 1986). In contrast, no correlations have been found between neuronal loss in the NB with age, duration, motor severity of PD, or associated tangles and plaques in the cerebral cortex (Arendt et al, 1983; Tagliavini et al, 1984; Gaspar and Gray, 1984; Nakano and Hirano, 1984; Mortimer et al, 1989). Thus, NB lesions appear to be a specific contributor to PD dementia.

Few studies have examined the interrelationship between lesions in the various subcortical nuclei. If the disease process affects all loci equally, it would be difficult to identify the unique contribution of each nucleus to resultant behavior. If, however, these various nuclei are differentially involved, specific brain–behavior correlations may be possible. In one study, the degree of neuronal loss in the LC, SN, and NB was compared for those patients with and without dementia (Gaspar and Gray, 1984). Patients with dementia tended to show greater neuronal loss in the LC and NB but showed no differential involvement of the SN. Our own studies specifically compared neuronal loss in the LC and NB (Fig. 13–2) (Chui et al, unpublished observations). Neuronal loss in the LC was uniformly severe and did not correlate with mental status. On the other hand, neuronal density was highly variable in the NB, with a strong trend showing an inverse relationship to dementia (Mortimer et al, unpublished observations). Taken together, these findings suggest that the NB, rather than the LC, may be a more specific contributor to the cognitive impairment in PD.

In summary, several preliminary relationships between behavioral deficits and underlying subcortical pathology may be posited. Correlations between CSF metabolites and behavior suggest that loss of neurons in the serotonergic median raphe may predispose to depression and that alterations in the noradrenergic system of the LC may contribute to bradyphrenia. Animal studies suggest that destruction of either dopaminergic mesostriatal or mesolimbic systems may lead to difficulty in shifting set, whereas neuronal loss in the NB may contribute to impairment of recent memory. In PD, overall severity of cognitive impairment has been correlated with the degree of neuronal loss in the mesolimbic dopaminergic system and the cholinergic NB. Thus, the characteristic features associated with PD dementia can be attributed to degeneration in multiple brainstem and subcortical nuclei.

CONCLUSIONS

In the final analysis, the specific constellation of symptoms in PD dementia may indicate the underlying pattern of pathology. The development of aphasia and apraxia in patients with PD may presage the occurrence of cortical lesions. This may include the plaques and tangles of AD or the cortical LB of DLBD. On the other hand, a symptom complex comprised of affective disturbance, bradyphrenia, and difficulty shifting set, most likely indicates classical PD lesions in the subcortex and brainstem. Thus, PD-associated dementia may not be a unitary disorder but rather an intricate mix of various concomitant pathologies.

ACKNOWLEDGMENT

This work was supported by NIH 1P50-AG05142, the California State Department of Health Services, and the Veteran's Administration. We would like to thank Chris Zarow and Edward Hsu for excellent technical assistance.

REFERENCES

Agid F, Ruberg M, Taquet H, et al. Biochemical neuropathology of Parkinson's disease. In: Hassler GR, Christ JF, eds. *Advances in Neurology,* vol 40: *Parkinson-Specific Motor and Mental Disorders.* New York: Raven Press; 1984a;189–198.

Agid Y, Ruberg M, Dubois B, Javoy-Agid F. Biochemical substrates of mental disturbances in Parkinson's disease. In: Hassler GR, Christ JF, eds. *Advances in Neurology,* vol 40: *Parkinson-Specific Motor and Mental Disorders.* New York: Raven Press; 1984b;211–218.

Albert ML. Subcortical dementia. In: Katzman R, Terry RD, Bick KL, eds. *Alzheimer's Disease: Senile Dementia and Related Disorders.* New York: Raven Press; 1978;173–180.

Alexander GE, DeLong MR, Strick PL. Parallel organization of functionally segregated circuits linking basal ganglia and cortex. *Annu Rev Neurosci.* 1986;9:357–381.

Arendt R, Bigl V, Arendt A, Tennstedt A. Loss of neurons in the nucleus basalis of Meynert in Alzheimer's disease, paralysis agitans, and Korsakoff's disease. *Acta Neuropathol.* 1983;61:101–108.

Azmita EC, Segal M. An autoradiographic analysis of the differential ascending projections of the dorsal and median raphe nuclei of the rat. *J Comp Neurol.* 1978;179:64–668.

Ball M. The morphologic basis of dementia in Parkinson's disease. *Can J Neurol Sci.* 1984;11:180–184.

Bartus RT, Flicker C, Dean RL, et al. Selective memory loss following nucleus basalis lesions: long-term behavioral recovery despite persistent cholinergic deficiencies. *Pharmacol Biochem Behav.* 1985;23:125–135.

Boller F, Mizutani T, Roesmann R, Gambetti P. Parkinson disease, dementia, and Alzheimer disease: clinicopathological correlations. *Ann Neurol.* 1980;7:329–335.

Boller F, Passafiume D, Keefe NC, et al. Visuospatial impairment in Parkinson's disease. *Arch Neurol.* 1984;41:485–490.

Braak H, Braak E. Cognitive impairment in Parkinson's disease: amyloid plaques, neurofibrillary tangles, and neuropil threads in the cerebral cortex. *J Neural Transm.* 1990;2:45–57.

Burkhardt CR, Filey CM, Kleinschmidt-DeMaster BK, et al. Diffuse Lewy body disease and dementia. *Neurology.* 1988;38:1520–1528.

Byrne E, Lennox G, Lowe J, Godwin-Austen RB. Diffuse Lewy body disease: clinical features in 15 cases. *J Neurol Neurosurg Psychiatry.* 1989;52:709–717.

Byrne EJ, Lowe JS, Godwin-Austen RB, et al. Dementia and Parkinson's disease associated with diffuse cortical Lewy bodies. *Lancet.* 1987;1:501.

Candy JM, Perry RH, Perry EK, et al. Pathologic changes in the nucleus of Meynert in Alzheimer's and Parkinson's diseases. *J Neurol Sci.* 1983;59:277–289.

Chan-Palay V, Asan E. Alterations in catecholamine neurons of the locus coeruleus in senile dementia of the Alzheimer type and in Parkinson's disease with and without dementia and depression. *J Comp Neurol.* 1989;287:373–392.

Chui HC. Dementia: A review emphasizing clinicopathologic correlations and brain–behavior relationships. *Arch Neurol.* 1989;46:806–814.

Chui HC, Mortimer JA, Slager U, et al. Pathologic correlates of dementia in Parkinson's disease. *Arch Neurol.* 1986;43:991–995.

Conrad L, Leonard C, Pfaff D. Connections of the median and dorsal raphe nuclei in the rat: an autoradiographic and degeneration study. *J Comp Neurol.* 1974;156:179–206.

Cools AR, Van Der Bercken JHL, Horstink MWI, et al. Cognitive and motor shifting aptitude disorder in Parkinson's disease. *J Neurol Neurosurg Psychiatry.* 1984;47:443–453.

Crystal H, Dickson D, Fuld P, et al. Clinico-pathologic studies in dementia: non-demented subjects with pathologically confirmed Alzheimer's disease. *Neurology.* 1988;38:1682–1687.

Crystal HA, Dickson DW, Lizardi JE, et al. Antemortem diagnosis of diffuse Lewy body disease. *Neurology.* 1990;40:1523–1528.

Cummings JL. Intellectual impairment in Parkinson's disease: clinical, pathologic, and biochemical correlations. *J Ger Psychiatry Neurol.* 1984;1:24–36.

Cummings JL, Benson DF. Subcortical dementia: Review of an emerging concept. *Arch Neurol.* 1984;41:874–879.

D'Amato RJD, Zweig RM, Whitehouse PJ, et al. Aminergic systems in Alzheimer's and Parkinson's disease. *Ann Neurol.* 1987;22:229–236.

Davies L, Wolska B, Hilbich C, et al. A4 amyloid protein deposition and the diagnosis of Alzheimer's disease: prevalence in aged brains determined by immunocytochemistry compared with conventional neuropathologic techniques. *Neurology.* 1988;38:1688–1693.

DeLong M. Activity of basal ganglia neurons during movement. *Brain Res.* 1972;40:127–135.

Dickson DW, Davies P, Mayeux R, et al. Diffuse Lewy body disease: neuropathological and biochemical studies of 6 patients. *Acta Neuropathol.* 1987;75:8–15.

Dickson DW, Mattiace LA, Crystal H, et al. Neuropathology of prospectively studied normal elderly humans. *Neurobiol Aging.* 1990;11:305.

Ditter SM, Mirra SS. Neuropathologic and clinical features of Parkinson's disease in Alzheimer's disease patients. *Neurology.* 1987;37:754–760.

Drachman DA. Memory and cognitive function in man: does the cholinergic system have a specific role? *Neurology.* 1977;27:783–790.

Drachman DA, Leavitt J. Human memory and the cholinergic system: a relationship to aging? *Arch Neurol.* 1974;30:113–121.

DuBois B, Pillon B, Sternic N, et al. Age-induced cognitive disturbances in Parkinson's disease. *Neurology.* 1990;40:38–41.

Ezrin-Water C, Resch L. The nucleus basalis of Meynert. *Can J Neurol Sci.* 1986;13:8–14.

Flowers KA, Robertson C. The effect of Parkinson's disease on the ability to maintain a mental set. *J Neurol Neurosurg Psychiatry.* 1985;48:517–529.

Galey D, Simon H, Le Moal M. Behavioral effects of lesions in the A10 dopaminergic area of the rat. *Brain Res.* 1977;124:83–97.

Gaspar P, Gray F. Dementia in idiopathic Parkinson's disease. *Acta Neuropathol.* 1984;64:43–52.

German DC, Manaye K, Smith WK, et al. Midbrain dopaminergic cell loss in Parkinson's disease: computer visualization. *Ann Neurol.* 1989;26:507–514.

Gibb WRG, Esiri MM, Lees AJ. Clinical and pathological features of diffuse cortical Lewy body disease (Lewy body dementia) *Brain.* 1987;110:1131–1153.

Gibb WRG, Luthert PJ, Janota I, Lantos PL. Cortical Lewy body dementia: clinical features and classification. *J Neurol Neurosurg Psychiatry.* 1989;52:185–192.

Goto A, Hirano A, Matsumoto S. Subdivisional involvement of nigrostriatal loop in idiopathic Parkinson's disease and striatonigral degeneration. *Ann Neurol.* 1989;26:766–770.

Graybiel AM, Hirsch E, Agid Y. The nigrostriatal system in Parkinson's disease. In: Streifler MB, Korczyn AD, Melamed E, Youdim MBH, eds. *Advances in Neurology,* vol 53. *Parkinson's Disease: Anatomy, Pathology, and Therapy.* New York: Raven Press; 1990;17–29.

Hakim AM, Mathiesen G. Dementia in Parkinson disease: a neuropathologic study. *Neurology.* 1979;29:1209–1214.

Halliday GM, Blumbergs PC, Cotton RGH, et al. Loss of brainstem serotonin- and substance P-containing neurons in Parkinson's disease. *Brain Res.* 1990a;510:104–107.

Halliday GM, Li YW, Blumbergs PC, et al. Neuropathology of immunohistochemically identified brainstem neurons in Parkinson's disease. *Ann Neurol.* 1990b;27:373–385.

Hansen L, Salmon D, Galasko D, et al. The Lewy body variant of Alzheimer's disease: a clinical and pathological entity. *Neurology.* 1990;40:1–8.

Heston LL. Dementia associated with Parkinson's disease: a genetic study. *J Neurol Neurosurg Psychiatry.* 1980;43:846–848.

Hornykiewicz O. Brain neurotransmitter changes in Parkinson's disease. In: Marsden D, Fahn S, eds. *Movement Disorders.* London: Butterworth Scientific; 1982;41–58.

Javoy-Agid F, Agid Y. Is the mesocortical dopaminergic system involved in Parkinson's disease? *Neurology.* 1980;30:1326–1330.

Jellinger K. Overview morphological changes in Parkinson disease. In: Yahr M, Bergmann KJ, eds. *Advances in Neurology,* vol 45. *Parkinson's Disease.* New York: Raven Press; 1986:1–18.

Joachim CL, Morris JH, Selko DJ. Clinically diagnosed Alzheimer's disease: autopsy results in 150 cases. *Ann Neurol.* 1988;24:50–56.

Johnston MV, McKinney M, Coyle J. Evidence for a cholinergic projection to neocortex from neurons in the basal forebrain. *Proc Natl Acad Sci USA.* 1979;76:5392–5396.

Katayama K, Veno Y, Tsukiyama T, Tsubokawa T. Long lasting suppression of timing of cortical neurones and decrease in cortical blood flow following train pulse stimulation of the locus coeruleus in the cat. *Brain Res.* 1981;216:173–179.

Katzman R, Terry R, DeTeresa R, et al. Clinical, pathological, and neurochemical changes in dementia: a subgroup with preserved mental status and numerous neocortical plaques. *Ann Neurol.* 1988;23:138–144.

Kemper T. Neuroanatomical and neuropathological changes in normal ageing and dementia. In: Albert E, ed. *Clinical Neurology of Aging.* Oxford: Oxford University Press; 1984:9–52.

Korofsky BE, Molliver ME. The serotonergic innervation of cerebral cortex: different classes of axon terminals arise from dorsal and median raphe nuclei. *Synapse.* 1987;1:153–168.

Khachaturian Z. Diagnosis of Alzheimer's disease. *Arch Neurol.* 1985;42:1097–1105.

Kosaka K. Diffuse Lewy body disease in Japan. *J Neurol.* 1990;237:197–204.

Kosaka K, Matsushita M, Oyanagi S, Mehraein P. A clinicopathological study of the "Lewy body disease." *Psychiatr Neurol.* 1980;82:292–311.

Kosaka K, Oyanagi S, Matsushita M, et al. Presenile dementia with Alzheimer-, Pick-, and Lewy body changes. *Acta Neuropathol.* 1976;36:221–233.

Kosaka K, Tsuchiya K, Yoshimura M. Lewy body disease with and without dementia: a clinicopathological study of 35 cases. *Clin Neuropathol.* 1988;7:299–305.

Lewy FH. Zur pathologischen Anatomie der Paralysis agitans. *Deutsch Z Nervenheilk.* 1913;50:50–55.

Lieberman AN. Parkinson's disease: a clinical review. *Am J Med Sci.* 1974;267:66–80.

Lieberman AN, Dziatolowski M, Kupersmith M, et al. Dementia in Parkinson disease. *Ann Neurol.* 1979;6:355–359.

Mann DMA. The locus coeruleus and its possible role in ageing and degenerative disease of the human CNS. *Mech Ageing Dev.* 1983;23:73–94.

Mann DMA, Yates PO. Pathological basis for neurotransmitter changes in Parkinson's disease. *Neuropathol Appl Neurobiol.* 1983;9:3–19.

Mann DMA, Yates PO, Hawkes J. The pathology of the human locus coeruleus. *Clin Neuropathol.* 1983;2:1–7.

Mason ST, Iversen SD. Reward, attention, and the dorsal noradrenergic bundle. *Brain Res.* 1978;150:135–148.

Mayeux R, Chen J, Mirabello E, et al. An estimate of the incidence of dementia in idiopathic Parkinson's disease. *Neurology.* 1990;40:1513–1517.

Mayeux R, Stern Y, Cote L, Williams JBW. Altered serotonin metabolism in depressed patients with Parkinson's disease. *Neurology.* 1984;34:642–646.

Mayeux R, Stern Y, Sano M, et al. Clinical and biochemical correlates of bradyphrenia in Parkinson's disease. *Neurology.* 1987;37:1130–1134.

Mesulam M-M. Large-scale neurocognitive networks and distributed processing for attention, language, and memory. *Ann Neurol.* 1990;28:597–613.

Mesulam M-M, Mufson EJ. Neural inputs into the nucleus basalis of the substantia innominata (Ch4) in the rhesus monkey. *Brain.* 1984;107:253–274.

Mesulam M-M, Mufson EJ, Levey A, Wainer BH. Cholinergic innervation of cortex by the basal forebrain: cytochemistry and cortical connections of the septal area, diagonal band nuclei, nucleus basalis (substantia innominata) and hypothalamus in the rhesus monkey. *J Comp Neurol.* 1983;214:170–197.

Mortimer JA, Christensen KJ, Webster DD. Parkinsonian dementia. In: Frederiks JAM, ed. *Handbook of Clinical Neurology,* vol 2. Amsterdam: Elsevier; 1985:371–384.

Mortimer JA, Chui HC, Slager UT, et al. Prospective clinicopathologic study of Parkinson's disease. *Neurology.* 1989;39(suppl 1):220.

Mortimer JA, Pirozzolo FJ, Hansch EC, Webster D. Relationship of motor symptoms to intellectual deficits in Parkinson disease. *Neurology.* 1982;32:133–137.

Murray CL, Fibiger HC. Learning and memory deficits after lesions of the nucleus basalis magnocellularis: reversal by physostigmine. *Neuroscience.* 1985;14:1025–1032.

Nakano I, Hirano A. Parkinson's disease: neuron loss in the nucleus basalis without concomitant Alzheimer's disease. *Ann Neurol.* 1984;15:415–418.

Ogren SO, Archer T, Ross SB. Evidence for a role of the locus coeruleus noradrenaline system in learning. *Neurosci Lett.* 1980;20:351–356.

Okazaki H, Lipkin LE, Aronson SM. Diffuse intracytoplasmic ganglionic inclusions (Lewy type) associated with progressive dementia and quadriparesis in flexion. *J Neuropathol Exp Neurol.* 1961;20:237–244.

Perry EK, Marshall E, Perry RH, et al. Cholinergic and dopaminergic activities in senile dementia of Lewy body type. *Alz Dis Asso Disor.* 1990;4:87–95.

Perry RH, Tomlinson BE, Candy JM, et al. Cortical cholinergic deficit in mentally impaired parkinsonian patients. *Lancet.* 1983;2:789–790.

Rafal RD, Posner MI, Walker JA, Friedrich FJ. Cognition and the basal ganglia: separating mental and motor components of performance in Parkinson's disease. *Brain.* 1984;107:1083–1094.

Raichle ME, Hartman BK, Eichling JO, Sharpe LG. Central noradrenergic regulation of cerebral blood flow and vascular permeability. *Proc Natl Acad Sci USA.* 1975;72:3726–3730.

Rinne JO, Rummukainen J, Paljarvi L, Rinne U. Dementia in Parkinson's disease is related to neuronal loss in the medial substantia nigra. *Ann Neurol.* 1989a;26:47–50.

Rinne JO, Rummakainen J, Paljarvi L, et al. Neuronal loss in the substantia nigra in patients with Alzheimer's disease and Parkinson's disease in relation to extrapyramidal symptoms and dementia. *Prog Clin Biol Res.* 1989b;317:325–332.

Rogers JD, Brogan D, Mirra SS. The nucleus basalis of Meynert in neurologic disease: a quantitative morphological study. *Ann Neurol.* 1985;17:163–170.

Rozenmuller JM, Eikenlenboom P, Stam FC, et al. A4 protein in Alzheimer's disease: primary and secondary cellular events in extracellular amyloid deposition. *J Neuropathol Exp Neurol.* 1989;48:674–691.

Simon H, Scatton B, Le Moal M. Dopaminergic A10 neurones are involved in cognitive functions. *Nature.* 1980;286:150–151.

Stern Y. Behavior and the basal ganglia. In: Mayeux R, Rosen WG, eds. *The Dementias.* New York: Raven Press; 1983:195–209.

Stern T, Mayeux R, Cote L. Reaction time and vigilance in Parkinson's disease: possible role of altered norepinephrine metabolism. *Arch Neurol.* 1984;41:1086–1089.

Tagliavini F, Pilleri G, Bouras C, Constantinidis J. The basal nucleus of Meynert in idiopathic Parkinson's disease. *Acta Neurol Scand.* 1984;69:20–28.

Taylor AE, Saint-Cyr JA, Lang AE. Frontal lobe dysfunction in Parkinson's disease. *Brain.* 1986;109:845–883.

Tiller-Borcich JK, Forno LS. Parkinson's disease and dementia with neuronal inclusions in the cerebral cortex: Lewy bodies or Pick bodies. *J Neuropathol Exp Neurol.* 1988;5:526–535.

Tomlinson BE, Blessed G, Roth M. Observations on the brains of nondemented old people. *J Neurol Sci.* 1968;7:331–356.

Tomlinson BE, Blessed G, Roth M. Observations on the brains of demented old people. *J Neurol Sci.* 1970;11:205–242.

Torack RM, Morris JC. Mesolimbocortical dementia: a clinicopathologic case study of a putative disorder. *Arch Neurol.* 1986;43:1074–1078.

Torack RM, Morris JC. The association of ventral tegmental area histopathology with adult dementia. *Arch Neurol.* 1988;45:497–501.

van Praag HM. Serotonin precursors in the treatment of depression. In: Ho BT, Schooler JS, Usdin E, eds. *Movement Disorders.* New York: Raven Press; 1982:259–286.

Villardita C, Smirni P, Le Pira F, et al. Mental deterioration, visuoperceptive disabilities and constructional apraxia in Parkinson's disease. *Acta Neurol Scand.* 1982;66:112–120.

Whitehouse PJ, Hedreen JC, White CL, Price DL. Basal forebrain neurons in the dementia of Parkinson's disease. *Ann Neurol.* 1983;13:243–248.

Wisniewski HM, Terry RD. Reexamination of the pathogenesis of the senile plaque. *Prog Neuropathol.* 1973;2:101–142.

Xuereb JH, Tomlinson BE, Irving D, et al. Cortical and subcortical pathology in Parkinson's disease: relationship to Parkinsonian dementia. In: Streifler MB, Korczyn AD, Melamed E, Youdim MBH, eds. *Advances in Neurology,* vol 53. *Parkinson's Disease: Anatomy, Pathology and Therapy.* New York: Raven Press; 1990:35–40.

Yoshimura M. Pathological basis for dementia in elderly patients with idiopathic Parkinson's disease. *Eur Neurol.* 1988;28(suppl 1):29–35.

Zetusky W, Jankovic J, Pirozzolo F. The heterogeneity of Parkinson's disease: clinical and prognostic implications. *Neurology.* 1985;35:522–526.

14

Biochemical Correlates of Cognitive Changes and Dementia in Parkinson's Disease

BRUNO DUBOIS AND BERNARD PILLON

During the past two decades, our knowledge concerning the frequency and nature of cognitive changes associated with Parkinson's disease (PD), on the one hand, and the type and extent of neuronal loss in the brains of patients, on the other, has progressed significantly. PD thus represents a unique model for studying the relationships between specific cognitive disorders and defined lesions of the CNS. Several attempts have been made to determine the neurochemical substrates that may underlie some of the behavioral deficits in PD. Before reviewing the data, however, we wish to make two general points. First, cognitive changes in PD do not comprise a monolithic picture that is identical in all patients. As reviewed in the preceding chapters, a spectrum of intellectual disorders can be observed, ranging from a few limited frontal signs to florid dementia with severe memory impairment. Nor can each of the various symptoms be attributed to pathology of one specific type of neuron or brain structure. Second, the identification of biochemical changes in PD is far from complete, and new data may well render present theories obsolete. Furthermore, neuronal interactions underlying brain functions are far too complex for such an approach to provide all the answers. They are, however, a place to start.

From the pathologist's point of view, PD is mainly characterized by degeneration of subcortical neuronal systems. In typical cases, cortical abnormalities (Chapter 13) consist essentially of numerous neurofibrillary tangles in the hippocampus (Hakim and Mathieson, 1979; Ball, 1984). For this reason, rare histological changes in extrahippocampal cortical neurons are not considered to play a significant role in the onset of cognitive disorders, at least in a great majority of cases.

Among the subcortical neuronal systems, nigrostriatal dopaminergic neurons are known to be the most affected by the disease, justifying the definition of PD as a "striatal dopamine deficiency" syndrome (Hornykiewicz, 1975). The dopaminergic avenue, therefore, is explored first and in greatest detail.

DOPAMINERGIC THEORY OF COGNITIVE DISORDERS IN PARKINSON'S DISEASE

What are the data? Most dopaminergic systems are affected in PD, as shown in Table 14–1. The findings can be summarized as follows: (1) the nigrostriatal dopaminergic system is the most severely affected; neuronal loss is thought to have reached 70 percent when the first PD symptoms appear (Bernheimer et al, 1973; Riederer and Wuketich, 1976), (2) dopamine depletion is greater in the putamen than in the caudate nucleus (Nyberg et al, 1983), probably because cell loss in the substantia nigra is greater in the caudal and internal portions of the structure that project preferentially to the putamen, (3) the surviving dopamine-containing neurons in the substantia nigra become overactive as a function of the severity of the lesion, but there is no definitive evidence for hypersensitivity of postsynaptic D1 and D2 dopamine receptors in the striatum (Agid et al, 1987), and (4) mesolimbic and mesocortical dopaminergic neurons degenerate in PD as well but to a lesser extent (Javoy-Agid and Agid, 1980).

Since degeneration of dopaminergic neurons constitutes the main biochemical abnormality found in PD, the dopamine depletion has been considered to account for most of the symptoms. This seems clearly to be the case for motor symptoms, such as akinesia, rigidity, and tremor, given the correlations between the extent of motor symptoms and lesions (Bernheimer et al, 1973), the response to levodopa treatment (Cotzias et al, 1969), and observations in cases of MPTP-induced parkinsonism where lesions are essentially limited to dopamine systems (Langston et al, 1983).

Table 14–1. Dopamine markers in brain of PD patients

	Dopamine depletion (%)	Decrease in TH activity (%)
Site of origin		
Substantia nigra		
Fahn et al, 1971	85	
McGeer and McGeer, 1976		70
Javoy-Agid et al, 1982	99	
Ventral tegmental area		
Ploska et al, 1982		
Area of projection		
Putamen		
Fahn et al, 1971	95	
McGeer and McGeer, 1976		77
Farley et al, 1977	91	
Rinne et al, 1979	76[a]	62
Caudate nucleus		
Fahn et al, 1971	87	
Rinne et al, 1979	71	83
Javoy-Agid et al, 1982	73	73
Frontal cortex		
Scatton et al, 1983	61[a]	
Hippocampus		
Scatton et al, 1983	68[a]	

[a]Levodopa treatment withdrawn before death.

Several attempts have been made to implicate dopaminergic lesions in cognitive symptoms. Some authors have tried to correlate intellectual changes with various indices of dopaminergic lesions, such as the severity of motor disability or concentrations of dopaminergic markers assayed postmortem. Others have tried to reverse cognitive impairment in patients by reestablishing normal central dopaminergic transmission through the administration of levodopa. The behavioral consequences of specific lesions of dopaminergic neuronal systems in experimental animals or in MPTP-intoxicated patients also may have provided some pertinent clues. For the sake of simplicity, the clinicopathological, experimental, and pharmacological data are discussed separately.

Cognitive Impairment and Motor Symptoms

One way to establish a relationship between dopamine depletion and cognitive disorders in PD is to find a correlation between the degree of motor disability, thought to reflect damage to the nigrostriatal dopaminergic system, and intellectual impairment. Such correlations have been found in large series of patients (Celesia and Wanamaker, 1972; Martilla and Rinne, 1976; Elizan et al, 1986; Growdon et al, 1990). Among the classic triad of motor symptoms, intellectual impairment usually correlated best with akinesia (Garron et al, 1972; Martilla and Rinne, 1976), even in untimed tests (Mortimer et al, 1982). At first glance, the correlation with akinesia might seem to have some pathophysiological significance, since this symptom is considered to be a marker of dopaminergic lesions for the following reasons: (1) a correlation has been found between the severity of akinesia and both the decrease in striatal dopamine content and neuronal loss in the substantia nigra (Bernheimer et al, 1973), and (2) akinesia, among all the PD symptoms, responds best to levodopa treatment (Cotzias et al, 1969). From these correlations with akinesia, it might be inferred that "cognitive impairment results from the same subcortical lesion that causes the motor symptoms" (Mortimer et al, 1982), that is, lesion of the nigrostriatal dopaminergic system.

It must be stressed, however, that correlations indicate nothing about causality. The severity of intellectual impairment, like that of motor disability, simply might be related to the duration or the stage of the disease (Celesia and Wanamaker, 1972). Furthermore, in young onset PD, characterized by severe akinesia and marked response to levodopa and considered to reflect pure degeneration of dopaminergic neurons, no significant cognitive impairment is observed even after long evolution of the disease (Quinn et al, 1987). These observations argue against a causal relationship between dopaminergic lesions and intellectual deterioration, and, a new approach to analysis by correlation was devised (Pillon et al, 1989a) in which the motor symptoms were distinguished according to their response to levodopa. In this case, cognitive dysfunction correlated strongly with motor symptoms that respond little, if at all, to levodopa, such as gait disorders or dysarthria, and weakly with motor symptoms that respond well, suggesting that cognitive disorders may be related to the dysfunction of nondopaminergic neuronal systems.

Additional evidence challenging a relationship between dopamine loss and cognitive dysfunction is provided by several other studies. In a longitudinal study on 52 PD patients, Portin and Rinne (1984) showed that both poor response to levodopa and absence of daily fluctuations in motor disability—considered to indicate the presence of additional nondopaminergic lesions in the brain—were associated with mental changes. In another study, the only PD patients impaired on all the neuropsychological tasks were those with a poor response to levodopa (Taylor et al, 1987). Granerus and colleagues (1979) also observed that patients who developed daily fluctuations under treatment early in the course of the disease, reflecting a rapid and pure degeneration of dopaminergic neurons, were less likely to develop dementia.

PD motor symptoms usually start on one side of the body and often remain lateralized during the early and middle stages of the disease (Hoehn and Yahr, 1967). This asymmetry is considered to reflect an asymmetrical striatal dopamine deficiency, which has been partially confirmed by position emission tomography (PET) (Garnett et al, 1984). If the striatal dopamine deficiency plays a role in cognitive disorders, specialized hemispheric functions contralateral to the motor symptoms should be altered selectively in patients with hemiparkinsonism, providing a unique opportunity to study the effect of asymmetrical subcortical degeneration on cognitive function (Direnfeld et al, 1984). The results of such studies have, however, been controversial. Some authors found specific differences. Spicer and associates (1988) observed that patients with right-sided motor involvement performed poorly on tasks sensitive to dominant hemisphere functions, such as serial digits, confrontation naming, and verbal association fluency. Accordingly, Starkstein and colleagues (1987) found that patients with right-sided PD performed less well than patients with left-sided symptoms on the WAIS verbal subtests and on verbal learning. Other authors were not able to find a specific pattern of differences between patients with right- and left-sided syndromes (Bentin et al, 1981; Boller et al, 1984; Huber et al, 1989; Riklan et al, 1990), and Direnfeld and co-workers (1984) observed that patients with predominantly left-sided symptoms were more impaired in all neuropsychological functions assessed, although no specific or distinctive pattern characterized this subgroup.

Methodological biases may account for some of these discrepancies. For example, the two groups of patients have to be matched for their overall level of cognitive impairment (Huber et al, 1989). This was not the case in all of the studies. In one study, adjustment for symptom severity resulted in the disappearance of differences between the groups (Ricklan et al, 1990). When methodological pitfalls are avoided, patterns of cognitive changes do not differ with respect to the lateralization of motor symptoms. Thus, correlational analyses with motor symptoms do not provide unequivocal evidence of a primary, isolated dopaminergic mechanism underlying cognitive changes in PD. Other avenues of investigation, however, continue to support a relationship between dopamine deficiency and certain aspects of intellectual impairment in PD.

Cognitive Changes and Biological Markers of Degeneration of Dopaminergic Neuronal Systems in Parkinson's Disease

Correlations between cognitive dysfunction and biochemical markers of dopaminergic neurons can be examined for evidence to support a dopamine theory of intellectual impairment in PD. In the first place, degeneration of the nigrostriatal dopaminergic system is massive in all patients—at least 70 percent cell loss before symptoms appear, reaching 90 percent by the time the patient dies. The extent of this phenomenon could easily mask a hypothetical relationship with more discrete cognitive disorders. Second, only a few pathological studies have been performed on selected populations of demented and nondemented PD patients. Furthermore, these studies generally are performed on atypical populations of hospitalized patients who have had the disease for many years. Cognitive impairment in these cases usually is severe, largely exceeding the subtle cognitive changes considered to be specific to the disease and related to loss of well-defined neuronal systems. The late-onset cognitive deterioration observed in these patients can result from additional lesions of other neuronal systems or histological changes in the cortex, which would obscure putative correlations between specific cognitive disorders and dopaminergic lesions. The principal correlations observed in postmortem studies are, indeed, with nondopaminergic lesions, since PD dementia has been attributed variously to (1) coexisting Alzheimer's disease (Alvord et al, 1974; Boller et al, 1980; De la Monte et al, 1989), (2) the presence of Alzheimer's disease type pathology primarily in the hippocampus (Hakim and Mathieson, 1979; Dubois et al, 1985a), (3) neuronal loss in the nucleus basalis of Meynert (Whitehouse et al, 1983), and (4) decreased choline acetyltransferase (CAT) activity (Ruberg et al, 1982; Dubois et al, 1983; Perry et al, 1985) or somatostatin-like immunoreactivity in the cerebral cortex (Epelbaum et al, 1983).

Several studies have focused on damage to dopaminergic systems in relation to cognitive impairment and have yielded contradictory results. Striatal dopamine concentrations were shown to decrease severely and to the same extent in demented and nondemented PD patients (Ruberg and Agid, 1988). Furthermore, a comparison of the neuronal loss in the substantia nigra of 18 demented and 14 nondemented PD patients showed no correlation with dementia (Gaspar and Gray, 1984). These observations suggest that mental impairment in PD is not related to the nigrostriatal dopaminergic deficiency (Marsden, 1982). However, in a study of 12 PD patients, Rinne and colleagues (1989) found a significant correlation between the degree of dementia and neuronal loss in the medial part of the substantia nigra, that is, the part that projects more specifically to the caudate nucleus, suggesting that degeneration of nigral projections may in itself contribute to dementia in PD via deafferentation of the caudate nucleus. This observation needs to be confirmed in a larger series of patients, as it contradicts previous studies. Degeneration of the mesocortical dopaminergic system also may be implicated in the cognitive changes (Agid et al, 1984), since the decrease in dopamine levels in neocortical areas is greater in demented than in nondemented PD patients (Scatton et al, 1983).

The few in vivo measurements performed on cerebrospinal fluid (CSF) have failed to clarify the issue. Levels of homovanillic acid (HVA), the principal metabolite of dopamine that mainly reflects dopamine use in the striatum, are reduced in the CSF of PD patients (Mann et al, 1983a), but attempts to detect a correlation between cognitive dysfunction and HVA concentrations in the CSF have been unsuccessful (Mayeux et al, 1985).

Experimental Evidence Implicating a Dopaminergic Mechanism in Cognitive Dysfunction

Two models have been used to study dopaminergic influences on cognition; lesions of the striatum and destruction of nigrostriatal neurons. It must be stressed that the former is not the best model for PD. Striatal neurons apparently are intact in PD patients but deafferented through loss of input from the nigrostriatal dopaminergic neurons.

However, experimental lesions in the striatum caused cognitive deficits in delayed alternation behavior and object reversal (reviewed in Divac and Oberg, 1979; Iversen, 1984). Interestingly, these deficits resemble those observed in PD. The behavioral consequences of lesions of the dopamine-containing neurons of the substantia nigra (Marshall et al, 1974) and of the striatal injection of 6-hydroxydopamine, an agent with neurotoxic properties specific to dopaminergic neurons (Annett et al, 1990), have been far less studied than the consequences of lesions of the striatum. Interestingly, the effects on motor function, characterized by impaired movement initiation and neglect of contralateral stimuli, are similar to those observed after striatal lesions. Cognitive changes are less well documented, but the lesions seem to interfere with acquisition of both active and passive avoidance, at least in rats (Fibiger et al, 1974).

The use of the neurotoxin MPTP in monkeys has given new impetus to the study of cognitive deficits after lesion of the nigrostriatal dopaminergic neurons. MPTP is known to destroy these neurons selectively, as shown by the dramatic reduction in dopamine levels in the substantia nigra, and in the caudate nucleus and putamen (Kitt et al, 1986; Elsworth et al, 1987). Taylor and colleagues (1990) have shown that MPTP-exposed monkeys exhibit cognitive deficits in an object retrieval task that tests planning ability. The treated animals made an increased number of perseverative errors that might be likened to a frontal-type deficit similar to that observed in PD patients. Although the magnitude of the striatal dopamine depletion was not determined postmortem, the cognitive changes were considered to result from lesions of the dopaminergic pathway. The reduction of HVA levels in the CSF of the monkeys to 20 percent of the baseline levels give weight to this assumption.

The influence of reduced dopaminergic transmission on cognition also might be mediated by the mesocorticolimbic dopaminergic pathway. Specific lesions of this system in experimental animals produced marked behavioral disturbances (Simon and Le Moal, 1984; Iversen, 1984): hypoexploration, disruption of behavioral inhibition, and delayed alternation, indicative of frontal dysfunction. This is not surprising given the target areas of these neurons that project to cortex (mainly prefrontal) and to limbic structures, such as the amygdala, hippocampus, and septal nuclei, known to be implicated in mental processes and behavioral regulation.

In conclusion, review of experimental studies supports the hypothesis that lesions of dopaminergic neuronal pathways can be responsible for cognitive changes by affecting the function of the deafferented structures.

MPTP in Humans

MPTP intoxication produces a parkinsonian syndrome in humans, provoked by specific damage to the nigrostriatal dopaminergic pathway. Study of the neuropsychological performance of these patients has provided a privileged source of information on cognitive disorders related specifically to dysfunction of dopaminergic neurons, without contamination by the effects of cholinergic or noradrenergic lesions present in patients with idiopathic PD. Patients with MPTP-induced parkinsonism, as well as six MPTP-exposed but relatively asymptomatic individuals, were compared to drug-addict controls (Stern and Langston, 1985; Stern et al, 1990). The patients with obvious parkinsonism performed less well in some memory tasks, drawing, category naming, and the Stroop-word color test. Although the battery used in this study was not extensive, the deficits observed in the patients resembled those of patients with idio-pathic PD, characterized by memory deficits and frontal lobelike symptoms, support-ing the idea that the dopaminergic system mediates a specific set of cognitive functions. Moreover, the fact that the same pattern of cognitive impairment was found in the relatively asymptomatic individuals suggests that the changes induced by dopamine depletion can occur at an early stage of the disease, even before motor symptoms appear.

Alleviation of Cognitive Disorders with Levodopa

If the cognitive functions that deteriorate in PD are mediated by a dopaminergic mechanism, improvement with levodopa analogous to the response of dopamine-dependent motor signs might be expected.

In initial reports, the global intellectual performance of PD patients improved after levodopa treatment on the Wechsler Adult Intelligence Scale (WAIS). There was a 4.5 full-scale IQ point improvement in the study of Blonsky (1969), although no infor-mation was given about the time elapsed between tests, a 9-point improvement in the study of Beardsley and Puletti (1971) in a group of 9 patients after 6 months of treat-ment, and a 10-point or greater improvement in the study of Loranger and co-workers (1972) in half of 40 patients assessed after a 5 to 13 month period. Apparently, levo-dopa has a beneficial effect. However, several observations reported by later investi-gators limit the significance of those observations. (1) Effects were observed only dur-ing short-term treatment (Beardsley and Puletti, 1971), (2) the response could have resulted from increased motivation: "the patient feels better physically, is psycholog-ically buoyed up, and is imbued with the 'magical' properties of this 'wonder' drug" (Blonsky, 1969), (3) the improvement may be adulterated by serious side effects (Lor-anger et al, 1972), such as confusion, delirium and psychosis (Barbeau, 1969; Celesia and Barr, 1970), although mainly in already demented patients (Sacks et al, 1972), that may preclude long-term use of the drug.

Subsequent studies have confirmed these apprehensions. Several authors reported that the initial improvement in mentation was followed by a gradual decline (Botez and Barbeau, 1975; Sweet et al, 1976; Halgin et al, 1977). Furthermore, an apparent increase in the frequency of dementia in PD raised the question of whether levodopa could aggravate the mental disorders in patients. It is now well established, however, that this increase results mainly from a prolongation of the course of the disease. The initial amelioration of cognitive performance under levodopa treatment has been con-firmed to be nonspecific, probably related to an awakening (Godwin-Austen et al, 1969) or antidepressant effect (Yahr et al, 1969). Shaw and colleagues (1980) reported an improvement in mood in 50 percent of patients treated with levodopa that was sustained in only two patients.

Besides these nonspecific effects on alertness, affect, and arousal (Brown et al, 1984), is there any evidence of additional specific improvements that might validate the concept of dopamine-dependent cognitive dysfunction? Marsh and associates (1971) demonstrated an isolated improvement in verbal learning (paired associated subtest) under levodopa, suggesting a specific effect on intermediate memory. Halgin and co-workers (1977) reported an improvement of recent memory but only in a group of PD patients treated for a short period (22 months or less). Patients on long-term levodopa regimens deteriorated specifically on verbal memory tests. On the other hand, an alleviation of frontal lobe-like symptomatology was observed in PD patients taking levodopa (Morel-Maroger, 1977), which was not confirmed by subsequent studies. In the Wisconsin Card Sorting Test (WCST), levodopa significantly reduced the number of errors, but without increasing the number of concepts (Bowen et al, 1975). The authors concluded that levodopa had a nonspecific effect on attention or arousal, since reactivation of dopaminergic transmission had no effect on the patients' overall conceptual ability. More recently, Gotham and colleagues (1988) found no significant effect of levodopa on WCST performance, confirming the observation of Taylor and associates (1987) with good and poor levodopa responders.

To avoid biases related to sampling of patients and progression of the disease, recent studies have compared cognitive functions of PD patients during on periods (when motor improvement, i.e., when striatal dopaminergic transmission under levodopa, is maximal) and off periods (when motor disability, i.e., reduction of striatal dopaminergic transmission, is maximal). These studies are summarized in Table 14–2 and show no definitive or reliable evidence that replenishment of dopamine concentrations in the striatum alleviates specific cognitive disorders.

In summary, it seems that levodopa has an awakening effect on patients starting

Table 14–2. Effects of levodopa on neuropsychological performance during on and off states

Studies	Results
Specific effect	
Delis et al, 1982	Decreased delayed retention and verbal fluency in off state in a single patient
Mohr et al, 1987, 1989	Decreased delayed recall of verbal materials in off state
Gotham et al, 1988	Decreased lexical fluency and Wisconsin CST performance in off state when compared to control; no significant difference, however, in patients themselves between on and off state
Pullman et al, 1988	Increased choice RT in off state when compared to controls
Nonspecific changes	
Brown et al, 1984	Mild cognitive worsening in off periods in only a proportion of patients, related to the level of affect and arousal
Huber et al, 1987, 1989	State-dependent memory performance with no influence of the absolute level of dopamine on memory
No effect	
Rafal et al, 1984	Increased overall reaction time in off state not associated with a concomitant slowing of purely cognitive components
Girotti et al, 1986	No variation in cognitive performance observed between on and off state in 21 patients, in spite of a worsening of mood
Pillon et al, 1989a	No alleviation of cognitive slowing with levodopa in 70 patients, although a 54% improvement of the motor score between on and off states
Starkstein et al, 1989	No significant differences on reaction time and neuropsychological tasks between on and off states

therapy. This initial effect frequently is accompanied by enhanced mood or cognitive functioning (Bachman and Albert, 1984). However, these gains in mood and cognition are not sustained indefinitely, and both depression and cognitive disorders can be observed in levodopa-treated patients. The mood of levodopa-treated patients may fluctuate in the course of a single day, as do motor symptoms, suggesting a common basis for their etiology. In contrast, there is no evidence that cognitive performance fluctuates in response to levodopa in patients with on/off phenomena. This may be interpreted in two ways: (1) cognitive changes are mediated by a dopaminergic mechanism but are unresponsive to levodopa for pharmacodynamic reasons that are not understood, or (2) cognitive changes are mediated, at least in part, by lesions of nondopaminergic neuronal systems, in which case, levodopa would not be expected to be effective.

ARGUMENTS IMPLICATING LESIONS OF NONDOPAMINERGIC NEURONS IN PD COGNITIVE DISORDERS

In addition to those of the nigrostriatal and mesocorticolimbic dopaminergic systems, other neuronal lesions have been described in PD, mainly confined to subcortical nuclei in the mesencephalic and diencephalic region: nucleus basalis of Meynert, locus ceruleus, and raphe nuclei (Jellinger, 1987). The neurons in these nuclei (cholinergic, noradrenergic, and serotoninergic, respectively) project to the cerebral cortex. Each of these neuronal systems have been implicated in cognitive processing by experimental and pharmacological studies.

Lesion of Cholinergic Neurons and Cognitive Changes

Decreases in the activity of CAT—an index of cholinergic innervation—in the cerebral cortex and in the substantia innominata support the contention that the innominatocortical cholinergic system is lesioned in PD patients (Candy et al, 1983; Ruberg et al, 1982; Dubois et al, 1985a; Perry et al, 1985). This assumption is confirmed by evidence of neuronal loss in the nucleus basalis of Meynert (Arendt et al, 1983; Whitehouse et al, 1983; Gaspar and Gray, 1984; Tagliavini et al, 1984), particularly in the middle and anterior portions of the structure. Neuronal loss was found to be greater in demented (60 percent to 77 percent) than in nondemented (34 percent to 49 percent) PD patients (Jellinger, 1987), in accordance with biochemical measures in the cortical projection areas. Furthermore, CAT activity was reduced even in nondemented PD patients in the frontal, parietal, and occipital cortex and in the hippocampus, although to a lesser extent than in patients with intellectual impairment (Dubois et al, 1985a; Perry et al, 1985). Like CAT activity, acetylcholinesterase activity is decreased in both nondemented and demented PD patients, but the decrease was greater in the latter (Perry et al, 1985; Ruberg et al, 1986). The density of muscarinic cholinergic receptors was increased in some areas of the cerebral cortex of PD patients but not in the caudate nucleus (Ruberg et al, 1982; Dubois et al, 1985a). Receptor hypersensitivity resulted in part from anticholinergic therapy administered before death, in accordance with animal experiments (Westlind et al, 1981). Nevertheless, a significant increase was observed also in the frontal cortex of patients who did not receive anticholinergics, suggesting that it may reflect denervation hypersensitivity as well. It is noteworthy, however, that receptor supersensitivity is not invariably associated with a cortical cholinergic deficit, since it was not observed in patients with Alzheimer's disease (Davies and Verth, 1978; Rinne et al, 1985), who also suffer a loss of cholinergic neurons in the basal forebrain. The main features of the pathology of cholinergic systems in PD are summarized in Table 14–3.

Pharmacological, pathological, and experimental data indicate that degeneration of the ascending cholinergic systems, the major source of cortical cholinergic innervation, may have an effect on cognition. Blockade of cholinergic transmission with anticholinergic drugs consistently results in learning and memory deficits in different species. Atropine and scopolamine, muscarinic receptor antagonists, have been shown to impair discrimination learning, passive and active avoidance, alternation behavior, T-maze and radial maze performance in rodents (Whitehouse, 1964; Buresova et al, 1964; Meyers 1965; Squire, 1969; Alpern and Mariott, 1973; Eckerman et al, 1980), delayed response tasks in primates (Bartus and Johnston, 1976), and memory acquisition, storage, retrieval, and free recall in humans (Drachmann and Leavitt, 1974; Kopelman and Corn, 1988; Sunderland et al, 1988). Interestingly, blockade of cholinergic transmission by scopolamine or hyoscine in healthy young human volunteers provoked memory and cognitive deficits that resemble those associated with aging (Drachmann and Leavitt, 1974) and with dementia of the Alzheimer's disease type (Broks et al, 1988; Kopelman and Corn, 1988). Even though the cholinergic depletion could not account for the full range of cognitive deficits observed in patients with Alzheimer's disease, the results indicate that a central cholinergic mechanism is implicated in some of the symptoms of the disease. This assumption is supported by loss of cholinergic neurons in the basal forebrain that has been repeatedly reported in dementia of the Alzheimer type (review in Hardy et al, 1985). The function of these neurons in cognitive processes has been studied in animal models. Ibotenic acid injections in the nucleus basalis, which resulted in a cortical cholinergic deficiency, induced a severe behavioral syndrome consisting of impaired spatial learning (in T-maze, radial maze, Morris water maze) and avoidance learning (Flicker et al, 1983; Dubois et al, 1985b; Hepler et al, 1985; Wishaw et al, 1985).

Studies on PD patients confirm that loss of these cholinergic neurons might play a role in their cognitive disorders. First, there is a tendency for the severity of intellectual

Table 14-3. Cholinergic systems in Parkinson's Disease

Innominatocortical and septohippocampal cholinergic neurons degenerate (Arendt et al, 1983; Whitehouse et al, 1983; Perry et al, 1985)
    Degeneration is severe in demented PD patients, similar to that of Alzheimer's disease (Jellinger, 1987)
    Degeneration is observed also in nondemented PD patients, indicating that cholinergic neurons are in the process of degeneration in all patients (Dubois et al, 1983)
Other cholinergic neurons of the CNS are differentially involved
    Striatal interneurons are spared, as suggested by
        Normal CAT activity in the striatum (Mc Geer and Mc Geer, 1976; Dubois et al, 1985a)
        Normal density of immunoreactive CAT-containing neurons in caudate and putamen (Hirsch et al, 1989)
        Tegmentopedunculopontine cholinergic neuron density is decreased in some patients (Hirsch et al, 1987; Jellinger, 1988)

decline to correlate with the magnitude of the cortical cholinergic deficiency (Dubois et al, 1983, 1985a). Second, cholinergic receptor antagonists regularly induce cognitive disorders in PD patients (Stephens, 1967), particularly when they are old (Doshay, et al, 1954) or already show intellectual impairment (De Smet et al, 1982). It was particularly interesting in this respect that PD patients without any sign of intellectual or memory impairment shared a selective vulnerability to low doses of scopolamine in a double-blind crossover study with matched controls (Dubois et al, 1987). To further investigate the contribution of cholinergic denervation to cognitive disorders in PD, the neuropsychological performance of patients treated with anticholinergics was compared to that of a group of patients matched for all the variables of parkinsonism, but who received no anticholinergic drugs (Dubois et al, 1990a). At the dose used, the performance of the two groups differed only on the frontal lobe tests, suggesting that the central cholinergic deficit demonstrated postmortem in PD may be implicated in the subcorticofrontal behavioral impairment characteristic of the disease.

LESION OF NORADRENERGIC AND SEROTONINERGIC SYSTEMS AND COGNITION

The noradrenergic and serotoninergic systems are of particular importance to cognition. The central noradrenergic pathways are not affected uniformly in PD, but the dorsal noradrenergic bundle that originates in the locus ceruleus is severely damaged. Both neuronal loss and noradrenaline depletion in the locus ceruleus were significantly more severe in demented patients (Mann et al, 1983b; Cash et al, 1987). Noradrenaline concentrations also were reduced in the neocortex and in limbic structures, such as the nucleus accumbens, amygdala, and hippocampus (Scatton et al, 1983), although in these structures, no difference between demented and nondemented PD patients could be detected. Neuronal damage in the locus ceruleus was accompanied by an increase in the number of beta$_1$ receptors and a decrease in the number of alpha$_2$ receptors in the frontal cortex of demented subjects. The activity of dopamine beta-hydroxylase (DBH), the enzyme catalyzing the synthesis of noradrenaline, was found to be unchanged in the frontal cortex. A similar dissociation between noradrenergic cell loss in the locus ceruleus and DBH activity in the cerebral cortex has been observed in Alzheimer's disease (Perry et al, 1981).

Degeneration of noradrenergic ceruleocortical neurons may contribute to cognitive changes in PD. Lesions of the locus ceruleus in animals have been reported to reduce selective attention, impairing learning, and memory (Iversen, 1984; Ogren et al, 1984). In Alzheimer's disease, noradrenergic markers were found to be decreased in the cortex and in the locus ceruleus, where severe neuronal loss has been demonstrated (review in Hardy et al, 1985). In PD, neuronal loss and a reduction in noradrenergic levels in the locus ceruleus were reported to be greater in demented than nondemented patients (Cash et al, 1987). MHPG levels in the CSF of PD patients were correlated with a measure of general intellectual ability and with performance on reaction time and attentional tasks (Stern et al, 1984). There are, however, no data from pharmacological studies using noradrenergic agonists or antagonists to support the hypothesis that altered noradrenergic transmission is implicated in the intellectual dysfunction of PD patients. In contrast, a role in the depression observed in PD patients is better substantiated. In accordance with the noradrenergic hypothesis of depression (Van Praag, 1982), tricyclic antidepressants that are potent noradrenaline uptake blockers have been shown to be efficacious in depressed PD patients (Strang, 1976).

The same analysis can be made for the ascending serotoninergic neurons. These neurons are partially destroyed in PD, judging from neuronal loss in the raphe nuclei and decreased serotonin concentrations in the striatopallidal complex and in certain cortical areas (Scatton et al, 1983). The decrease was greatest in the hippocampus and frontal cortex. No difference between demented and nondemented patients was observed. Serotonin receptors do not seem markedly affected in the cerebral cortex, as the density of 5HT1 and 5HT2 receptors was not modified (Perry et al, 1984).

The central serotoninergic deficiency may be implicated in cognitive processes. Serotoninergic systems have been shown to influence learning behavior in animals (Green and Heal, 1985). Similar decreases in cortical and hippocampal serotonin and 5-HIAA concentrations have been observed in patients with Alzheimer's disease (review in Hardy et al, 1985). It seems, however, that, like the noradrenergic deficiency, the serotoninergic deficit is more likely to be implicated in depressive states in PD patients: 5-HIAA concentrations in the CSF are lower in depressed PD patients than in the others (Mayeux et al, 1984), and imipramine-like drugs, which are inhibitors of serotonin uptake, have significant antidepressant activity in PD patients.

In addition to massive involvement of the nigrostriatal dopaminergic pathway and partial degeneration of the long ascending subcorticocortical systems, dysfunction of other neuronal circuitry also may be implicated directly or indirectly in the genesis of cognitive symptomatology in PD. Examples include loss of neurons both in the basal ganglia, as suggested by the dysfunction of various peptidergic and amino acid-containing neurons (review in Agid et al, 1989) and in the brainstem, where cell loss in the pedonculopontine tegmental nucleus has been found in some patients (Hirsch et al, 1987; Jellinger, 1988). Alterations of neurons in the cerebral cortex—i.e., diffuse Lewy body inclusions and Alzheimer's disease-like histological changes—probably occur in a sizable number of cases, suggesting that intrinsic cortical pathology may account for some of the cognitive disorders in demented patients. The identity of the affected cortical neurons is not well known. The best-documented deficit concerns somatostatin-containing neurons. Somatostatin concentrations are decreased in some regions of the cerebral cortex of severely demented PD patients (Epelbaum et al, 1983) as well as in patients with Alzheimer's disease (review in Hardy et al, 1985). The role of the somatostatin-containing neurons is unknown, although the distribution of their processes suggests that they ensure communication between different regions of the cortex. Furthermore, there may be a relationship between somatostatin-containing and CAT-containing structures in the human cerebral cortex, since they have similar distributions, and reciprocal regulations of acetylcholine and somatostatin release have been reported (Nemeth and Cooper, 1979).

TENTATIVE SYNTHESIS

It is hazardous to attempt a theory of the neuronal basis of cognitive disorders in the absence of prospective anatomoclinical studies. The main problem is to distinguish the roles of dopaminergic and nondopaminergic brain lesions. The dopamine hypothesis is certainly attractive because it takes into account the most severe lesion reported in the disease. Indeed, dopamine depletion, which is the first biochemical deficiency to appear, probably plays a primary role in the genesis of the frontal lobe dysfunction observed in the early stages of the disease. Impaired performance on the Wisconsin Card Sort, Stroop, and Trail-Making tests have been reported in the beginning of the disease, even in untreated de novo patients (Lees and Smith, 1983; Hietanen and Teravainen, 1986), that is, in patients with isolated lesions of the nigrostriatal dopaminergic pathway. This assumption is consistent with the presence of frontal lobe-like cognitive disorders in MPTP-induced parkinsonism.

What is the anatomical substrate for the dopamine theory? Recent anatomical data provide a coherent description of the interaction between dopaminergic innervation of the striatum and frontal lobe. The striatum, particularly the caudate nucleus, and various associative areas of the frontal cortex are linked by at least two parallel and independent neuronal circuits (Alexander et al, 1986) distinguished by their origin in distinct regions of the frontal cortex, the dorsolateral prefrontal and lateral orbifrontal circuits. The circuits have yet to be fully characterized from a functional standpoint, but their projection sites suggest that they participate in cognitive processes. Experimental studies in animals support this hypothesis. Striatal lesions cause disturbances resembling those observed after damage to the frontal lobes (review in Divac and Oberg, 1979). Furthermore, lesion studies show functional specialization within the striatum consistent with this anatomical evidence for independent neuronal circuits. Interestingly, all these circuits are dependent on a dopaminergic mechanism via the nigrostriatal or the mesocorticolimbic dopaminergic neurons. Disruption of caudate outflow (resulting from involvement of the nigrostriatal dopaminergic system) would be expected to alter the functioning of these circuits, as would depletion of dopamine (resulting from involvement of the mesocorticolimbic dopaminergic system) within the frontal cortex or limbic structures.

In conclusion, it may be postulated that striatal dopaminergic depletion plays a role in the frontal lobe-like syndrome observed in early stages of the disease. The lack of a reliable correlation with motor symptoms may result from the fact that the dopamine depletion in the caudate is not as great as in the putamen, as shown in vivo by PET (Nahmias et al, 1985).

During the course of the disease, patients become increasingly handicapped as motor symptoms unresponsive to levodopa—gait disorders or dysarthria—appear and cognitive disorders worsen. All these symptoms may correspond to the development of nondopaminergic lesions, notably of the ascending cholinergic, noradrenergic, and serotoninergic ascending systems. The respective role of each of these additional pathological alterations remains, however, difficult to establish. These systems are thought to regulate cell activity in regions of projection involved in specific functions, rather than transmitting specific information themselves. Furthermore, they do not act separately but contribute in parallel or by mutual interaction to the expression of integrated behaviors. On the other hand, each of the cognitive syndromes commonly found in PD (namely, changes in linguistic, visuospatial, mnesic, and executive abilities, as well as bradyphrenia) involves a variety of overlapping processes that depend on the distribution of the lesions, their severity, and the order of their appearance in the course of the disease. Despite these precautions, one is tempted to propose that cholinergic lesions, which denervate the hippocampus and cerebral cortex, affect memory function, attention, and frontal lobe activity (Dubois et al, 1990a) and that the noradrenergic lesion of the locus ceruleus may contribute to attentional disorders and, together with serotoninergic dysfunction, to depressive mood.

If, as the evidence suggests, cognitive disorders in PD result mainly from lesions of subcortical origin, cognitive programs intrinsic to the cortex are not necessarily damaged but rather deactivated. Deactivation may occur beyond a certain threshold of denervation when a single neuronal system is involved or when more than one system is damaged (Terry et al, 1978). For example, it has been shown that degeneration of cholinergic neurons, which is severe in mentally impaired patients, is present in all patients even in the absence of intellectual and memory disorders. This suggests that there are two phases in the degeneration of cholinergic input to the cerebral cortex: a moderate and asymptomatic phase and a second period where neuronal loss becomes sufficient for memory disorders to appear. Intellectual impairment will occur when synaptic adjustments (hyperactivity of the remaining neurons or supersensitivity of muscarinic receptors) are no longer sufficient to compensate for neuronal loss. At this point, inappropriate administration of anticholinergic drugs can provoke confusional states (De Smet et al, 1982).

Alternatively, deactivation may occur only when destruction of several ascending neuronal pathways reaches the necessary threshold. This has been demonstrated in experimental studies. Simultaneous disruption of the nigrostriatal and mesocortico-limbic dopaminergic systems causes marked impairment of the conditioned avoidance response in rats, whereas selective disruption of one or the other of these systems has no effect (Koob et al, 1984). Destruction of the ascending cholinergic system increases the behavioral consequences of damage to serotoninergic neurons (Nilsson et al, 1988). If these results can be transposed to humans, they suggest that disorders of cognition mediated by ascending subcorticocortical systems may be observed in PD, either when there is sufficient partial destruction of several ascending neuronal pathways, or when there is a severe and selective lesion of one of them (Dubois et al, 1991).

Age of onset of the disease may influence the threshold at which neuronal lesions become symptomatic. The compounding effect of aging on cognitive disturbances has been demonstrated by comparing the neuropsychological performance of early-onset and late-onset PD patients to age-matched controls (Dubois et al, 1990b), suggesting that additional age-related brain lesions may adversely affect compensatory mechanisms, revealing underlying neuronal degeneration associated with PD. This could explain the high frequency of dementia in older PD patients.

In a small number of patients, dementia defined according to DSM-III criteria is observed. In these cases, neuronal loss or Alzheimer's disease-like histological changes in the cerebral cortex may play a crucial role in the intellectual deterioration, in addition to subcortical lesions. The role of cortical lesions in PD is not, however, clearly established. Furthermore, some cases of this type of dementia have been reported in the absence of apparent cortical lesions (Dubois et al, 1985a; Perry et al, 1985), suggesting that subcortical lesions may be sufficiently severe to cause overt dementia, at least in some patients. Conversely, Alzheimer's disease-like changes have been observed in the cortex of PD patients without evidence of dementia.

The foregoing hypotheses based on clinical, pathological, and experimental observations are certainly oversimplifications. Nevertheless, they may have the merit of stimulating further experiments, particularly longitudinal studies aimed at establishing objective correlates of the clinical observations.

ACKNOWLEDGMENTS

The authors wish to express their gratitude to Merle Ruberg and Yves Agid for helpful discussion and comments and for their correction of the manuscript.

REFERENCES

Agid Y, Cervera P, Hirsch EC, et al. Biochemistry of Parkinson's disease 28 years later: a critical review. *Mov Disord.* 1989;4(Suppl 1):126–144.

Agid Y, Javoy-Agid F, Ruberg M. Biochemistry of neurotransmitters in Parkinson's disease. In: Marsden CD, Fahn S, eds. *Movement Disorders 2. Neurology,* vol 7. London: Butterworths; 1987:166–230.

Agid Y, Ruberg M, Dubois B, Javoy-Agid F. Biochemical substrates of mental disturbances in Parkinson's disease. In: Hassler RG, Christ JF, eds. *Advances in Neurology,* vol 40. New York: Raven Press; 1984:211–218.

Alexander GE, De Long MR, Strick PL. Parallel organization of functionally segregated circuits linking basal ganglia and cortex. *Annu Rev Neurosci.* 1986;9:357–381.

Alpern HP, Marriott JG. Short-term memory: facilitation and disruption with anticholinergic agents. *Physiol Behav.* 1973;11:571–575.

Alvord EC, Forno LS, Kusske JA, et al. The pathology of parkinsonism: a comparison of degeneration in cerebral cortex and brainstem. In: McDowell F, Barbeau A, eds. *Advances in Neurology,* vol 5. New York: Raven Press; 1974:175–193.

Annett LE, Rogers DC, Dunnett B. Unilateral 6-OHDA lesions in marmosets: a primate model for neural transplantation in Parkinson's disease. In: Franks AJ, Ironside JW, Mindham RHS, et al, eds. *Studies in Neuroscience—Function and dysfunction in the basal ganglia.* Manchester: University Press; 1990;9:181–197.

Arendt T, Bigl V, Arendt A, Tennestedt A. Loss of neurons in the nucleus basalis of Meynert in Alzheimer's disease, paralysis agitans and Korsakoff's disease. *Acta Neuropathol.* 1983;61:101–108.

Bachman DL, Albert ML. The dopaminergic syndromes of dementia. In: Pilleri G, Tagliavini F, eds. *Brain pathology,* vol I. Bern: Brain Anatomy Institute Ostermundigen; 1984:91–119.

Ball MJ. The morphological basis of dementia in Parkinson's disease. *Can J Neurol Sci.* 1984;11:180–184.

Barbeau A. L-Dopa therapy in Parkinson's disease: a critical review of nine year's experience. *Can Med Assoc J.* 1969;101:799–800.

Bartus RT, Johnston HR. Short-term memory in the rhesus monkey: disruption from the anticholinergic scopolamine. *Pharmacol Biochem Behav.* 1976;5:39–46.

Beardsley J, Puletti F. Personality (MMPI) and cognitive (WAIS) changes after levodopa treatment. *Arch Neurol.* 1971;25:145–150.

Bentin S, Silverberg R, Gordon HW. Asymmetrical cognitive deterioration in demented and Parkinson patients. *Cortex.* 1981;17:533–544.

Bernheimer H, Birkmayer W, Hornykiewicz O, et al. Brain dopamine and the syndromes of Parkinson and Huntington. *J Neurol Sci.* 1973;20:415–455.

Blonsky ER. *Proceedings of the Second Annual Symposium.* Chicago: The United Parkinson's Foundation; 1969:10–19.

Boller F, Mizutani T, Roessmann U, et al. Parkinson disease, dementia and Alzheimer disease: clinicopatholical correlations. *Ann Neurol.* 1980;7:329–335.

Boller F, Passafiume D, Keefe NC, et al. Visuospatial impairments in Parkinson's disease. *Arch Neurol.* 1984;41:485–490.

Botez MI, Barbeau A. Neuropsychological findings in Parkinson's disease: a comparison between various tests during long-term L-dopa therapy. *Int J Neurol.* 1975;10:222–232.

Bowen FP, Kamienny RS, Burns MM, et al. Parkinsonism: effects of levodopa on concept formation. *Neurology.* 1975;25:701–704.

Broks P, Preston GC, Traub M, et al. Modelling dementia: effects of scopolamine on memory and attention. *Neuropsychologia.* 1988;26,5:685–700.

Brown RG, Marsden CD, Quinn N, et al. Aterations in cognitive performance and affect arousal state during fluctuations in motor function in Parkinson's disease. *J Neurol Neurosurg Psychiatry.* 1984;47:454–465.

Buresova O, Bures J, Bohdanecky Z, Weiss T. Effect of atropine on learning, extinction, retention and retrieval in rats. *Psychopharmacologia.* 1964;5:255–263.

Candy JM, Perry RH, Perry EK, et al. Pathological changes in the nucleus of Meynert in Alzheimer's and Parkinson's diseases. *J Neurol Sci.* 1983;54:277–289.

Cash R, Dennis T, Lheureux R, et al. Parkinson's disease and dementia: norepinephrine and dopamine in locus coeruleus. *Neurology.* 1987;37:42–46.

Celesia GG, Barr AN. Psychosis and other psychiatric manifestations of levodopa therapy. *Arch Neurol.* 1970;23:193–200.

Celesia GG, Wanamaker WM. Psychiatric disturbances in Parkinson's disease. *Dis Nerv Syst.* 1972;33:577–583.

Cotzias GC, Papavasiliou PS, Gellene R. Modification of parkinsonism: chronic treatment with L-dopa. *N Engl J Med.* 1969;280:337–345.

Davies P, Verth AH. Regional distribution of muscarinic acetylcholine receptor in normal and Alzheimer's type dementia brains. *Brain Res.* 1978;138:385–392.

De la Monte SM, Wells SE, Hedley-White T, Growdon JH. Neuropathological distinction between Parkinson's dementia and Parkinson's plus Alzheimer's disease. *Ann Neurol.* 1989;26:309–320.

Delis D, Direnfeld L, Alexander MP, Kaplan E. Cognitive fluctuations associated with on-off phenomenon in Parkinson's disease. *Neurology.* 1982;32:1049–1052.

De Smet Y, Ruberg M, Serdaru M, et al. Confusion, dementia and anticholinergics in Parkinson's disease. *J Neurol Neurosurg Psychiatry.* 1982;45:1161–1164.

Direnfeld LK, Albert ML, Volicer L, et al. Parkinson's disease: the possible relationship of laterality to dementia and neurochemical findings. *Arch Neurol.* 1984;41:935–941.

Divac I, Oberg RG. *The Neostriatum.* Oxford: Pergamon Press; 1979:323 pp.

Doshay LJ, Constable K, Zeir A. Five year follow-up of treatment with trihexyphenidyl (Artane). *JAMA.* 1954:1334–1336.

Drachman DA, Leavitt J. Human memory and the cholinergic system. *Arch Neurol.* 1974;30:113–121.

Dubois B, Boller F, Pillon B, Agid Y. Cognitive deficits in Parkinson's disease. In: Boller F, Grafman J, eds. *Handbook of Neuropsychology,* vol 5. Amsterdam: Elsevier; 1991:195–240.

Dubois B, Danzé F, Pillon B, et al. Cholinergic-dependent cognitive deficits in Parkinson's disease. *Ann Neurol.* 1987;22:26–30.

Dubois B, Hauw JJ, Ruberg M, et al. Démence et maladie de Parkinson: corrélations biochimiques et anatomo-cliniques. *Rev Neurol.* 1985a;141:184–193.

Dubois B, Mayo W, Agid Y, et al. Profound disturbances of spontaneous and learned behaviors following lesions of the nucleus basalis magnocellularis in the rat. *Brain Res.* 1985b;338:249–258.

Dubois B, Pillon B, Lhermitte F, Agid Y. Cholinergic deficiency and frontal dysfunction in Parkinson's disease. *Ann Neurol.* 1990a;28:117–121.

Dubois B, Pillon B, Sternic N, et al. Age-induced cognitive disturbances in Parkinson's disease. *Neurology.* 1990b;40:38–41.

Dubois B, Ruberg M, Javoy-Agid F, et al. A subcortico-cortical cholinergic system is affected in Parkinson's disease. *Brain Res.* 1983;288:213–218.

Eckerman DA, Winford AG, Edwards JD, et al. Effects of scopolamine, pentobarbital and amphetamine on radial arm maze performance in the rat. *Pharmacol Biochem Behav.* 1980;12:595–602.

Elizan TS, Sroka H, Maker H, et al. Dementia in idiopathic Parkinson's disease. Variables associated with its occurrence in 203 patients. *J Neural Transm.* 1986;65:285–302.

Elsworth JD, Deutch AY, Redmond DE Jr, et al. Differential responsiveness to 1-methyl-4-phenyl-1,2,3,6-tetrahydropyridine toxicity in subregions of the primate substantia nigra and striatum. *Life Sci.* 1987;40:193–202.

Epelbaum J, Ruberg M, Moyse E, et al. Somatostatin and dementia in Parkinson's disease. *Brain Res.* 1983;278:376–379.

Fahn S, Libsch LR, Cutler RW. Monoamines in the human neostriatum: topographic distribution in normals and in Parkinson's disease and their role in akinesia, rigidity, chorea and tremor. *J Neurol Sci.* 1971;14:427–455.

Farley IJ, Price KS, Hornykiewicz O. Dopamine in the limbic regions of the human brain: normal and abnormal. *Adv Biochem Psychopharmacol.* 1977;16:57–64.

Fibiger HC, Phillips AG, Zis AP. Deficits in instrumental responding after 6-hydroxydopamine lesions of the nigro-neostriatal dopaminergic projection. *Pharmacol Biochem Behav.* 1974;2,1:87–96.

Flicker C, Dean RC, Watkins DL, et al. Behavioral and neurochemical effects following neurotoxic lesions of a major cholinergic input to the neocortex in the rat. *Pharmacol Biochem Behav.* 1983;18:973–981.

Garnett ES, Nahmias C, Firnau G. Central dopaminergic pathways in hemiparkinsonism examined by positron emission tomography. *Can J Neurol Sci.* 1984;11:174–179.

Garron DC, Klawans HL, Narin F. Intellectual functioning of persons with idiopathic parkinsonism. *J Nerv Ment Dis.* 1972;154:445–452.

Gaspar P, Gray F. Dementia in idiopathic Parkinson's disease: a neuropathological study on 32 cases. *Acta Neuropathol.* 1984;64:43–53.

Girotti F, Carella F, Grassi MP, et al. Motor and cognitive performances of Parkinsonian patients in the on and off phases of the disease. *J Neurol Neurosurg Psychiatry.* 1986;49:657–660.

Godwin-Austen RB, Tomlinson EB, Frears CC, Kok HWL. Effects of L-dopa in Parkinson's disease. *Lancet.* 1969;2:165–168.

Gotham AM, Brown RG, Marsden CD. "Frontal" function and levodopa in Parkinson's disease, "on" and "off" levodopa. *Brain.* 1988;111:299–321.

Granerus AK, Carlsson A, Svanbord A. The aging neuron—influence on symptomatology and therapeutic response in Parkinson's disease. In: Poirier LJ, Sourkas PL, Bédard PJ, eds. *Advances in Neurology,* vol 24. New York: Raven Press; 1979:327–334.

Green AR, Heal DJ. The effects of drugs on serotonin-mediated behavioural model. In: Green AR, ed. *Neuropharmacology of Serotonin.* Oxford: Oxford University Press; 1985:326–365.

Growdon JH, Corkin S, Rosen JT. Distinctive aspects of cognitive dysfunction in Parkinson's disease. In: Streifler AM, Korczyn AM, Melamed E, Youdim MBH, eds. *Advances in Neurology,* vol 53. New York: Raven Press; 1990:365–376.

Hakim AM, Mathieson G. Dementia in Parkinson disease: a neuropathologic study. *Neurology.* 1979;29:1209–1214.

Halgin R, Riklan M, Mishiak H. Levodopa, parkinsonism and recent memory. *J Nerv Ment Dis.* 1977;164:268–272.

Hardy J, Adolfsson R, Alafuzoff I, et al. Transmitter deficits in Alzheimer's disease. *Neurochem Int.* 1985;7:545–563.

Hepler DJ, Wenk GJ, Cribbs BJ, et al. Memory impairments following basal forebrain lesions. *Brain Res.* 1985;346:8–14.

Hietanen M, Teravainen H. Cognitive performance in early Parkinson's disease. *Acta Neurol Scand.* 1986;73:151–159.

Hirsch EC, Graybiel AM, Duyckaerts C, Javoy-Agid F. Neuronal loss in the pedunculopontine tegmental nucleus in Parkinson's disease and in progressive supranuclear palsy. *Proc Natl Acad Sci USA.* 1987;84:5976–5980.

Hirsch EC, Graybiel AM, Hersh LB, et al. Striosomes and extrastriosomal matrix contain different amounts of immunoreactive-choline acetyltransferase in the human striatum. *Neurosci Lett.* 1989;96:145–150.

Hoehn MM, Yahr MD. Parkinsonism: onset, progression and mortality. *Neurology.* 1967;17:427–442.

Hornykiewicz O. Parkinson's disease and its chemotherapy. *Biochem Pharmacol.* 1975;24:1061–1065.

Huber SJ, Freidenberg DL, Shuttleworth EC, et al. Neuropsychological similarities in lateralized parkinsonism. *Cortex.* 1989;25:461–470.

Huber SJ, Shulman HG, Paulson GW, Shuttleworth EC. Fluctuations in plasma dopamine level impair memory in Parkinson's disease. *Neurology.* 1987;37:1371–1375.

Huber SJ, Shulman HG, Paulson GW, Shuttleworth EL. Dose dependent memory impairment in Parkinson's disease. *Neurology.* 1989;39:438–440.

Iversen S. Cortical monoamines and behavior. In: Descarries L, Reader TA, Jasper HH, eds. *Monoamine Innervation of Cerebral Cortex.* New York: Alan R Liss; 1984:321–349.

Javoy-Agid F, Agid Y. Is the mesocortical dopaminergic system involved in Parkinson's disease? *Neurology.* 1980;30:1326–1330.

Javoy-Agid F, Ruberg M, Taquet H, et al. Biochemical neuroanatomy of the human substantia nigra (pars compacta) in normal and parkinsonian subjects. In: Friedhoff AJ, Chase TN, eds. *Gilles de la Tourette Syndrome.* New York: Raven Press; 1982:151–163.

Jellinger K. The pathology of parkinsonism. In: Marsden CD, Fahn S, eds. *Movement Disorders 2. Neurology,* vol 7. London: Butterworths; 1987:124–165.

Jellinger K. The pedunculopontine nucleus in Parkinson's disease, progressive supranuclear palsy and Alzheimer's disease. *J Neurol Neurosurg Psychiatry.* 1988;51:540–543.

Kitt CA, Cork LC, Eidelberg F, et al. Injury of nigral neurons exposed to 1-methyl-4-phenyl-1,2,3,6-tetrahydropyridine: a tyrosine hydroxylase immunocytochemical study in monkey. *Neuroscience.* 1986;17:1089–1103.

Koob GF, Simon H, Herman JP, Le Moal M. Neuroleptic-like disruption of the conditioned avoidance response requires destruction of both the mesolimbic and nigrostriatal dopamine systems. *Brain Res.* 1984;303:319–329.

Kopelman MD, Corn TH. Cholinergic "blockade" as a model for cholinergic depletion. *Brain.* 1988;111:1079–1110.

Langston JW, Ballard P, Tetrud JW, Irwin I. Chronic parkinsonism in humans due to a product of mepedrine analogue synthesis. *Science.* 1983;219:979–980.

Lees AJ, Smith E. Cognitive deficits in the early stages of Parkinson's disease. *Brain.* 1983;106:257–270.

Loranger AW, Goodell H, Lee JE, McDowell F. Levodopa treatment of Parkinson's syndrome. Improved intellectual functioning. *Arch Gen Psychiatry.* 1972;26:163–168.

Mann DMA, Yates PO. Pathological basis for neurotransmitter changes in Parkinson's disease. *Neuropathol Appl Neurobiol.* 1983a;9:3–19.

Mann DMA, Yates PO, Hawkes J. The pathology of the human locus coeruleus. *Clin Neuropathol.* 1983b;2:1–7.

Marsden CD. The mysterious motor function of the basal ganglia: the Robert Wartenberg lecture. *Neurology.* 1982;32:514–539.

Marsh GG, Markham CM, Ansel R. Levodopa's awakening effect on patients with parkinsonism. *J Neurol Neurosurg Psychiatry.* 1971;34:209–218.

Marshall JP, Richardson JS, Teitelbaum P. Nigrostriatal bundle damage and the lateral hypothalamic syndrome. *J Comp Physiol Psychol.* 1974;87:808–830.

Martilla RJ, Rinne UK. Dementia in Parkinson's disease. *Acta Neurol Scand.* 1976;54:431–441.

Mayeux R, Stern Y, Cote L, Williams JBW. Altered serotonin metabolism in depressed patients with Parkinson's disease. *Neurology.* 1984;34:642–646.

Mayeux R, Stern Y, Williams JBW, et al. Clinical and biochemical features of depression in Parkinson's disease. *Am J Psychiatry.* 1985;143:756–759.

McGeer PL, McGeer EG. Enzymes associated with the metabolism of catecholamines, acetylcholine and GABA in human controls and patients with Parkinson's disease and Huntington's chorea. *J Neurochem.* 1976;26:65–76.

Meyers B. Some effects of scopolamine on a passive avoidance response in rats. *Psychopharmacologia.* 1965;8:111–119.

Mohr E, Fabbrini G, Ruggieri S, et al. Cognitive concomitants of dopamine system stimulation in Parkinsonians patients. *J Neurol Neurosurg Psychiatry.* 1987;50:1192–1196.

Mohr E, Fabbrini G, Williams J, et al. Dopamine and memory function in Parkinson's disease. *Movement Disorders.* 1989;4:113–120.

Morel-Maroger A. Effects of levodopa on "frontal" signs in parkinsonism. *Br Med J.* 1977;2:1543–1544.

Mortimer JA, Pirozzolo FJ, Hansch EC, Webster DD. Relationship of motor symptoms to intellectual deficits in Parkinson's disease. *Neurology.* 1982;32:133–137.

Nahmias C, Garnett ES, Firnav G, Lang A. Striatal dopamine distribution in parkinsonian patients during life. *J Neurol Sci.* 1985;69:223–230.

Nemeth EF, Cooper JR. Effect of somatostatin on acetylcholine release from rat hippocampal synaptosomes. *Brain Res.* 1979;165:166–170.

Nilsson OE, Strecker RE, Daszuta A, Bjorklund A. Combined cholinergic and serotoninergic denervation of the forebrain produces severe deficits in a special learning task in the rat. *Brain Res.* 1988;453:235–246.

Nyberg P, Nordberg A, Webster P, Winblad B. Dopaminergic deficiency is more pronounced in putamen than in nucleus caudatus in Parkinson's disease. *Neurochem Pathol.* 1983;1:193–202.

Ogren SO, Archer T, Ross CB. Norepinephrine in learning and memory—the status of cognitive deficit. In: Usdin E, Carlsson A, Dahlstrom A, Engel J, eds. *Catecholamines: Neuropharmacology and Central Nervous System—Theoretical Aspects.* New York: Alan R Liss; 1984:285–292.

Perry EK, Tomlinson BE, Blessed G, et al. Neuropathological and biochemical observations on the noradrenergic system in Alzheimer's disease. *J Neurol Sci.* 1981;51:279–287.

Perry EK, Perry RH, Candy JM, et al. Cortical serotonin-S2 receptor binding abnormalities in Alzheimer's disease—comparison with Parkinson's disease. *Neurosci Lett.* 1984;51:353–357.

Perry EK, Curtis M, Dick DJ, et al. Cholinergic correlates of cognitive impairment in Parkinson's disease: comparisons with Alzheimer's disease. *J Neurol Neurosurg Psychiatry.* 1985;48:413–421.

Pillon B, Dubois B, Bonnet AM, et al. Cognitive "slowing" in Parkinson's disease fails to respond to levodopa treatment: the "fifteen objects test." *Neurology.* 1989a;39:762–768.

Pillon B, Dubois B, Cusimano G, et al. Does cognitive impairment in Parkinson's disease result from non-dopaminergic lesions? *J Neurol Neurosurg Psychiatry.* 1989b;52:201–206.

Ploska A, Taquet H, Javoy-Agid F, et al. Dopamine and methionine-enkephalin in human brain. *Neurosci Lett.* 1982;33:191–196.

Portin R, Rinne UK. Predictive factors for dementia in Parkinson's disease. *Acta Neurol Scand.* 1984;69 (suppl 98):57–58.

Pullman SL, Watts RL, Juncos JL, et al. Dopaminergic effects on simple and choice reaction time performance in Parkinson's disease. *Neurology.* 1988;38:249–254.

Quinn N, Critchley P, Marsden CD. Young onset Parkinson's disease. *Movement Disord.* 1987;2:73–91.

Rafal RD, Posner MI, Walker JA, Friedrich FJ. Cognition and the basal ganglia: separating mental and motor components of performance in Parkinson's disease. *Brain.* 1984;107:1083–1094.

Riederer P, Wuketich S. Time course of nigrostriatal degeneration in Parkinson's disease. *J Neural Transm.* 1976;38:277–301.

Riklan M, Stellar S, Reynolds C. The relationship of memory and cognition in Parkinson's disease to lateralisation of motor symptoms. *J Neurol Neurosurg Psychiatry.* 1990;53:359–360.

Rinne JO, Rummukainen J, Paljärui L, Rinne UK. Dementia in Parkinson's disease is related to neuronal loss in the medial substantia nigra. *Ann Neurol.* 1989;26:47–50.

Rinne JO, Laakso K, Lönnberg P, et al. Brain muscarinic receptors in senile dementia. *Brain Res.* 1985;336:19–25.

Rinne UK, Sonninen V, Laaksonen H. Responses of brain neurochemistry to levodopa treatment in Parkinson's disease. In: Poirier LJ, Sourkes TL, Bédard PJ, eds. *Advances in Neurology.* New York: Raven Press; 1979;24:259–274.

Ruberg M, Agid Y. Dementia in Parkinson's disease. In: Iversen L, Iversen SD, Snyder SH, eds. *Psychopharmacology of Aging Nervous System—Handbook of Psychopharmacology,* vol 20. New York: Plenum Press; 1988:157–205.

Ruberg M, Ploska A, Javoy-Agid F, Agid Y. Muscarinic binding and choline acetyltransferase in parkinsonian subjects with reference to dementia. *Brain Res.* 1982;232:129–139.

Ruberg M, Rieger F, Villageois A, et al. Acetylcholinesterase and butylcholinesterase in frontal cortex and cerebrospinal fluid of demented and non-demented patients with Parkinson's disease. *Brain Res.* 1986;362:83–91.

Sacks OW, Kohl MS, Messeloff CR, et al. Effects of levodopa in parkinsonian patients with dementia. *Neurology.* 1972;22:516–519.

Scatton B, Javoy-Agid F, Rouquier L, et al. Reduction of cortical dopamine, noradrenaline, serotonin and their metabolites in Parkinson's disease. *Brain Res.* 1983;275:321–328.

Shaw KM, Lees AJ, Stern GM. The impact of treatment with levodopa on Parkinson's disease. *Q J Med.* 1980;49:283–293.

Simon H, Le Moal M. Mesencephalic dopaminergic neurons: functional role. In: Usdin E, Carlsson A, Dahlstrom A, Engel J, eds. *Catecholamines: Neuropharmacology and Central Nervous System—Theoretical Aspects.* New York: Alan R Liss; 1984:293–308.

Spicer KB, Robert RJ, Le Witt PA. Neuropsychological performance in lateralized parkinsonism. *Arch Neurol.* 1988;45:429–432.

Squire LR. Effects of pretrial and postrial administration of cholinergic and anticholinergic drugs on spontaneous alternation. *J Comp Physiol Psychol.* 1969;69:69–75.

Starkstein SE, Esteguy M, Berthier ML, et al. Evoked potentials reaction time and cognitive performance in on and off phases of Parkinson's disease. *J Neurol Neurosurg Psychiatry.* 1989;52:338–340.

Starkstein S, Leiguarda R, Gershanik O, Berthier M. Neuropsychological disturbances in hemiparkinson's disease. *Neurology.* 1987;37:1762–1764.

Stephens DA. Psychotoxic effects of benzhexol hydrochloride (Artane). *Br J Psychiatry.* 1967;113:213–218.

Stern Y, Langston JW. Intellectual changes in patients with MPTP-induced parkinsonism. *Neurology.* 1985;35:1506–1509.

Stern Y, Mayeux R, Cote L. Reaction time and vigilance in Parkinson's disease: possible role of norepinephrine metabolism. *Arch Neurol.* 1984;41:1086–1089.

Stern Y, Tetrud JW, Martin WR, et al. Cognitive changes following MPTP exposure. *Neurology.* 1990;40:261–264.

Strang RR. Imipramine in treatment of parkinsonism: a double-blind placebo study. *Br Med J.* 1976;2:33–34.

Sunderland R, Tariot P, Newhouse P. Differential responsivity of mood, behavior, and cognition to cholinergic agents in elderly neuropsychiatric population. *Br Res Rev.* 1988;13:371–389.

Sweet RD, McDowell FH, Feigenson JS, et al. Mental symptoms in Parkinson's disease during chronic treatment with levodopa. *Neurology.* 1976;26:305–310.

Tagliavini F, Pilleri G, Bouras G, Constantidinis J. The basal nucleus of Meynert in idiopathic Parkinson's disease. *Acta Neurol Scand.* 1984;69:20–28.

Taylor JR, Elsworth JD, Roth RH, et al. Cognitive and motor deficits in the acquisition of an object retrieval/detour task in MPTP-treated monkeys. *Brain.* 1990;113:617–637.

Taylor AE, Saint-Cyr JA, Lang AE. Parkinson's disease: cognitive changes in relation to treatment response. *Brain.* 1987;110:35–51.

Terry RD. Aging, senile dementia and Alzheimer's disease. In: Katzman R, Terry RD, Bick KL, eds. *Alzheimer's Disease: Senile Dementia and Related Disorders.* New York: Raven Press; 1978.

Van Praag HM. Depression. *Lancet.* 1982;2:1259–1264.

Westlind A, Grynfarb M, Hedlund B, et al. Muscarinic supersensitivity induced by septal lesion or chronic atropine treatment. *Brain Res.* 1981;225:131–141.

Whitehouse JM. Effects of atropine on discrimination learning in the rat. *J Comp Physiol Psychol.* 1964;57:13–15.

Whitehouse PJ, Hedreen JC, White CL, Price DL. Basal forebrain neurons in the dementia of Parkinson disease. *Ann Neurol.* 1983;13:243–248.

Wishaw IS, O'Connor WT, Dunnett SB. Disruption of central cholinergic mechanisms in the rat by basal forebrain lesions or atropine: effects on feeding, sensorimotor behaviour, locomotor activity and spatial navigation. *Behav Brain Res.* 1985;17:103–115.

Yahr MD, Duvoisin RC, Schear MJ, et al. Treatment of parkinsonism with levodopa. *Arch Neurol.* 1969;21:343–354.

15

Electrophysiological Correlates of Dementia in Parkinson's Disease

DOUGLAS S. GOODIN

In his monograph, *An Essay on the Shaking Palsy,* James Parkinson (1817) stressed that the intellect is preserved in this condition. Even in the early part of this century it was still generally believed that dementia is not an important symptom of Parkinson's disease (PD). Thus, Wilson (1940) stated that "on the intellectual side there may be noted some bradyphrenia or slowness of thought yet it is probably more apparent than real, being due to retarded execution but not perception." More recently, there has been a growing appreciation of the fact that abnormalities of cognitive function do occur in PD, both as an intrinsic part of the condition and also as a side effect of anti-parkinsonian medication (Pollock and Hornabrook, 1966; Meier and Martin, 1970; Garron et al, 1972; Loranger et al, 1972; Botez and Barbeau, 1973; Marttila and Rhinne, 1976; Lieberman et al, 1979; Delis et al, 1982; Beardsley and Puletti, 1971; Rafal et al, 1984).

The nature of the cognitive disturbance, however, has been a matter of considerable controversy. Some authors have attributed the intellectual decline to a slowness of thought (bradyphrenia) analogous to the slowness of movement (bradykinesia) that is characteristic of this condition and possibly related to similar neuropathological mechanisms (Wilson, 1940; Hoehn and Yahr, 1967; Marsh et al, 1971; Garron et al, 1972; Loranger et al, 1972; Mortimer et al, 1982). In this view, bradyphrenia is thought to occur without actual dementia in the same manner that bradykinesia occurs without actual weakness. This implies that patients with PD may take longer to perform a task, because of either bradykinesia or bradyphrenia or both, but that if given enough time, they will complete it successfully. Other authors have argued that an organic dementia does occur in such diseases as PD, where the primary pathology is subcortical and have suggested that this dementia can be distinguished from the dementia syndrome that occurs in such conditions as Alzheimer's disease, where the pathological changes are predominantly cortical (Albert et al, 1974; Benson, 1984; Cummings and Benson, 1984; Huber et al, 1986; de la Monte et al, 1989). Some authors have emphasized the clinical similarities of the dementia syndrome produced by either Alzheimer's disease or PD (possibly related to the combination of cortical and subcortical pathology seen in both conditions), whereas others have suggested that dementia may not even be an intrinsic part of PD but may reflect the codevelopment of

Alzheimer's disease (Hakim and Mathieson, 1979; Boller, 1980; Boller et al, 1980; Whitehouse et al, 1981, 1982; Mayeux et al, 1983).

Electrophysiological methods, particularly the technique of recording averaged evoked potentials, have been used to investigate disorders of both the central and peripheral nervous systems (for review, see Starr, 1978). This technique relies on averaging of the electroencephalogram (EEG) and uses a computer to synchronize the average with the occurrence of a particular sensory event. This method permits the recording of electrical potentials arising from both cortical and subcortical neural structures that are activated by repetitive visual, auditory, or somatosensory stimuli and, unlike such structural imaging techniques as computed tomography (CT), is able to assess function within the human nervous system.

Two distinct classes of evoked potential can be recorded in response to a sensory stimulus. The evoked potentials commonly used for clinical purposes—the visual evoked potential (VEP), the brainstem auditory evoked potential (BAEP), and the somatosensory evoked potential (SEP)—belong to a class called stimulus-related or exogenous evoked potentials (SRPs). In general, SRPs are obligate responses of the nervous system to a stimulus and are sensitive to the physical characteristics of the stimulus that elicits them. For example, stimulus features, such as intensity in the somatosensory system, check size in the visual system, and loudness in the auditory system, are important determinants of the amplitude and latency of these responses. SRPs, however, usually are not affected by the attention of the subjects or whether the sensory information is actually used by the subject. In contrast, components of the other class of evoked potentials—the event-related or endogenous evoked potentials (ERPs)—are relatively insensitive to the physical characteristics of the eliciting stimulus (Donchin et al, 1978; Tueting, 1978; Hillyard and Woods, 1979; Hillyard and Kutas, 1983; Goodin, 1986). As an example of this insensitivity to stimulus features, ERPs can even be recorded in response to a missing stimulus if its occurrence was anticipated by the subject. ERPs are, however, dependent on attention of the subject and the context in which the stimulus occurs. Thus, ERPs are not recorded when a subject is inattentive to the stimuli (Fig. 15–1). Also, if the target stimuli are made harder to discriminate from nontarget stimuli or if the complexity of the task is increased, the peak latencies of the ERP components are prolonged compared to when the task requirements are easier (Ford et al, 1976; Duncan-Johnson and Donchin, 1977; Kutas et al, 1977; Squires et al, 1977; McCarthy and Donchin, 1981; Goodin et al, 1983a).

Because ERPs have been linked experimentally to such cognitive variables as selective attention, expectancy, task difficulty, and memory, they have been used in clinical situations to study patients with intellectual impairment (for review, see Goodin, 1986). In these studies, the general finding is that the peak latencies of certain ERP components are abnormally prolonged in organic dementias or confusional states, whereas these ERP component latencies are normal in patients with depression or other nondementing illnesses in which there may be an apparent deterioration in cognitive function. Also, unlike SRPs, which often remain abnormal despite the recovery of function in the sensory pathways being tested, ERPs vary in parallel with the cognitive state and can, therefore, be used to follow the course of dementing illnesses (Goodin et al, 1983b). The recording of these potentials thus provides an objective measure of cognitive function that is well suited to the study of dementia in PD.

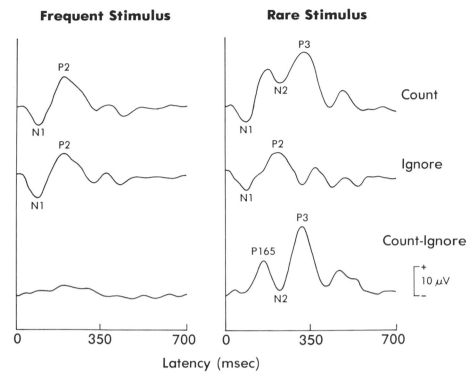

Figure 15–1. Long-latency evoked potentials recorded from a normal 28-year-old subject. Electrodes were placed at the vertex (C_z) and referenced to linked mastoid electrodes. Waveforms on the left show the responses to a frequent tone (1000 Hz; 85 percent of trials). Waveforms on the right show the responses to a rare tone (2000 Hz; 15 percent of trials). The average of 340 responses to the frequent tone and 60 responses to the rare tone are shown in each condition. The sequence of tones (50 msec duration, 60 dBHL, 1.5 sec ISI) was pseudorandom, with the constraint that no two rare tones occurred consecutively. Responses to the rare and frequent stimuli when the subject was required to count the rare tones as they occurred (Count condition) are shown in the top row. Waveforms representing the responses to the same stimuli when the subject ignores the tone sequence and reads a magazine during the test procedure (Ignore condition) are shown in the middle row. Waveforms obtained by the subtraction of the Ignore waveforms from the Count waveforms for the rare and frequent tones, are shown in the bottom row (see text for further details). (From Goodin, Squires, Henderson, Starr. Psychophysiology. 1978;15:360.)

METHODOLOGY

ERPs can be recorded with a variety of different experimental arrangements, although the simplest and most widely used clinically is the so-called odd-ball paradigm. In this experimental design, a subject is presented with a sequence of two distinguishable stimuli, one of which occurs on 70 percent to 90 percent of the trials (the frequent stimulus), whereas the other (the rare stimulus) occurs randomly on the rest of the trials. Unlike SRPs, these responses tend to habituate at short interstimulus intervals

(ISIs), and, therefore, ERPs usually are recorded at ISIs of 1 second or more. Similar ERPs can be recorded to stimuli of any sensory modality, although the auditory modality is used most often in clinical practice. Because ERPs depend on selective attention, it is important that the subject actually listen to the sequence of stimuli, and this is accomplished by having the subject count or otherwise respond to the rare stimulus. Cerebral responses are recorded from different scalp locations, and responses to the rare and the frequent stimuli are averaged separately. Each average is time-locked to the onset of its respective stimulus. The peak latencies and amplitudes of the different components of the response are then measured and compared to the amplitude and latency of these components in control subjects. Because age is an important factor in determining the amplitude and latency of these responses, the usual practice is to construct age-latency regression lines from the responses in control subjects and to measure the extent to which an individual's response deviates from these normal regression lines (Goodin et al, 1978c; Syndulko et al, 1982; Brown et al, 1983; Pfefferbaum et al, 1984; Picton et al, 1984).

Figure 15–1 shows the evoked potentials recorded from a normal subject in response to a sequence of auditory stimuli. The frequent tone in these recordings had a pitch of 1000 Hz and occurred on 85 percent of the trials, whereas the rare tone had a pitch of 2000 Hz and occurred randomly on the remaining 15 percent of the trials. At the top are shown the responses recorded when the subject was asked to keep a mental record of the number of rare stimuli (Count condition). The cerebral response to the frequent tone consists of a negative (N1)–positive (P2) complex, comprising the vertex potential. The response to the rare tone is more complex because the ERP components have been superimposed on the vertex potential. The N1 component is followed by a positive wave referred to as the "apparent P2" because it represents the sum of the stimulus-related P2 and the event-related P165 (Goodin et al, 1978b). Following these components, there is a negative (N2)–positive (P3) complex representing the principal components of the ERP. Figure 15–1 (middle) shows waveforms that were recorded using the same experimental arrangements except that the subject was instructed to read a magazine and to ignore the sequence of auditory stimuli (Ignore condition). In this circumstance, the ERPs are absent, and the response to both the frequent and the rare tones consists of only the vertex potential. At bottom are shown the difference waveforms obtained by subtraction of the waveforms obtained in the Ignore condition from the corresponding waveforms obtained in the Count condition. This difference waveform is a flat line for the frequent tone because in both conditions only the vertex potential is obtained. For the rare tone, the vertex potential has been similarly subtracted out, and the P165, N2, and P3 components of the ERP can be seen clearly.

The neural generators of these long-latency evoked potentials are not fully understood. For example, some authors have attributed the vertex potential to activity in unimodal sensory association cortex (Vaughan and Ritter, 1970). However, because similar appearing vertex potentials can be elicited by visual, auditory, or somatosensory stimuli and because the vertex potential elicited by one sensory modality habituates the vertex potential elicited by another, it must relate, at least in part, to activity in multimodal cortex (Davis and Zerlin, 1966; Davis et al, 1972). ERPs are similarly elicited by stimuli in any sensory modality and, thus, are also believed to relate to activity in multimodal association cortex. Some authors have attributed these ERPs to neural activity in the hippocampus or other limbic structures (Wood et al, 1980; Halgren et al, 1980; Yingling and Hosobuchi, 1984), but the actual neuroanatomical basis of these potentials is still uncertain.

ELECTROPHYSIOLOGICAL ACCOMPANIMENTS OF DEMENTIA IN PARKINSON'S DISEASE

Stimulus-Related Potentials

Several different electrophysiological abnormalities have been described in PD patients. For example, some patients with this disease have a slowing of central conduction time or a delay in the peak latency of the different components of the BAEP and SEPs or a prolongation in the latency of the major occipital positivity of the VEP (Tartaglione et al, 1984; O'Donnell et al, 1987; Onofrj et al, 1986; Bodis-Wollner et al, 1987; Tachibana et al, 1988). In the visual system, where dopaminergic mechanisms are thought to be important in sensory processing, attempts have been made to use changes in the VEP both for diagnostic purposes and as a measure of therapeutic response (Tartaglione et al, 1984; Onofrj et al, 1986; Bodis-Wollner et al, 1987). There has, however, been no attempt to relate these SRP changes either to the presence of a clinically apparent dementia or to the likelihood that an individual patient will develop cognitive difficulties in the future. Consequently, it is not known whether these evoked potential changes have any relationship to the cognitive decline that occurs in PD. However, as mentioned earlier, because SPPs are relatively insensitive to cognitive variables, it seems unlikely that changes in these potentials will prove to be reliable electrophysiological accompaniments of an intellectual decline in PD.

Event-Related Potentials

The recording of ERPs has been applied more directly to the study of cognition in PD. Hansch and colleagues (1982) studied 20 patients with idiopathic PD (only some of whom had clinically evident cognitive impairment) and compared the findings with 20 age-matched, normal control subjects. They reported a delay in the latency of both the P2 and P3 components of the ERP in the patients compared to the normal controls. They also found that 4 of the 20 patients had abnormally delayed N1 latencies, although, as a group, patients were not significantly different from controls in this regard. These authors also reported a correlation between the P3 latency and the Symbol Digit Modalities Test (SDMT) score and thereby provided a link between the ERP changes and the altered cognitive function. They interpreted these findings as supportive evidence of bradyphrenia in PD. This conclusion, however, is unwarranted, at least as bradyphrenia was defined earlier. A prolongation of the P3 latency has been found in dementia of many different etiologies that are not characterized clinically by bradykinesia (for review, see Goodin, 1986), and thus this finding is nonspecific. O'Donnell and colleagues (1987) also studied an unselected group of PD patients and reported a prolongation of the N2 and P3 component latencies in this group compared to normal controls. They too found a delay of the N1 latency in the PD patients, although this did not reach statistical significance. The findings of both of these studies, however, are difficult to interpret because there was no attempt to relate the electro-physiological abnormalities to either the presence of a clinically apparent cognitive disturbance or the severity of the PD symptoms. Nonetheless, these considerations are important if the aim is to shed light on the nature of the cognitive disturbance in PD. For example, if bradyphrenia (rather than dementia) accounts for the apparent mental slowing in PD, patients with comparable motor manifestations of the disease should show comparable electrophysiological changes. If, by contrast, a true dementia occurs, the electrophysiological changes should be correlated with the presence of a clinically apparent dementia. Also, if it is possible to distinguish the PD dementia syndrome from those syndromes resulting from more cortically based pathology (e.g., Alzheimer's disease), electrophysiological differences between these conditions might be anticipated.

Goodin and Aminoff (1987) studied 28 patients with idiopathic Parkinson's disease, 14 of whom met diagnostic criteria for dementia (American Psychiatric Association, 1980) and 14 of whom had clinically normal mental function. The patients in these two groups were well matched for age, stage of disease (Hoehn and Yahr, 1967), duration of illness, and the amount and type of antiparkinsonian medication (Table 15–1). These authors found a significant prolongation in the latencies of the N1, N2, and P3 components of the ERP in the demented patients with PD. These ERP changes were specific for the cognitive disturbance in the PD patients because each was significant compared both with nondemented patients and with age-matched normal control subjects (Table 15–2, Fig. 15–2).

The finding of clear electrophysiological differences between demented and nondemented patients despite a comparable motor disturbance in each group (as measured by the Hoehn and Yahr stage, Table 15–1) suggests that dementia and bradykinesia are not tightly coupled. These ERP changes thus relate to the dementia and

Table 15–1. Clinical features of demented and nondemented patients with Parkinson's Disease

Feature	Demented group	Nondemented group	Significance of difference between groups
Age (years)	71.4 (7.5)[a]	67.2 (4.8)	NS
Hoehn and Yahr stage	2.5 (0.5)	2.7 (0.5)	NS
Duration of illness (years)	4.8 (2.9)	5.0 (2.7)	NS
Medications[b]			
Carbidopa (mg/day)[c]	87.2 (101.9)	58.4 (52.7)	NS
Levodopa (mg/day)[c]	826.9 (1018.7)	450.0 (418.3)	NS
Mini-Mental State score	23.2 (3.8)	27.9 (1.2)	$p < 0.0005$

[a]Mean values are given with SD in parentheses.

[b]Amantadine was taken by 1 nondemented patient and 2 demented patients in standard doses of 200 mg daily or less. Bromocriptine was taken by 4 nondemented patients (in doses of 37.5, 20, 7.5, and 5 mg daily, respectively) and by 1 demented patient (27.5 mg daily). Anticholinergic medication was taken by 5 nondemented patients and by 3 demented patients. There was no significant difference in the mean dose of any of these medications between the two groups.

[c]The difference between the demented and nondemented groups was not significant. The mean difference appears large because one of the demented patients was taking 400 mg of carbidopa and 4000 mg of levodopa per day, without apparent evidence of toxicity.

From Goodin and Aminoff. Ann Neurol. 1987; 21:90–94.

Table 15-2. Mean component latencies (msec) for demented and nondemented patients with Parkinson's Disease

	Evoked Potential Component			
	N1	P2	N2	P3
Nondemented PD patients	90 (6)[a]	182 (20)	245 (23)	361 (28)
Demented PD patients	103 (10)	186 (13)	293 (25)	399 (40)
Significance of difference between demented and nondemented patients	$p = 0.001$	NS	$p < 0.0005$	$p = 0.019$
Expected latency[b]	90	178	242	340

[a]Numbers in parentheses are SD; clinical characteristics of the demented and nondemented patients with Parkinson's disease are provided in Table 15-1.

[b]The expected latency of each component for a subject of comparable age (69 years) computed from normal age-latency regression lines (Goodin and Aminoff, 1986).

From Goodin and Aminoff. Ann Neurol. 1987; 21:90–94.

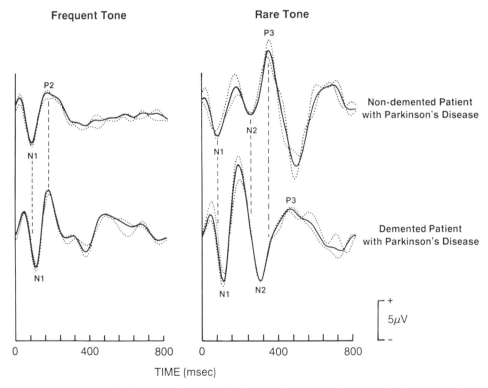

Figure 15-2. Evoked potentials, recorded at C_z, from a nondemented subject aged 59 years (top trace) and a demented subject aged 69 years (bottom trace), both with Parkinson's disease. Traces on the left are the responses to the frequent tone and those on the right are responses to the rare tone. Individual trials are shown in dotted lines, and the sum of the trials is shown in a solid line. (From Goodin and Aminoff. *Ann Neurol.* 1987;21:90–94.)

not to the motor disturbance, indicating that bradyphrenia, as defined earlier, does not account for the intellectual decline that sometimes occurs in PD. The dementia of PD is, however, electrophysiologically different from the dementia that occurs in patients with Alzheimer's disease, where a prolongation of the N1 latency is not seen (Goodin et al, 1978c; Neshige et al, 1988; Patterson et al, 1988; Ball et al, 1989; Polich et al, 1990). Additionally, the N1 latency, but not the N2 or P3 latency, was correlated with the Mini-Mental State (MMS) score (Folstein et al, 1975) in the demented patients, underscoring the close relationship between the N1 latency change and the cognitive decline in PD. In contrast, no correlation between N1 latency and MMS score was found in patients with Alzheimer's disease, further indicating the difference between the dementia syndromes produced by the two conditions.

These findings require confirmation, but it is of note that Verma and colleagues (1989) have reported a prolongation of the N1 latency in a group of patients with "subcortical dementia," the majority of whom had PD. These findings, together with those of Goodin and Aminoff (1987), suggest that an organic dementia (distinct from either bradyphrenia or coincidental Alzheimer's disease) does occur in PD and that it may be possible to distinguish this dementia syndrome from those that occur in other diseases.

COMPARISON OF ELECTROPHYSIOLOGICAL CHANGES IN PARKINSONIAN DEMENTIA WITH OTHER DEMENTIA SYNDROMES

The concept of subcortical dementia was introduced by Albert and associates (1974) and has been supported subsequently by others (Benson, 1984; Cummings and Benson, 1984; Huber et al, 1986). In particular, it has been proposed that the dementia that occurs in the course of diseases where the pathology is predominantly subcortical (e.g., Parkinson's disease and Huntington's disease) is clinically different from the dementia that occurs in diseases where the pathology is principally in the neocortex (e.g., Alzheimer's disease). Some authors have challenged the notion that clinically different syndromes exist (Mayeux et al, 1983), whereas others have reported anatomical changes in both cortical and subcortical structures in all three conditions (Hakim and Mathieson, 1979; Bruyn et al, 1979; Boller, 1980; Boller et al, 1980; Whitehouse et al, 1981, 1982).

As mentioned previously, the observation that the N1 latency is prolonged in PD dementia but not in the dementia of Alzheimer's disease suggests that an electrophysiological distinction can be made between cortical and subcortical dementias. Huntington's disease is an inherited condition that begins in midlife and is characterized clinically by both a choreiform movement disorder and a progressive dementia. The pathology, like that in PD, is predominantly subcortical, and if the concept of a subcortical dementia syndrome is valid, patients with this disease might be electrophysiologically similar to demented patients with PD.

Hömberg and colleagues (1986) studied 30 patients with Huntington's disease and 60 normal control subjects and reported a delay in latency of not only the N1 component but also the P2, N2, and P3 components in this condition. These authors also reported prolongations in the N2 and P3 latencies in asymptomatic persons at risk to develop Huntington's disease because they had an affected parent, thereby providing evidence of subclinical cognitive impairment in at least some members of this group of people. These authors also reported significant correlations between the ERP findings and scores on several neuropsychological tests, linking these ERP changes to the cognitive decline. These correlations were, however, only significant for the P2, N2, and P3 components of the ERP, and thus the relationship of the N1 latency change to the dementia was uncertain.

Goodin and Aminoff (1986) compared the electrophysiological findings in 22 patients with Alzheimer's disease, 13 patients with Huntington's disease, 13 demented patients with PD, and 40 normal control subjects. All three groups of demented patients had delayed latencies of the N2 and P3 components of the ERP compared to normal controls (Fig. 15–3, Table 15–3). In contrast, only the groups with subcortical dementia (PD and Huntington's disease) had a delay in the N1 latency. These differences in N1 latency were significant compared with both normal control subjects and patients with Alzheimer's disease but were not significantly different between the two subcortical groups (Table 15–3). However, even within the subcortical category, there were electrophysiological differences because, as Hömberg and colleagues (1986) also reported, the patients with Huntington's disease had a significant delay in the P2 latency compared to all other groups, including the PD group (Table 15–3). Using electrophysiological criteria alone, it was possible to correctly categorize patients into each of the three diagnostic groups in over 60 percent of instances.

As another example, patients who are infected with the human immunodeficiency virus (HIV) often complain of cognitive difficulties, and in patients who meet other diagnostic criteria for the acquired immunodeficiency syndrome (AIDS), dementia is quite prevalent (Snider et al, 1983; Levy et al, 1985; Navia et al, 1986b; Navia and Price, 1987). The nature of the cognitive deficit in HIV encephalopathy is not yet fully characterized, although the pathological changes are predominantly subcortical (Navia et al, 1986a), and it might be anticipated that the resulting dementia would be of the subcortical type. Goodin and associates (1990) studied demented patients with AIDS, and, as in other subcortical dementias, they found significant ERP latency delays that were especially marked for the N1, N2, and P3 component latencies. They also reported similar but less marked changes in asymptomatic patients seropositive for HIV, suggesting the presence of a subclinical cognitive disturbance in these subjects.

Taken together, these findings suggest that subcortical varieties of dementia can be distinguished from cortical dementia on the basis of changes in the early components of the ERP, particularly by a delay in the latency of the N1 component, which is seen only in the former circumstance. Nonetheless, it is not possible to make a simple division between cortical and subcortical dementia syndromes because electrophysiological distinctions can be drawn between different conditions even within the broad category of subcortical dementia.

COMMENTS

Electrophysiological techniques have been used to assess cognitive function in a wide variety of clinical and experimental contexts and are well suited to serve both as an aid

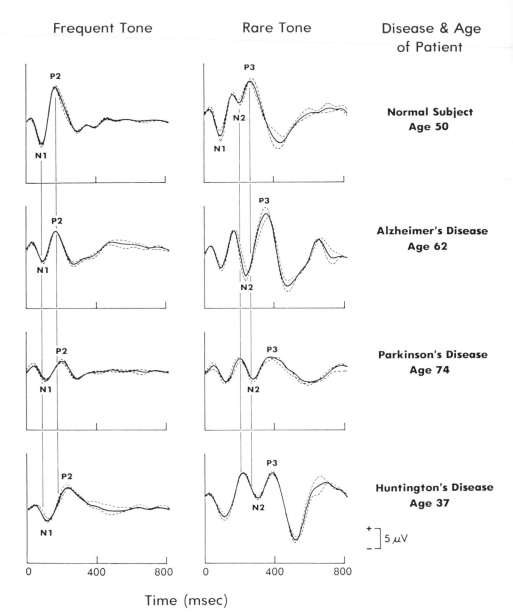

Figure 15-3. Evoked potential waveforms recorded from the vertex in a normal subject and in individual patients with Alzheimer's, Parkinson's, and Huntington's diseases. Waveforms on the left are in response to the frequent tone and consist of the N1–P2 vertex potential. Waveforms on the right are to the rare tone and, in addition to the earlier components, consist of N2 and P3 components. The patient with Alzheimer's disease shows a prolongation in latency of the N2 and P3 components relative to the normal subject, but normal N1 and P2 latencies. The patients with Parkinson's disease and Huntington's disease, in contrast, show not only a greater delay in the N2 and P3 latency but also a prolongation of the N1 and P2 latencies. (From Goodin and Aminoff. *Brain.* 1986;109:1103–1113.

Table 15–3. Statistical significance of observed intergroup differences in latency of evoked potential components for demented patients with Huntington's Disease, Parkinson's Disease, or Alzheimer's Disease and normal nondemented control patients

	Age-adjusted latency (msec)	Significance of Intergroup Latency Differences		
		Normal	Alzheimer's Disease	Huntington's Disease
N1 component				
Normal	90			
Alzheimer's disease	90	$p = 0.9573$		
Huntington's disease	100	$p = 0.0023$	$p = 0.0107$	
Parkinson's disease	104	$p = 0.0004$	$p = 0.0001$	$p = 0.4522$
P2 component				
Normal	173			
Alzheimer's disease	173	$p = 0.9624$		
Huntington's disease	203	$p = 0.0001$	$p = 0.0001$	
Parkinson's disease	184	$p = 0.1054$	$p = 0.0648$	$p = 0.0136$
N2 component				
Normal	232			
Alzheimer's disease	268	$p = 0.0001$		
Huntington's disease	284	$p = 0.0001$	$p = 0.1893$	
Parkinson's disease	289	$p = 0.0001$	$p = 0.0243$	$p = 0.7016$
P3 component				
Normal	321			
Alzheimer's disease	368	$p = 0.0001$		
Huntington's disease	382	$p = 0.0001$	$p = 0.3695$	
Parkinson's disease	395	$p = 0.0001$	$p = 0.0315$	$p = 0.4574$

From Goodin and Aminoff. Brain. 1986; 109:1103–1113.

in the evaluation of PD patients and as a method to answer some of the neurobehavioral questions that have arisen about this condition. Although evidence that addresses these questions can be derived from findings using other experimental methods (as discussed in Chapter 11), the use of evoked potentials and, in particular the recording of ERPs have documented that dementia (not bradyphrenia) occurs as an intrinsic part of PD. In addition, these techniques have demonstrated clear differences between the dementia of PD and that of Alzheimer's disease, indicating that PD dementia is not the result of concomitant Alzheimer's disease. Finally, the observation that there are changes in the early components of the ERP that are specific to dementing illnesses with subcortical pathology suggests that an electrophysiological distinction between cortical and subcortical dementia is possible. In the future, possibly with the use of new experimental arrangements, it seems likely that the recording of evoked potentials can continue to shed light on the many evolving controversies in the neurobehavior of PD.

REFERENCES

Albert ML, Feldman RG, Willis AL. The subcortical dementia of supranuclear palsy. *J Neurol Neurosurg Psychiatry.* 1974;37:121–130.

American Psychiatric Association. *Diagnostic and Statistical Manual of Mental Disorders,* 3rd ed. Washington, DC: APA; 1980.

Ball SS, Marsh JT, Schubarth G, et al. Longitudinal P300 latency changes in Alzheimer's disease. *J Gerontol.* 1989;44:M195–200.

Beardsley JV, Puletti F. Personality (MMPI) and cognitive (WAIS) changes after levodopa treatment. Occurrence in patients with Parkinson's disease. *Arch Neurol.* 1971;25:145–150.

Benson DF. Clinical differences among types of dementia. *Ann Neurol.* 1984;15:403–404.

Bodis-Wollner I, Marx MS, Mitra S, et al. Visual dysfunction in Parkinson's disease: loss in spatiotemporal contrast sensitivity. *Brain.* 1987;110:1675–1698.

Boller F. Mental status of patients with Parkinson disease. *J Clin Neuropsychol.* 1980;2:157–172.

Boller F, Mizutani T, Roessmann U, Gambetti P. Parkinson disease, dementia and Alzheimer disease: clinicopathological correlations. *Ann Neurol.* 1980;7:329–335.

Botez MI, Barbeau A. Long-term mental changes in levodopa treated patients. *Lancet.* 1973;2:1028–1029.

Brown WS, Marsh JT, La Rue A. Exponential electrophysiological aging: P3 latency. *Electroencephalogr Clin Neurophysiol.* 1983;55:277–285.

Bruyn GW, Bots TAM, Dom R. Huntington's chorea: current neuropathological status. *Adv Neurol.* 1979;23:83–93.

Cummings JL, Benson DF. Subcortical dementia. Review of an emerging concept. *Arch Neurol.* 1984;41:874–879.

Davis H, Zerlin S. Acoustic relations of the human vertex potential. *J Acoust Soc Am.* 1966;39:109–116.

Davis H, Osterhammel RA, Weit CC, Gjerdijen DB. *Electroencephalogr Clin Neurophysiol.* 1972;33:537–545.

de la Monte SM, Wells SE, Hedley-Whyte ET, Growdon JH. Neuropathological distinction between Parkinson's dementia and Parkinson's plus Alzheimer's disease. *Ann Neurol.* 1989;26:309–320.

Delis D, Direnfeld L, Alexander MP, Kaplan E. Cognitive fluctuation associated with an on–off phenomenon in Parkinson's disease. *Neurology.* 1982;32:1049–1052.

Donchin E, Ritter W, McCallum WC. Cognitive psychophysiology: the endogenous components of the ERP. In: Callaway E, Tueting P, Koslow S, eds. *Brain Event-Related Potentials in Man.* New York: Academic Press; 1978:349–411.

Duncan-Johnson CC, Donchin E. On quantifying surprise: the variation of event-related potentials with subjective probability. *Psychophysiology.* 1977;14:456–467.

Folstein MF, Folstein SE, McHugh PR. "Mini-Mental State": a practical method for grading the cognitive state of patients for the clinician. *J Psych Res.* 1975;12:189–198.

Ford JM, Roth WT, Kopell BS. Auditory evoked potentials to unpredictable shifts in pitch. *Psychophysiology.* 1976;13:32–39.

Garron DC, Klawans HL, Narin F. Intellectual functioning of persons with idiopathic parkinsonism. *J Nerv Ment Dis.* 1972;154:445–452.

Goodin DS. Event-related (endogenous) potential. In: Aminoff MJ, ed. *Clinical Neurology.* New York: Churchill Livingstone; 1986:575–595.

Goodin DS, Aminoff MJ. Electrophysiological differences between demented and nondemented patients with Parkinson's disease. *Ann Neurol.* 1987;21:90–94.

Goodin DS, Aminoff MJ. Electrophysiological differences between subtypes of dementia. *Brain.* 1986;109:1103–1113.

Goodin DS, Aminoff MJ, Chernoff DN, Hollander H. Long latency event-related potentials in patients infected with human immunodeficiency virus. *Ann Neurol.* 1990;27:414–419.

Goodin DS, Squires KC, Henderson BH, Starr A. An early event-related cortical potential. *Psychophysiology.* 1978b;15:360–365.

Goodin DS, Squires KC, Starr A. Long latency event-related components of the auditory evoked potential in dementia. *Brain.* 1978c;101:635–648.

Goodin DS, Squires KC, Starr A. Variations in early and late event-related components of the auditory evoked potential with task difficulty. *Electroencephalogr Clin Neurophysiol.* 1983a;55:680–686.

Goodin DS, Starr A, Chippendale T, Squires KC. Sequential changes in the P3 component of the auditory evoked potential in confusional states and dementing illnesses. *Neurology.* 1983b;33:1215–1218.

Hakim AM, Mathieson G. Dementia in Parkinson disease: a neuropathologic study. *Neurology.* 1979;29:1209–1214.

Halgren E, Squires NK, Wilson CL, et al. Endogenous potentials generated in the human hippocampal formation amygdala by infrequent events. *Science.* 1980;210:803–805.

Hansch EC, Syndulko K, Cohen SN, et al. Cognition in Parkinson's disease: an event-related potential perspective. *Ann Neurol.* 1982;11:599–607.

Hillyard SA, Kutas M. Electrophysiology of cognitive processing. *Annu Rev Psychol.* 1983;34:33–61.

Hillyard SA, Woods DL. Electrophysiological analysis of human brain function. In: Gazzaniga MS, ed. *Handbook of Behavioral Neurobiology.* New York: Plenum Press; 1979:345–378.

Hoehn MM, Yahr MD. Parkinsonism: onset, progression and mortality. *Neurology.* 1967;17:427–442.

Hömberg V, Hefter H, Granseyer G, et al. Event-related potentials in patients with Huntington's disease and relatives at risk in relation to detailed psychometry. *Electroencephalogr Clin Neurophysiol.* 1986;63:552–569.

Huber SJ, Shuttleworth EC, Paulson GW, et al. Cortical vs subcortical dementia: neuropsychological differences. *Arch Neurol.* 1986;43:392–394.

Kutas M, McCarthy G, Donchin E: Augmenting mental chronometry: the P300 as a measure of stimulus evaluation time. *Science.* 1977;197:792–795.

Levy RM, Bredesen DE, Rosenblum ML. Neurological manifestations of the acquired immunodeficiency syndrome (AIDS): experience at UCSF and review of the literature. *J Neurosurg.* 1985;6:475–495.

Lieberman A, Dziatolowski M, Kupersmith M, et al. Dementia in Parkinson's disease. *Ann Neurol.* 1979;6:355–359.

Loranger AW, Goodell H, McDowell FH, et al. Intellectual impairment in Parkinson's disease. *Brain.* 1972;95:405–412.

Marsh GG, Markham CM, Ansel R. Levodopa's awakening effect on patients with parkinsonism. *J Neurol Neurosurg Psychiatry.* 1971;34:209–218.

Marttila RH, Rhinne UK. Dementia in Parkinson's disease. *Acta Neurol Scand.* 1976;54:431–444.

Mayeux R, Stern Y, Rosen J, Benson DF. Is "subcortical dementia" a recognizable clinical entity? *Ann Neurol.* 1983;14:278–283.

McCarthy G, Donchin E. A metric for thought: a comparison of P300 latency and reaction time. *Science.* 1981;211:77–80.

Meier M, Martin W. Intellectual changes associated with levodopa therapy. *JAMA.* 1970;213:465–466.

Mortimer JA, Pirozzolo FJ, Hansch EL, Webster DD. Relationship of motor symptoms to intellectual deficits in Parkinson's disease. *Neurology.* 1982;32:133–137.

Navia BA, Price RW. The acquired immunodeficiency syndrome dementia complex as the presenting or sole manifestation of human immunodeficiency virus infection. *Arch Neurol.* 1987;44:65–69.

Navia BA, Cho E-S, Petito CK, Price RW. The AIDS dementia complex: II. neuropathology. *Ann Neurol.* 1986a;19:525–535.

Navia BA, Jordan BD, Price RW. The AIDS dementia complex: I. clinical features. *Ann Neurol.* 1986b;19:517–524.

Neshige R, Barrett G, Shibasaki H. Auditory long latency event-related potentials in Alzheimer's disease and multi-infarct dementia. *J Neurol Neurosurg Psychiatry.* 1988;51:1120–1125.

O'Donnell BF, Squires NK, Martz MJ, et al. Evoked potential changes and neuropsychological performance in Parkinson's disease. *Biol Psychol.* 1987;24:23–37.

Onofrj M, Ghilardi MF, Basciani M, Gambi D. Visual evoked potentials in parkinsonism and dopamine blockade reveal a stimulus-dependent dopamine function in humans. *J Neurol Neurosurg Psychiatry.* 1986;49:1150–1159.

Parkinson J. *An Essay on the Shaking Palsy.* London: Sherwood, Neely, and Jones; 1817.

Patterson JV, Michalewski HJ, Starr A. Latency variability of the components of auditory event-related potentials to infrequent stimuli in aging, Alzheimer-type dementia, and depression. *Electroencephalogr Clin Neurophysiol.* 1988;71:450–460.

Pfefferbaum A, Ford JM, Wenegrat BG, et al. Clinical applications of the P3 component of event-related potentials: I. Normal aging. *Electroencephalogr Clin Neurophysiol.* 1984;59:85–103.

Picton TW, Stuss DT, Champagne SC, Nelson RF. The effects of age on the human event-related potential. *Psychophysiology.* 1984;21:312–325.

Polich J, Ladish C, Bloom FE. P300 assessment of early Alzheimer's disease. *Electroencephalogr Clin Neurophysiol.* 1990;77:179–189.

Pollock M, Hornabrook RW. The prevalence, natural history and dementia of Parkinson's disease. *Brain.* 1966;89:429–488.

Rafal RD, Posner MI, Walker JA, Friedrich FJ. Cognition and the basal ganglia: separating mental and motor components of performance in Parkinson's disease. *Brain.* 1984;107:1083–1094.

Snider WD, Simpson DM, Nielsen S, et al. Neurological complications of acquired immune deficiency syndrome: analysis of 50 patients. *Ann Neurol.* 1983;14:403–418.

Squires NK, Donchin E, Squires KC, Grossberg S. Bisensory stimulation: inferring decision related processes from the P300 component. *J Exp Psychol.* 1977;2:299–315.

Starr A. Sensory evoked potentials in clinical disorders of the nervous system. *Annu Rev Neurosci.* 1978;1:1103–1127.

Syndulko K, Hansch EC, Cohen SN, et al. Long latency event-related potentials in normal aging and dementia. In: Courjon J, Mauguiere F, Revol M, eds. *Clinical Application of Evoked Potentials in Neurology.* New York: Raven Press; 1982:279–285.

Tachibana H, Takeda M, Sugita M. Electrophysiological differences between Parkinson's disease and vascular parkinsonism. *Jpn J Med.* 1988;27:261–266.

Tartaglione A, Pizio N, Bino G, et al. VEP changes in Parkinson's disease are stimulus dependent. *J Neurol Neurosurg Psychiatry.* 1984;47:305–307.

Tueting P. Event-related potentials, cognitive events and information processing. In: Otto D, ed. *Multidisciplinary Perspectives in Event-related Brain Potential (ERP) Research.* Washington, DC: US Government Printing Office; 1978:159–169.

Vaughan HG Jr, Ritter W. The sources of auditory evoked responses recorded from the human scalp. *Electroencephalogr Clin Neurophysiol.* 1970;28:360–367.

Verma NP, Nichols CD, Greiffenstein MF, et al. Waves earlier than P_3 are more informative in putative subcortical dementias: a study with mapping and neuropsychological techniques. *Brain Topogr.* 1989;1:183–191.

Whitehouse PJ, Price DL, Clark AW, et al. Alzheimer disease: evidence for selective loss of cholinergic neurons in the nucleus basalis. *Ann Neurol.* 1981;10:122–126.

Whitehouse PJ, Price DL, Struble RG, et al. Alzheimer's disease and senile dementia: loss of neurons in the basal forebrain. *Science.* 1982;215:1237–1239.

Wilson SAK. In: Bruce AN, ed. *Neurology,* vols 1 and 2. London: Butterworths; 1940.

Wood CC, Allison T, Goff WR, et al. On the neural origins of P300 in man. In: Kornhuber HH, Deecke L, eds. *Progress in Brain Research,* Vol 54. Amsterdam: Elsevier; 1980:51–56.

Yingling CD, Hosobuchi Y. A subcortical correlate of P300 in man. *Electroencephalogr Clin Neurophysiol.* 1984;59:72–76.

IV
DEPRESSION

16

Clinical Subtypes of Parkinson's Disease and Depression

JOAN SANTAMARIA AND EDUARDO TOLOSA

Mental depression is common in Parkinson's disease (PD); 30 percent to 60 percent of patients become depressed at some point in the course of the disease. Some authors have seen nothing special in this association given the natural tendency of chronic disabling illnesses to induce reactive depression. Several findings, however, do not fit this view. For example, the prevalence of depression is higher in PD than in other chronic disorders, and its severity is not related reliably to the severity of motor signs. In addition, some patients develop depression months or years before the onset of PD. In these depressed patients, the motor disability and mood disorder may follow an independent course after treatment with levodopa. Finally, there are similarities between the clinical and biochemical findings in PD and depression. Some clinical manifestations of PD, including akinesia and psychomotor retardation, are typical of mental depression and may overlap clinically. In both disorders, abnormalities in dopaminergic, noradrenergic, and serotonergic transmission have been reported. These findings suggest that at least in some PD patients, depression might be a manifestation of the pathological process causing the disease. We review evidence supporting both views and discuss whether the occurrence of depression may help in delineating different PD subgroups.

The first section of this chapter deals with some methodological issues related to the examination of depression in PD. The following sections summarize information in the literature regarding prevalence, correlates of depression in untreated PD, the effects of treatment with levodopa on depression, depression in chronically treated PD, clinical subtypes of PD and depression, and comparison of PD depression with other neurological illnesses.

METHODOLOGICAL CONSIDERATIONS

It is difficult to compare the results of studies in the literature because there are considerable differences in selection criteria and in the methods of assessing depression (Gotham et al, 1986). These methodological differences can be summarized as follows.

Selection Criteria

Some authors have studied consecutive patients seen in an ambulatory clinic (Mayeux et al, 1981; Santamaria et al, 1986; Starkstein et al, 1989), consecutive patients referred for thalamotomy (Warburton, 1967), inpatients in a general hospital (Brown and Wilson, 1972), inpatients in a psychiatric hospital (Mindham, 1970), a group of letter-recruited volunteer outpatients from a movement disorders clinic (Huber et al, 1990), a mixture of letter-recruited volunteer outpatients and members of a PD society (Gotham et al, 1986; Brown et al, 1988), or mainly a group of residents in homes for the aged (Robins, 1976). In some studies, the method of inclusion was not specified (Celesia and Wanamaker, 1972; Marsh and Markham, 1973; Mindham et al, 1976; Huber et al, 1988).

   Duration of PD also has been variable. Recent-onset patients were studied by some (Vogel, 1982; Santamaria et al, 1986), and nonrecent-onset patients or a mixture of both were examined by most other authors.

   Treatment of depression and PD also has varied. In some studies, only untreated (both PD and depression) patients were included (Warburton, 1967; Celesia and Wanamaker, 1972; Brown and Wilson, 1972; Robins, 1976; Vogel, 1982; Santamaria et al, 1986). Most authors studied a mixture of patients with treated or untreated PD or depression, and some studies did not specify the treatment of patients (Horn, 1974; Gotham et al, 1986; Brown et al, 1988).

   Patients meeting DSM III criteria for dementia (Huber et al, 1988) or overt dementia (Mayeux et al, 1981, 1984, 1986) were excluded in some but not other studies. Patients with postencephalitic, arteriosclerotic, and drug-induced PD were excluded in most articles as well as patients who had undergone thalamotomy, whereas they were included in other studies (Mindham, 1970; Brown et al, 1972; Marsh and Markham, 1973; Robins, 1976; Mindham et al, 1976). Most studies included only personally examined patients with two or more of the main PD signs (tremors, rigidity, akinesia, or postural impairment). A few, however, included patients not examined by the authors, with the diagnosis of PD based on hospital records or on the patient's adherence to a Parkinson's disease society (Gotham et al, 1986; Brown et al, 1988).

Assessment of Depression

In the early publications, depression was diagnosed using unstructured interviews, with severity rated by clinical impression. Some authors assessed depression retrospectively by searching for its symptoms in clinical records (Brown and Wilson, 1972). More recently, the diagnosis of depression has been made according to DSM III criteria, and severity has been rated using standardized depression scales [Beck Depression Inventory (BDI), Hamilton Depression Rating Scale (HDRS), Zung scale, Minnesota Multiphasic Personality Inventory (MMPI)]. In some studies, diagnosis of depression was based mainly or solely on scores from a depression scale (Mayeux et al, 1981; Gotham et al, 1986; Brown et al, 1988; Huber et al, 1988; Starkstein et al, 1990a). On occasion, these inventories were filled out by the patients (or their relatives) at home without supervision (Gotham et al, 1986; Brown et al, 1988). Depression, PD signs, or functional impairment were rated in some studies by the same author (Robins, 1976; Huber et al, 1988), whereas in other studies, different investigators assessed these symptoms independently (Santamaria et al, 1986; Starkstein et al, 1989, 1990a, b), or they were self-assessed by the patients at home (Gotham et al, 1986; Brown et al, 1988).

Some authors compared the severity of depressive symptoms in patients with a group of healthy subjects (Marsh and Markham, 1973; Mayeux et al, 1981; Santamaria et al, 1986) or with a group of neurological, psychiatric, or medical patients with other chronic diseases (Warburton, 1967; Mindham, 1970; Horn, 1974; Robins, 1976; Gotham et al, 1986). Many studies did not use a control group.

In summary, because of these methodological differences, it is not surprising that general conclusions about PD and depression have not been achieved. Resolution of these methodological issues should be a primary concern of future research. This would facilitate comparison of different studies and allow more generalized conclusions to be drawn. The following sections are organized with respect to severity of PD, treatment, and type of study design.

UNTREATED PARKINSON'S DISEASE

Depression in Recent-Onset Parkinson's Disease

Only two studies have been published on the subject. Vogel (1982) reported that in 20 recent-onset PD patients (less than 2 years since symptom onset and stages I or II of Hoehn and Yahr), the mean HDRS score was high (12.3 points). The number of patients actually depressed was not given, and a control group was not studied. Five patients (25 percent) had been treated before PD onset for a "compulsive or depressive neurosis." Total depression scores did not correlate with severity of motor disability. However, some depressive symptoms were positively correlated with motor impairment, including retarded thinking, lack of initiative, inhibited drive and thinking, and feelings of affective coldness ("apathic syndrome"). Other depressive symptoms, including feelings of being ill, sleep difficulties, decreased appetite, reduced sex drive, and suicidal ideation ("somatic-depressive syndrome"), were unrelated to motor disability. Patients with predominant tremor were less depressed than those with akinesia.

Santamaria and colleagues (1986) studied 34 recent-onset (mean duration of 1.8 years), mild to moderately impaired, untreated PD patients (17 patients were on low doses of anticholinergics). They found that 32 percent of the patients were depressed (10 with a dysthymic disorder and 1 with major depression by DSM III criteria), whereas only 4 of the 23 (17 percent) healthy controls (spouses of the patients) were depressed (major depression absent, dysthymic disorder in 1, adaptive disorder in 2, and atypical depression in 1). Neither the presence nor the severity of depression was related to severity of motor signs or functional disability. In 90 percent of the depressed patients, mood changes had started before the first PD symptom. Patients with depression antedating the beginning of PD had a younger age at onset, fewer PD signs, and a more frequent family history of PD.

In summary, depression is common in recent-onset and untreated PD patients. It occurs in about a third of the patients, and its appearance or severity is not related to the motor symptoms or functional impairment, although some symptoms of depression may be related. In 20 percent to 90 percent of the patients with depression, mental symptoms appeared before onset of the motor disorder.

Depression in Advanced Parkinson's Disease

There are only a few studies that addressed this subject, and all were conducted in the pre-levodopa era. Warburton (1967) studied 140 patients referred for thalamotomy, with a mean disease duration of approximately 10 years and moderate to severe disability. This group may have included mostly patients with predominant tremor or rigidity, since these are the symptoms more likely to be improved by thalamotomy. Depressive symptoms were found in 88 (63 percent), 61 (44 percent) had "a sustained feeling of depression for weeks or months before the interview . . . never reaching the point of suicidal contemplation" (grade II of his scale), 17 (12 percent) had "a sustained feeling of depression severe enough to contemplate suicide and warranting psychiatric treatment at the time of the interview" (grade III), and 10 (7 percent) had mild nonsustained symptoms of depression (grade I). A control group of 140 patients with 30 different conditions also was evaluated, and depression was found in 49 (35 percent). Only 8 were classified as grade II, 0 as grade III, and 41 as grade I. In the PD patients, depression was not related to degree of physical handicap, duration of illness, or age at onset of the disease.

Celesia and Wanamaker (1972) studied a group of 153 patients with a disease duration of 5 years or less in 42, 6 to 10 years in 52, and more than 10 years in 47. Nine of 41 (22 percent) patients in Hoehn and Yahr stages I or II, 29 of 69 (42 percent) in stage III, 17 of 34 (50 percent) in stage IV, and 2 of 9 (22 percent) in stage V were depressed. Severity of depression, according to a three-degree scale modified from Warburton (1967), was not different between the groups, and its presence was unrelated to the age of onset or duration of the motor symptoms. This pattern was in contrast to dementia, which was related to both severity and PD duration. Simultaneous occurrence of dementia and depression was not reported.

Robins (1976) studied 45 patients (3 with parkinsonism from other causes), 10 of whom had undergone thalamotomy or pallidectomy. The number of patients actually depressed was not specified, although it was higher than in a control group of 45 hemiplegics, paraplegics, and a mixture of other conditions even though physical disability was lower in the PD patients. Horn (1974) compared 24 PD patients with 22 paraplegics and 20 healthy controls. There was no mention on the treatment of the patients or of the actual number of subjects who were depressed. Similar to the findings of Robins (1976), MMPI depression scores were highest in the PD group. Depression scores in the PD patients were unrelated to severity of physical handicap, duration of illness, age, or sex.

In conclusion, in advanced and untreated PD, depression occurs in 40 percent to 60 percent of patients, is moderate to severe in the majority of cases, and is unrelated to age at onset and duration or degree of physical disability. Prevalence of depression in this group is higher than in other chronic disabling conditions, although this subject has not been completely clarified.

EFFECTS OF LEVODOPA TREATMENT ON DEPRESSION

Celesia and Wanamaker (1972) followed 35 PD patients for 1 to 2 years who were depressed at the initial examination and subsequently placed on levodopa. In 25 (71 percent) there was a "recurrence of depression," even though the motor signs presumably had improved with treatment. Only 2 nondepressed patients at first examination developed depression during the course of levodopa treatment.

Marsh and Markham (1973) studied 27 patients before and after 3 months and 15 months of levodopa treatment. They found significantly higher depression scores using the MMPI in PD patients compared with a group of healthy controls or physiotherapy patients without neurological disease. These results did not change after levodopa treatment even though the PD patients had a significant improvement in disability scores. Similar results were reported by Shaw and colleagues (1980) after a longer follow-up (6 years) of a large group of PD patients started on levodopa. Although 50 percent of the depressed PD patients had a transient improvement of mood, it was sustained only in a minority. Most patients, however, derived stable benefit from levodopa for motor symptoms. Most of the patients remaining depressed after 6 years of levodopa treatment had a history of pretreatment depression.

Cherington (1970) reported that 6 of 12 PD patients started on levodopa developed depression after several months, necessitating a decrease in the dose. Two of the patients with a previous history of depression attempted suicide. Mindham and associates (1976) reported a low positive correlation between depression and functional disability in a group of 50 untreated PD patients (3 with postencephalitic PD, 8 with unilateral or bilateral thalamotomy). Twenty-four of the patients were depressed. Six months later, after improvement of the physical signs with levodopa, this relationship persisted. A high rate of depression (55 percent) developed during this period, occurring more frequently and requiring lower doses in patients with a history of prior depression.

In summary, despite an initial improvement of mood symptoms, most PD patients with depression continue to be depressed 1 to 6 years after starting levodopa despite improved disability status. A small number of nondepressed patients started on levodopa may develop depression after several months. This is more common in patients with prior depressive episodes and requires lower doses of levodopa.

DEPRESSION IN PD PATIENTS UNDER CHRONIC LEVODOPA TREATMENT

Most recent studies of depression and PD have included patients receiving chronic levodopa treatment, some of them with depression treated using antidepressant drugs. These confounding variables make it difficult to know which symptoms are due to PD and which have been modified by levodopa or antidepressants. Two types of studies have been published. Some evaluated the prevalence of depression in PD patients only once (cross-sectional), and others performed a follow-up evaluation after a variable period of time (longitudinal studies).

Cross-Sectional Studies

Mayeux and colleagues (1981) studied depression and cognitive impairment in a group of 55 PD patients treated with stable doses of levodopa. Ten patients also were treated with antidepressants. Thirty-one healthy controls (spouses of the patients) also were evaluated. Mean duration of disease was 9 years, and patients with overt dementia were excluded. Using the Beck criteria, 47 percent of the patients and 12 percent of the controls rated themselves as significantly depressed (a score on the BDI higher than 10). In addition, 43 percent had depression before the onset of PD. The authors found significant correlations between scores on the BDI and the modified Mini-Mental State examination (MMS) and between the MMS and a PD evaluation form (PDE) (more specifically with bradykinesia and rigidity) but not between the BDI and the PDE. Further, in the 10 patients on antidepressants there was a negative correlation between the BDI and PDE. Depressed patients tended to be younger and to have less physical impairment.

Mayeux and associates (1984) reported two types of depressive disorders (major depression and dysthymia) in a group of 43 PD patients subjected to a dopaminergic drug holiday. Depressed PD patients had low levels of serotonin metabolites in the CSF. Patients with major depression had the lowest levels, and this was most closely related to psychomotor retardation and loss of self-esteem (Mayeux et al, 1986).

Sano and co-workers (1989) reported the coexistence of depression and dementia in 6 of 110 PD patients. Dementia alone was present in 31 (28 percent) and depression alone in 27 (25 percent). Patients with dementia and those with depression-dementia were older, and depressed patients were similar in age to PD patients without any of these disorders. Patients with coexisting depression and dementia had the lowest levels of CSF serotonin metabolites, followed by patients with depression or dementia alone.

Starkstein and associates (1989, 1990b) examined a group of 105 PD patients with a mean disease duration of approximately 10 years. All were treated with levodopa and 13 with antidepressants. The prevalence of depression (major depression and dysthymia) was 41 percent. Patients with onset of PD symptoms before 55 years of age were less motorically impaired, had a longer duration of the disease, and were more often depressed than those with the onset of PD symptoms after age 55. Late-onset patients had significantly more tremor, akinesia, and rigidity than younger patients even though duration of disease was shorter. In early-onset PD patients, depression correlated with cognitive impairment (MMSE), and in late-onset PD patients, depression correlated with functional disability. In 29 percent of the PD patients with major depression, there was a history of depressive symptoms before PD onset.

Hietanen and Terävänen (1988) compared the BDI scores and neuropsychological performance of 49 early-onset PD patients (onset before 60 years of age) with 59 late-onset patients (onset after 60). Mean duration of the disease was 3.5 years. Most patients (68 percent) were untreated. Late-onset patients were more impaired and were more likely to be demented than early-onset patients, but the mean BDI scores did not differ between the two groups (6.2 and 6.3, respectively).

Huber and colleagues (1988) studied 50 levodopa-treated PD patients with a mean disease duration of 5 years. The number of patients actually depressed was not specified. None of the patients met DSM III criteria for dementia. Analysis of the scores on a PD symptom scale, the MMSE, and the HDRS showed that depression scores were unrelated to severity of motor signs or intellectual impairment. The degree of intellectual impairment was positively correlated with severity of bradykinesia and rigidity but negatively correlated with tremor. Subsequently, Huber and colleagues (1990) compared the characteristics of depression as evaluated by the BDI in 53 treated mild PD patients (stages I or II of Hoehn and Yahr) with 50 patients who had moderate to severe disease (stages III or IV). None were taking antidepressants, as in the previous study. Depressive symptoms related to mood and self-reproach appeared to be independent of the severity of PD, whereas vegetative and somatic symptoms generally increased as a function of PD severity.

In summary, studies of patients under long-term levodopa treatment suggest that depression occurs in 40 percent to 65 percent and consists basically of two types: major depression and dysthymia. A history of depression before PD has been reported in 30 percent to 40 percent of the depressed patients. In one study, depression was found more often in patients with an early onset of PD (under 55 years of age) than in patients with later onset of disease, but in another, it occurred similarly among patients with PD onset under and over 60. Generally, there is no relationship between depression and PD signs or functional disability. Breaking down depression into its different symptoms suggests that vegetative and somatic symptoms may be more related to disability than to mood symptoms.

Longitudinal Studies

There are only three studies on this issue. Mayeux and colleagues (1988b) reevaluated depression in a group of 49 chronic levodopa-treated PD patients after a mean follow-up of 2.5 years. One of the 49 patients was lost and 13 died before follow-up. Another 17 could not be examined by the authors, and information was obtained from other sources. They found that depression was still present in 17 of the 21 patients originally depressed.

Brown and associates (1988) reevaluated a group of 132 PD patients 1 year after initial examination. Speed of progression of PD and severity of initial disability were determinants of the course of depression. That is, mildly affected and stable patients had the lowest depression scores initially and at follow-up, whereas severely impaired patients had the highest depression scores on both occasions, even though functional disability had stabilized or slightly improved. Patients with moderate disability and high BDI scores had an improvement of depression if the disease remained stable, whereas in patients with moderate disability and low BDI scores, depression increased if disability worsened.

Starkstein and colleagues (1990a) followed 70 PD patients who had been evaluated at the same institution 3 to 4 years before. Ten patients were taking antidepressants. Depression was defined as a score of 7 or higher on the HDRS. According to the authors, this criterion has an 88 percent specificity for the diagnosis of depression. At follow-up, 14 patients had died, 4 were in nursing homes, and 3 were lost. Patients who were depressed initially (18/49) had a higher risk of developing dementia than those who were not depressed (31/49), even though 10 of the 18 were no longer depressed at follow-up. Eight of the 31 initially nondepressed were depressed at follow-up. Depressed patients showed a faster progression of PD signs, particularly tremor. It was speculated that depression in PD may herald a rapid cognitive decline and a shorter life expectancy. This hypothesis is not consistent with cross-sectional studies that found patients with depression to have the longest duration of PD symptoms (Starkstein et al, 1990b).

In summary, although there is information on the natural history of depression in PD patients under chronic levodopa treatment, results are somewhat inconsistent because of methodological differences in the few reported studies.

CLINICAL SUBTYPES OF PARKINSON'S DISEASE AND DEPRESSION

Several factors suggest that there are distinct clinical subtypes of PD. Age at onset, different patterns of progression and response to medications, variability of cognitive impairment, and involvement of different motor symptoms have suggested that distinct PD groups can be identified. Information on the role of depression in identifying such subgroups is sparse.

Age at Onset of Parkinson's Disease

It has been accepted generally that PD patients with an old age at onset (for most studies, older than 55 to 70 years) have a faster progression, greater cognitive impairment, greater functional disability, more severe bradykinesia and gait impairment, and a generally poorer prognosis than patients with young-onset PD (Lieberman et al, 1979; Zetusky et al, 1985; Mayeux et al, 1988a; Hietanen and Teräväinen, 1988; Starkstein et al, 1989; Diamond et al, 1989; Jankovic et al, 1990). Some authors, however, have not found such differences either clinically or pathologically (Gibb and Lees, 1988).

The relationship between depression and age at onset of PD is more controversial. Two studies found a higher frequency of depression in patients with a younger age at onset (Santamaria et al, 1986; Starkstein et al, 1989), and Mayeux and colleagues (1981) had the same impression. Other studies did not find this difference (Celesia and Wanamaker, 1972; Vogel, 1982; Hietanen and Teräväinen, 1988; Gibb and Lees, 1988; Jankovic et al, 1990) or did not comment on this issue. Thus, age at onset does not appear to be a reliable predictor of depression in PD.

Severity of Motor Involvement

In recent-onset untreated PD patients, disability and PD signs are not related to depression, or they are negatively correlated. In advanced untreated PD patients, most studies have reported no relationship between severity of motor signs and presence or severity of depression, whereas a few found the contrary. Most studies found that improvement of disability with levodopa does not modify the prevalence of depression in PD patients. In chronic levodopa-treated PD patients, there is no relationship between severity of PD motor signs and depression, although some authors reported that this could be different in early and late stages of the disease. Thus, severity of motor symptoms also does not appear to be a reliable predictor of depression in PD.

Family History

A genetic etiology for PD has fallen into some discredit since the publication of very low concordance rates among twins (Ward et al, 1983) and of MPTP-induced parkinsonism (Langston et al, 1983). Although simple mendelian genetic factors do not appear to have a major role, however, more complex genetic factors may be involved. In very young onset PD patients (onset before age 21), there is a frequent family history (Quinn et al, 1987). Zetusky and colleagues (1985) found that 22.5 percent of PD patients have a close relative with the disease. A family history of PD was correlated with younger age at onset, presence of tremor, preservation of mental status, and slower progression of the disease. Depression was not explored in this study, however. Santamaria and associates (1986) found that patients with depression antedating PD clinical signs were more likely to have a family history of PD, a younger age at onset, and relatively less disability.

Prior Depressive Episodes

Depression antedating the onset of PD has been reported often, and its frequency has ranged between 3.2 percent to 20 percent of the patients and 30 percent to 90 percent of those who were depressed at initial interview. Some studies have suggested that when depressed PD patients are followed up after starting levodopa, depression tends to persist, whereas very few of the initially nondepressed patients become depressed. On the other hand, cross-sectional studies of patients under chronic levodopa treatment or with advanced, untreated PD, do not specify when depression started in the 40 percent to 65 percent of patients who are depressed at the time of the study, although 30 percent to 43 percent of them had a previous history of depression.

Although there is some suggestion that depression is helpful in classifying subtypes of PD, subgroups based on family history or prior depressive episodes appear most promising.

COMPARISON WITH OTHER NEUROLOGICAL ILLNESSES

Joffe and colleagues (1987) examined patients with multiple sclerosis (MS) using a systematic psychiatric evaluation. They found past or present major depression (lifetime depression) in 42 percent of the patients, and 13 percent had a bipolar disorder, a figure several times higher than that expected in the general population. The mean BDI score was 11.1, and the mean HDRS score was 8.4. As in PD, severity of depression was unrelated to physical disability, and in the group with lifetime depression, it was negatively correlated. In 7 of the 42 patients with major depression (17 percent), mood changes preceded the clinical onset of MS by more than 2 years, in 25 (60 percent), depression followed the onset of MS by 2 or more years, and in 10 (24 percent), it appeared within the first 2 years after the onset of MS. According to Schiffer (1987), the depressive episodes tend to occur with exacerbations of the disease, but they also can be independent. Patients with MS and bipolar disorders had significantly more relatives with an affective disorder or MS than did unipolar probands with MS or MS patients without an affective disorder (Schiffer et al, 1988). Schiffer and Wineman (1990) also found a weak relationship between neurological disability and BDI scores in a group of 28 MS patients.

Depression has been studied in Alzheimer's disease (AD). Estimates of depression range from 0 to 87 percent (Fischer et al, 1990). The degree of depressed mood in multiinfarct dementia and AD was comparable when assessed by the HDRS (80 percent and 70 percent with a HDRS score higher than 9, respectively). Whereas the HDRS was similar in mild, moderate, and severe cases of multiinfarct dementia, it was significantly lower in severe AD patients, suggesting that as the severity of dementia increases, the severity of depression decreases. Reding and co-workers (1985) performed a prospective study of patients with probable cognitive impairment and found that 57 percent of depressed nondemented elderly patients had developed dementia at a follow-up evaluation 3 years later. Depression was less common when AD was clinically well defined (19 percent). They suggested that depression may be an early manifestation in diseases where dementia later develops.

In summary, depression occurs frequently in progressive CNS disorders, such as MS or AD, and there are differences and similarities between depression in these diseases and PD. Bipolar disorder is practically unseen in PD, contrary to MS, and a decrease in the frequency of depression as the severity of disease increases has been reported only in AD. In all three disorders, depression may antedate the onset of neurological signs.

SUMMARY

There are many unanswered questions regarding depression in PD. Study limitations have prevented definitive conclusions regarding the prevalence of depression in PD compared to other chronic neurological illnesses, the role played by psychological reactions compared to neurobiologic alterations, and the natural history of depression in PD. There is a suggestion that patients in whom depression precedes PD tend to be younger and less impaired and are more likely to have a family history of PD. The natural history of depression in untreated PD is unknown, and this information will not be available since the advent of dopaminergic drugs. Studies evaluating this issue are few, have used old methodology to assess depression, and probably have included about 20 percent of patients who do not have PD at necropsy. Recent studies have included patients treated with dopaminergics as well as antidepressant drugs. Finally, the natural history of mental depression in PD patients under chronic levodopa treatment also is unknown. A detailed prospective study is needed to answer these questions.

REFERENCES

Brown GL, Wilson WP. Parkinsonism and depression. *South Med J.* 1972;65:540–545.
Brown RG, MacCarthy B, Gotham A-M, et al. Depression and disability in Parkinson's disease: a follow-up of 132 cases. *Psychol Med.* 1988;18:49–55.
Celesia GG, Wanamaker WM. Psychiatric disturbances in Parkinson's disease. *Dis Nerv Syst.* 1972;33:577–583.
Cherington M. Parkinsonism, L-dopa and mental depression. *J Am Geriatr Soc.* 1970;18:513–516.
Diamond SG, Markham CH, Hoehn MM, et al. Effect of age at onset on progression and mortality in Parkinson's disease. *Neurology.* 1989;39:1187–1190.
Fischer P, Simanyi M, Danielczyk W. Depression in dementia of the Alzheimer type and in multi-infarct dementia. *Am J Psychiatry.* 1990;147:1484–1487.

Gibb WRG, Lees AJ. A comparison of clinical and pathological features of young- and old-onset Parkinson's disease. *Neurology.* 1988;38:1402–1406.

Gotham A-M, Brown RG, Marsden CD. Depression in Parkinson's disease: a quantitative and qualitative analysis. *J Neurol Neurosurg Psychiatry.* 1986;49:381–389.

Hietanen M, Teräväinen H. The effect of age of disease onset on neuropsychological performance in Parkinson's disease. *J Neurol Neurosurg Psychiatry.* 1988;51:244–249.

Horn S. Some psychological factors in parkinsonism. *J Neurol Neurosurg Psychiatry.* 1974;37:27–31.

Huber SJ, Freidenberg DL, Paulson GW, et al. The pattern of depressive symptoms varies with progression of Parkinson's disease. *J Neurol Neurosurg Psychiatry.* 1990;53:275–278.

Huber SJ, Paulson GW, Shuttleworth EC. Relationship of motor symptoms, intellectual impairment, and depression in Parkinson's disease. *J Neurol Neurosurg Psychiatry.* 1988;51:855–858.

Jankovic J, McDermott M, Carter J, et al. Variable expression of Parkinson's disease: a base-line analysis of the DATATOP cohort. *Neurology.* 1990;40:1529–1534.

Joffe RT, Lippert GP, Gray TA, et al. Mood disorder and multiple sclerosis. *Arch Neurol.* 1987;44:376–378.

Langston JW, Ballard P, Tetrud JW, Irwin I. Chronic parkinsonism in humans due to a product of meperidine analogue synthesis. *Science.* 1983;219:979–980.

Lieberman A, Dziatolowski M, Kuppersmith M, et al. Dementia in Parkinson's disease. *Ann Neurol.* 1979;6:355–359.

Marsh GG, Markham CH. Does levodopa alter depression and psychopathology in parkinsonism patients? *J Neurol Neurosurg Psychiatry.* 1973;36:925–935.

Mayeux R, Stern Y, Côté L, Williams JBW. Altered serotonin metabolism in depressed patients with Parkinson's disease. *Neurology.* 1984;34:642–646.

Mayeux R, Stern Y, Rosen J, Leventhal J. Depression, intellectual impairment, and Parkinson's disease. *Neurology.* 1981;31:645–650.

Mayeux R, Stern Y, Rosenstein R, et al. An estimate of the prevalence of dementia in idiopathic Parkinson's disease. *Arch Neurol.* 1988a;45:260–262.

Mayeux R, Stern Y, Sano M, et al. The relationship of serotonin to depression in Parkinson's disease. *Movement Disord.* 1988b;3:237–244.

Mayeux R, Stern Y, Williams JBW, et al. Clinical and biochemical features of depression in Parkinson's disease. *Am J Psychiatry.* 1986;143:756–759.

Mindham RHS. Psychiatric symptoms in parkinsonism. *J Neurol Neurosurg Psychiatry.* 1970;33:188–191.

Mindham RHS, Marsden CD, Parkes JD. Psychiatric symptoms during L-dopa therapy for Parkinson's disease and their relationship to physical disability. *Psychol Med.* 1976;6:23–33.

Quinn N, Critchley P, Marsden CD. Young onset Parkinson's disease. *Movement Disord.* 1987;2:73–91.

Reding M, Haycox J, Blass J. Depression in patients referred to a dementia clinic: a three-year prospective study. *Arch Neurol.* 1985;42:894–896.

Robins AH. Depression in patients with parkinsonism. *Br J Psychiatry.* 1976;128:141–145.

Sano M, Stern Y, Williams J, et al. *Arch Neurol.* 1989;46:1284–1286.

Santamaria J, Tolosa E, Vallés A. Parkinson's disease with depression: a possible subgroup of idiopathic parkinsonism. *Neurology.* 1986;36:1130–1133.

Schiffer RB. The spectrum of depression in multiple sclerosis: an approach for clinical management. *Arch Neurol.* 1987;44:596–599.

Schiffer RB, Wineman NM. Antidepressant pharmacotherapy of depression associated with multiple sclerosis. *Am J Psychiatry.* 1990;147:1493–1497.

Schiffer RB, Weitkamp LR, Wineman NM, Guttormsen S. Multiple sclerosis and affective disorder. Family history, sex, and HLA-DR antigens. *Arch Neurol.* 1988;45:1345–1348.

Shaw KM, Lees AJ, Stern GM. The impact of treatment with levodopa on Parkinson's disease. *Q J Med.* 1980;49:283–293.

Starkstein SE, Berthier ML, Bolduc PL, et al. Depression in patients with early versus late onset of Parkinson's disease. *Neurology.* 1989;39:1441–1445.

Starkstein SE, Bolduc PL, Mayberg HS, et al. Cognitive impairments and depression in Parkinson's disease: a follow-up study. *J Neurol Neurosurg Psychiatry.* 1990a;53:597–602.

Starkstein SE, Preziosi TJ, Bolduc PL, Robinson RG. Depression in Parkinson's disease. *J Nerv Ment Dis.* 1990b;178:27–31.

Vogel H-P. Symptoms of depression in Parkinson's disease. *Pharmacopsychiatry.* 1982;15:192–196.

Warburton JW. Depressive symptoms in Parkinson patients referred for thalamotomy. *J Neurol Neurosurg Psychiatry.* 1967;30:368–370.

Ward CD, Duvoisin RC, Ince SE, et al. Parkinson's disease in 65 pairs of twins and in a set of quadruplets. *Neurology.* 1983;33:815–824.

Zetusky WJ, Jankovic J, Pirozzolo RJ. The heterogeneity of Parkinson's disease: clinical and prognostic implications. *Neurology.* 1985;35:522–526.

17

Biochemistry of Depression in Parkinson's Disease

MARY SANO AND RICHARD MAYEUX

Depression is a serious and frequent problem for patients with Parkinson's disease (PD). The range of severity of affective disturbance is broad, with both transient mood swings and major depression reported in PD patients. There is much evidence to support a biochemical basis of depression in PD. Involvement of the dopamine system is responsible for the hallmark movement disorders in PD, but it is recognized that degeneration also occurs in other biochemical systems, including the serotonergic and noradrenergic systems. The serotonergic system is important in major depression in general and may have a particular role in PD depression. The catecholamine systems also may be associated with symptoms of depression, such as mood swings and sleep disturbance.

Reports of the frequency of depression in PD vary greatly, perhaps due to the ways in which it is assessed. Different biochemical mechanisms may underlie different aspects of depression, so it is important to define the specific behaviors and to establish criteria for diagnosis. This chapter begins with an overview of the techniques used to assess depression. It then considers the evidence for a biochemical basis of depression and depressive symptoms in PD. Mechanisms that may underlie these disturbances are postulated.

METHODOLOGICAL ISSUES IN ASSESSING DEPRESSION

Several methodological issues must be considered when assessing research on depression in PD. First, it is important to distinguish between specific diagnostic entities (such as major depression or dysthymia) and symptoms of depression, since they may reflect different biochemical mechanisms. This distinction can be made by establishing operational criteria for symptoms and syndromes. The criteria for a diagnosis of major depression require persistent depressed mood or anhedonia. A diagnosis of dysthymia requires intermittent depression or anhedonia (for most of the day) for a period of at least 2 years. These diagnoses require the presence of a subset of other symptoms, including anxiety, feelings of guilt, and vegetative signs, such as sleep and appetite disturbance. Symptoms of depression may be present even when one does not meet criteria for a diagnosis of major depression or dysthymia. These symptoms can be bothersome, even incapacitating. However, they may not reflect the same processes as major depression.

A second issue in assessment is the type of instrument used to gather information about depression. Standardized instruments are required for reliability. However, some instruments are most useful for assessing the presence of symptoms and establishing a diagnosis, whereas others assess symptom severity. Unfortunately, both types of instruments often are used interchangeably. The importance of this issue is illustrated by Gotham and colleagues (1986), who reviewed 14 studies that used different instruments and included over 100 PD patients. The variety of different instruments yielded estimates of depression ranging from 20 percent to 90 percent.

Table 17–1 provides a description of several instruments that can be used to assess aspects of depression. To establish a diagnosis of depressive disorders, the clinical meaningfulness and the persistence of the symptoms must be evaluated. These dimensions typically are not assessed with symptom checklists or symptom scales. Standardized assessments of depression can be achieved with good reliability with semistructured interviews using trained interviewers. Such instruments permit an interactive format and allow the interviewer to ask additional questions to determine if a given response conforms to the intent of diagnostic criteria. The Structured Clinical Interview for DSM III diagnosis-Revised (SCID-R) is a semistructured interview that can be used to assess depressive episodes through out life (Spitzer et al, 1990). This technique is important for the assessment of incidence of depression.

Depression scales, such as the Hamilton Depression Rating Scale (Hamilton, 1960) and the Beck Depression Inventory (Beck et al, 1961), assess the presence and severity of depressive symptoms usually over a brief period of time (i.e., the past week or month). Checklists, such as the Profile of Mood States (POMS) (Guy, 1976) and the 90-item Symptom Checklist (SCL-90) (Derogatis and Cleary, 1977), assess immediate mood. These instruments are sensitive to acute or transient features of depression.

A third issue to consider when assessing studies of depression in PD is the source material. Chart reviews may provide different prevalence estimates than patient interviews because of the different quality of information and may suffer from selection biases. In a retrospective chart review study of 339 patient seen over an 18-month period, 47 percent met criteria for major depression or dysthymia (Sano et al, 1989). However, in-person interviews of patients seen during the same prevalent period yielded a rate of major depression of 37 percent. One explanation for this difference maybe that those with major depression may have been less willing to participate in the interview study. Despite these discrepancies it is evident that depression is common in PD.

ROLE OF SEROTONIN

Serotonin and Depression

Alterations in serotonin have been associated with depression in the absence of PD. Depressed patients have lower cerebrospinal fluid (CSF) concentrations of 5-hydroxy-indoleacetic acid (5-HIAA), a serotonin metabolite, than nondepressed patients (Van Praag and de Haan, 1979; Van Praag, 1982). 5-HIAA also is reduced in the CSF of

Table 17–1. Description of instruments used to assess depression in Parkinson's Disease

Name of Instrument	Type	Utility	Limitations
Schedule for Affective Disorders and Schizophrenia (Endicott and Spitzer, 1978)	Semistructured interview	Derives diagnosis	Time consuming; requires training
Structured Clinical Interview for DSMIIIR (Spitzer et al, 1990)	Semistructured interview	Derives diagnosis	Time consuming (less than SADS); requires training (less than SADS)
Present State Exam (PSE) (Wing et al, 1967)	Structured interview	Derives diagnosis	Assesses past month only; requires training
Hamilton Depression Rating Scale (HDRS) (Hamilton, 1960; Williams, 1988)	Open interview (guide available)	Quantifies severity of depression	Not diagnostic (rates physical symptoms)
Beck Depression Inventory (BDI) (Beck et al, 1961)	Interviewer or self-administered	Quantifies severity of depression	Not diagnostic
Symptom Checklist (SCL-90) (Derogatis and Cleary, 1977)	Self-administered checklist	Measures domains including depression	Not diagnostic
Center for Epidemiological Studies Depression Scale (CES-D) (Raloff, 1977)	Self-administered	Measures symptoms in nonpatient groups	Not diagnostic
Profile of Mood States (POMS) (Guy, 1976)	Self-administered checklist	Measures mood change over brief intervals	Not diagnostic

schizophrenic "suicide attempters" (Ninan et al, 1984) and in the brains of suicide victims (Lloyd et al, 1974). Further, an improvement in depression after treatment with L-5-hydroxytryptophan (5-HTP), the serotonergic precursor, has been reported (Van Praag, 1982). There is a reduction of imipramine binding sites, a presynaptic marker of serotonin, in the brains of patients committing suicide (Stanley et al, 1982).

Parkinson's Disease, Serotonin, and Depression

Serotonin depletion also appears to be related to depression in PD. Patients with PD and depression have lower CSF 5-HIAA than age-matched controls (Mayeux et al, 1984; Kostic et al, 1987). This finding has been reported in both the presence and absence of dopamine agonists (Mayeux et al, 1984, 1988). An alleviation of depression in PD has been observed with oral administration of 5-HTP (Mayeux et al, 1988). These effects were specific, in that treatment was associated with improvements in depression in the absence of changes in parkinsonian symptoms or changes in activities of daily living. Concomitant increases in CSF 5-HIAA (Mayeux et al, 1988) also were observed with this agent. Lowered CSF 5-HIAA has been observed in nondepressed PD patients (Mayeux et al, 1984). This may indicate that an underlying loss of serotonin predisposes some PD patients to depression.

Similar trends can be observed in the results from imipramine binding studies that measure presynaptic serotonergic receptor sites in both platelets and brain (Langer et al, 1987). Correlations between the number of platelet-binding and brain-binding sites in animal studies (Arbilla et al, 1980), suggest that platelet binding may reflect CNS activity. In addition, a study demonstrated that the number of platelet-binding sites correlated with CSF 5-HIAA. Schneider and co-workers (1988) found a 22 percent decrease in the number of imipramine binding sites in PD patients compared to controls. Four of the nine PD patients had either major depression or dysthymic disorder, which may have contributed to the reported difference. Other studies (Raisman et al, 1986) found a lower number of imipramine binding sites in the brains of PD patients even in the absence of depression. We recently reported that imipramine binding sites were reduced in depressed PD patients compared with age-matched controls (Sano et al, 1990). Although not significantly different, nondepressed PD patients had fewer binding sites than controls but more than those in the depressed group. This finding adds further support to the idea of a deficit in the serotonergic system in PD.

Neuroanatomical Correlates of Serotonergic System

CSF levels of metabolites usually are thought to reflect nonspecific changes in brain chemistry, but in suicide victims there is a correlation between CSF 5-HIAA and imipramine binding sites in the frontal cortex (Stanley et al, 1985). Positron emission tomography (PET) studies have suggested the presence of hypometabolism in prefrontal cortex in patients with major depression (Baxter et al, 1989). The frontal lobes may play a role in mood and emotional regulation. Subcortical structures, including the caudate and thalamus, have established connections to frontal cortex, including orbital frontal and prefrontal regions (Alexander et al, 1986), and these connections have been implicated in the cognitive and behavioral changes found in PD and in other basal ganglia diseases (Laplane et al, 1989). Mayberg and colleagues (1990) examined PET activity using 2- [^{18}F]-fluoro-2-deoxy-D-glucose in PD patients with depression. Lower metabolism was found in the caudate and in the inferior orbital–frontal cortex of the depressed PD patients than in the nondepressed PD patients or the control group. Others have reported a relative prefrontal hypometabolism in patients with bilateral lesions of the basal ganglia (Laplane et al, 1989). Many of these cases were initially thought to be depressed, but further examination revealed a picture of apathy with a denial of depressed mood.

Neuropathological studies provide evidence of damage to serotonergic pathways in PD. The dorsal raphe and the median raphe primary ascending serotonergic pathways project to diencephalic and limbic structures (Azmitia and Gannon, 1985) involved in emotion and motivation in both animal models and humans. Postmortem studies indicate a 50 percent loss of large neurons in the dorsal raphe nucleus in PD patients (Jellinger, 1986). In addition, decreased serotonin concentrations have been reported in cortical projection areas from these brainstem structures. Serotonin pathways are present at the level of the locus ceruleus, in and around the interpeduncular nucleus, projecting posteriorly toward the spinal cord (Azmitia and Gannon, 1985; Cooper et al, 1986). Zweig and colleagues (1989) have reported deterioration in this area. However, serotonergic neuron damage is not as pervasive as dopaminergic system damage, and at least in the interpeduncular system, damage is not significantly correlated with dopamine system changes (Zweig et al, 1989).

Other animal studies suggest that levodopa may have a direct effect on regional serotonin turnover. Unilateral lesions of the ascending dopaminergic pathway in rats produced by 6-hydroxydopamine yielded a twofold increase in serotonin turnover in the ipsilateral striatum. Treatment with L-dopa resulted in a 50 percent decrease in turnover of striatal serotonin on the lesioned side (Kerasidis et al, 1990). Deterioration of dopamine pathways presumably is the common pathology in all PD patients. The rat model may explain the small but significant changes in serotonergic activity in PD patients who are not depressed. The serotonin system, particularly the raphe nuclei, degenerates in some PD patients. Damage to multiple serotonergic systems might yield additive effects that can be observed in CSF studies, and depression may occur as a result of these changes.

ROLE OF OTHER NEUROTRANSMITTER SYSTEMS

Role of Dopamine in Mood Fluctuations

Motor fluctuations in Parkinson's disease range from severe PD symptoms (off state) to relatively normal motor function (on state) and presumably are related to striatal dopamine. Patients often report mood swings associated with these on/off phenomena. These shifts in mood are transient and, therefore, different from those seen in major affective disorder. There is some controversy as to whether these disturbances reflect an endogenous response or a reaction to the disability of PD.

Major depression appears unrelated to brain dopamine levels, since there is no correlation between the dopamine metabolite, homovanilic acid (HVA), in CSF and depression in PD patients regardless of treatment status with respect to dopamine agonists (Mayeux et al, 1984, 1988). Transient improvement in depressed mood may accompany the initiation of levodopa treatment in PD patients. Cantello and associates (1986) describe mood fluctuations in PD patients who are taking dopamine agonists. Since these mood changes occur toward the end of the dose interval, when motor function is poor, a role for dopamine in depression was postulated. However, plasma levels of levodopa remain near 50 percent of peak concentrations even when the motor response has worn off, suggesting that the time courses of mood changes and dopamine levels are not associated (Lees, 1989). Stimulation of the dopamine system with methylphenidate causes transient euphoria in controls and in nondepressed PD patients. However, no improvement in mood with methylphenidate occurred in patients with depression and PD matched for duration of illness and disease severity (Cantello et al, 1989).

Others have examined mood shift in PD patients who experience on/off and dyskinesias (Menza et al, 1990) Using a checklist to evaluate mood during these phases, patients tended to report higher levels of depression, anxiety, hostility, and confusion in the off phase, when dopamine levels are low, than in the on phase when dopamine is relatively high. However, the negative symptoms reappeared when the patients experienced dyskinesias, when presumably dopamine levels also are high. This suggests that these mood shifts may be reactions to the motor disturbances in PD and are not linked to dopaminergic fluctuations.

Role of Noradrenaline in Depression

Disturbances in noradrenergic systems have been noted in depression. The dexamethasone suppression test (DST) is considered a biological index of noradrenergic function and may be a biological marker for depression. Depressed patients demonstrate a failure to suppress plasma cortisol after dexamethasone administration, reflecting a disturbance in the hypothalamic-pituitary-adrenal axis. This response is assumed to reflect reduction in noradrenergic regulation of this pathway.

Several reports have indicated dexamethasone suppression in PD patients both with and without behavioral disturbances. Table 17-2 summarizes six studies that examined the dexamethasone suppression test in PD patients. Reports of nonsuppression in PD patients without other behavioral disturbances range from 10 percent to 44 percent. In addition, two separate studies found higher baseline cortisol in the nonsuppressors (Mayeux et al, 1986; Rabey et al, 1990). An underlying alteration in noradrenergic regulation could predispose one to affective disturbance. Higher rates of suppression in depressed than in nondepressed patients with PD have been noted (Pfeiffer et al, 1987; Frochtengaten et al, 1987; Kostic et al, 1990), although this finding is not consistent across studies (Mayeux et al, 1986; Rabey et al, 1990). In a case report of a patient with PD and depression (not included in Table 17-2), Jaeckle and Dilsaver (1986) describe an association between dexamethasone response and symptoms of depression and PD. Before treatment, the patient demonstrated significant depression, moderate to severe extrapyramidal signs, and an abnormal response to the DST. After electroconvulsive therapy (9 bilateral frontotemporal treatments), depressive symptoms and extrapyramidal signs were reduced, and the DST response was normalized. The same pattern was found with treatment with lithium. Overall, it appears that DST is an inconsistent marker of noradrenergic functioning and may not be useful in delineating the role of this transmitter in depression and PD.

Table 17–2. Summary of six studies using Dexamethasone Suppression Test in patients with Parkinson's Disease

Authors	Patient group	Nonsuppressors	Comment
Pfeiffer et al, 1987	15 PD + depression	6 (40%)	
	31 PD only	4 (12%)	
	46 PD total	10 (22%)	
	19 Controls	0	
Mayeux et al, 1986	21 PD + depression	4	Baseline cortisol higher
	28 PD only	11 (39%)	in nonsuppressors
	49 PD total	22 (45%)	
Frochtengarten et al, 1987	35 PD + depression	5 (14%)	
	21 PD only	0	
	56 PD total	5 (9%)	
	27 Controls	1 (4%)	
Kawamura et al, 1987	9 PD total	4 (44%)	Depression not assessed
	8 Controls	0	
Kostic et al, 1990	16 PD + depression	12 (75%)	
	18 PD only	5 (28%)	
	34 PD total	17 (50%)	
	16 Controls	1 (6%)	
Rabey et al, 1990	14 PD + dementia	8 (57%)	Baseline cortisol higher
	18 PD only	9 (50%)	in nonsuppressors
	32 PD total	17 (53%)	
	20 Controls	4 (20%)	

Noradrenergic disturbances are well documented in PD. Postmortem findings in PD patients demonstrate significant changes in the locus ceruleus (LC), the major source of noradrenaline. LC neuron loss in these patients is severe, even among those who have no other behavioral manifestations (Gaspar and Gray 1984; Chan-Pallay and Assan, 1989). LC degeneration has been implicated in the on/off phenomenon after levodopa administration. Reduced CSF dopamine beta-hydroxylase activity has been reported in patients with freezing episodes and PD (Narabayashi et al, 1986). In his review, Sandyk (1989) has proposed that LC degeneration creates a hypersensitivity of noradrenergic receptors, which, in turn, triggers the switch between on and off and indirectly plays a role in associated mood swings and sleep disorders that may accompany depression.

COEXISTING DEPRESSION AND DEMENTIA

Depression and cognitive impairment may coexist in patients with PD. In a retrospective chart review of 339 PD patients, 5.4 percent were noted to have both major depression and dementia. These patients tended to be older and have a later onset of PD (Sano et al, 1989). A prospective study of 115 patients found a similar rate for the coexistence of these two syndromes. Starkstein and colleagues (1989) compared the nature of the cognitive deficits of patients with major depression and PD to a nondepressed PD group matched for age. These authors found poorer performance primarily in timed tasks and in tasks associated with frontal lobe function. These deficits are consistent with finding of decreased measures of metabolism in the frontal cortex

(Mayberg et al, 1990). Depressed patients also had lower Mini-Mental State score and a longer duration of illness.

Several biochemical abnormalities have been noted in both depression and dementia in PD. CSF concentrations of the serotonergic metabolite 5-HIAA are lower in patients with both conditions (Sano et al, 1989). Postmortem studies demonstrate significant neuron loss in the LC, suggesting noradrenergic involvement, in both demented and depressed PD patients (Chan-Pallay and Assan, 1989). However, noradrenergic system changes do not parallel changes in dopaminergic systems, which presumably reflect disease severity. Perhaps in some patients, behavioral disturbances, including depression and dementia, occur with increasing duration of illness because of concomitant disturbances in other biochemical systems rather than because of the severity of the dopaminergic deficit.

CONCLUSIONS AND IMPLICATIONS FOR TREATMENT

Depression is a frequent and serious problem for patients with PD. There is strong biochemical and neuroanatomical evidence to suggest that serotonergic dysfunction plays an important role in major depression. These findings support pharmacological intervention targeted toward this biochemical system. Serotonergic agents, such as fluoxetine, may be particularly useful for the treatment of depression in PD and are worthy of systematic clinical trials. In addition, PD patients may experience significant depressive symptomatology related to their physical condition. These symptoms are less persistent and often respond with improved motor signs. To address these transient, reactive complaints, treatment of the motor signs should be reviewed to determine if the patient is receiving maximum benefit with minimal side effects. Patients might be asked to determine whether there is an association between the severity of motor symptoms and depressive symptoms. They may be able to identify a specific sign or symptom that is most bothersome and that could provide guidance in choosing pharmacological treatment. Unfortunately, depression recurs. In fact, the progressive, degenerative nature of PD predisposes patients to changes in affective state and mood. The effectiveness and need for any treatment strategy must, therefore, be reviewed periodically.

ACKNOWLEDGMENTS

The authors would like to thank their colleagues, Drs. Lucien Coté, Karen Marder, Michael Stanley, Yaakov Stern, and Janet Williams, for their generous contributions to the preparation of this manuscript.

REFERENCES

Alexander GE, Delong MR, Strick PL. Parallel organization of functionally segregated circuits linking basal ganglia and cortex. *Annu Rev Neurosci.* 1986;9:357–381.
Arbilla S, Briley M, Cathala F, et al. Parallel changes in [³H]-imipramine binding sites in cat

brain and platelets following chronic treatment with imipramine. *Proc Biol Psychiatry Soc.* 1980;35:154–155.

Azmitia EC, Gannon P. The serotonergic system: a review of human and animal studies and a report on Macaca fascicularis. In: Fahn S, ed. *Myoclonus.* New York: Raven Press; 1985.

Baxter LR, Schwartz JM, Phelps ME, et al. Reduction of pre-frontal cortex glucose metabolism common to three types of depression. *Arch Gen Psychiatry.* 1989;46:243–250.

Beck AT, Ward CH, Mendelson M, et al. An inventory for measuring depression. *Arch Gen Psychiatry.* 1961;4:53–61.

Cantello R, Aguggia M, Gilli M, et al. Major depression in Parkinson's disease and the mood response to intravenous methylphenidate: possible role of the "hedonic" dopamine system. *J Neurol Neurosurg Psychiatry.* 1989;52:724–731.

Cantello R, Gilli M, Riccio A, Bergamasco B. Mood changes associated with "end-of-dose deterioration" in Parkinson's disease: a controlled study. *J Neurol Neurosurg Psychiatry.* 1986;49:1182–1192.

Chan-Pallay V, Assan E. Alterations in catecholamine neurons of the locus coeruleus in senile dementia of the Alzheimer type and in Parkinson's disease with and without dementia and depression. *J Comp Neurol.* 1989;287:373–392.

Cooper JR, Bloom FE, Roth RH. *The Biochemical Basis of Neuropharmacology,* 5th ed. New York: Oxford University Press; 1986.

Derogatis L, Cleary P. Confirmation of the dimensional structure of the SCL-90: a study in construct validity. *J Clin Psychol.* 1977;33:981–989.

Endicott J, Spitzer RL. A diagnostic interview: the schedule for affective disorders and schizophrenia. *Arch Gen Psychiatry.* 1978;35:837–844.

Frochtengarten ML, Villares JC, Maluf E, Carlini EA. Depressive symptoms and the dexamethasone suppression test in parkinsonian patients. *Biol Psychiatry.* 1987;22:386–389.

Gaspar P, Gray F. Dementia in idiopathic Parkinson's disease. *Acta Neuropathol.* 1984;64:43–52.

Gotham AM, Brown RG, Marsden CD. Depression in Parkinson's disease: a quantitative and qualitative analysis. *J Neurol Neurosurg Psychiatry.* 1986;49:381–389.

Guy W. *ECDEU Assessment Manual for Psychopharmacology,* rev., NIMH Psychopharmacology Research Branch. DHEW pub. no. (ADM) 76-338. Washington, DC: Government Printing Office; 1976.

Hamilton M. A rating scale for depression. *J Neurol Neurosurg Psychiatry.* 1960;23:56–62.

Jaeckle RS, Dilsaver SC. Covariation of depressive symptoms, parkinsonism, and post-dexamethasone plasm cortisol levels in a bipolar patient: simultaneous response to ECT and lithium carbonate. *Acta Psychiatry Scand.* 1986;74:68–72.

Jellinger K. Overview of morphological changes in Parkinson's disease. In: Yahr MD, Bergmann KJ, eds. *Advances in Neurology: Parkinson's disease.* New York: Raven Press; 1986:1–19.

Kawamura T, Kinoshita M, Iwasaki Y, Nemoto H. Low-dose dexamethasone suppression test in Japanese patients with Parkinson's disease. *J Neurol.* 1987;234:264–265.

Kerasidis H, Karstaedt P, Pincus J, et al. Effects of levodopa on regional brain serotonin metabolism in rats with unilateral destruction of the dopamine pathways. *Ann Neurol.* 1990;28:265.

Kostic VS, Djuricic BM, Covickovic-Sternis N, et al. Depression and Parkinson's disease: possible role of serotonergic mechanisms. *J Neurol.* 1987;234:94–96.

Kostic VS, Covickovic-Sternic N, Beslac-Bumbasirevic L, et al. Dexamethasone suppression test in patients with Parkinson's disease. *Movement Disord.* 1990;5:23–26.

Langer SZ, Galzin AM, Poirier MF, et al. Association of the (^{3}H)-imipramine and (^{3}H)-paroxetine binding with the 5HT transporter in brain and platelets: relevance to studies in depression. *J Recept Res.* 1987;7:499–521.

Laplane D, Levasseur M, Pillon B, et al. Obsessive-compulsive and other behavioral changes with bilateral basal ganglia lesions. *Brain.* 1989;112:699–725.

Lees AJ. The on-off phenomenon. *J Neurol Neurosurg Psychiatry.* 1989;(suppl):29–38.

Lloyd KJ, Farley IJ, Deck JHN, Hornykiewicz O. Serotonin and 5-hydroxyindoleacetic acid in discrete areas of the brainstem of suicide victims and control patients. *Adv Biochem Psychopharmacol.* 1974;11:387–397.

Mayberg HS, Starkstein SE, Sadzot B, et al. Selective hypometabolism in the inferior frontal lobe of depressed patients with Parkinson's Disease. *Ann Neurol.* 1990;26:57–64.

Mayeux R, Stern Y, Cote L, Williams JBW. Altered serotonin metabolism in depressed patients with Parkinson's disease. *Neurology.* 1984;34:642–646.

Mayeux R, Stern Y, Sano M, et al. The relationship of serotonin to depression in Parkinson's disease. *Movement Disord.* 1988;3:237–244.

Mayeux R, Stern Y, Williams JBW. Clinical and biochemical features of depression in Parkinson's disease. *Am J Psychiatry.* 1986;143:756–759.

Menza M, Sage J, Marshall E, et al. Mood changes and "On-Off" phenomena in Parkinson's disease. *Movement Disord.* 1990;5:148–151.

Narabayashi H, Kondo T, Yokochi F, Nagatsu T. Clinical effects of L-threo-3,4-dihydroxyphenylserine in cases of parkinsonism and pure akinisia. In: Yahr MD, Bergman KJ, eds. *Advances in Neurology.* New York: Raven Press; 1986;45:593–602.

Ninan PT, Kammen DT van, Schenin M. SF 5-hydroxyindoleacetic acid levels in suicide schizophrenic patients. *Am J Psychiatry.* 1984;141:566–569.

Pfeiffer RF, Hsieh HH, Diercks MJ, et al. Dexamethasone suppression test in Parkinson's disease. *Adv Neurology.* 1987;45:439–442.

Rabey JM, Scharf M, Oberman Z, et al. Cortisol, ACTH, and beta-endorphin after dexamethasone administration in Parkinson's dementia. *Biol Psychiatry.* 1990;27:581–591.

Raisman R, Cash R, Agid Y. Parkinson's disease: decreased density of ^{3}H-imipramine and ^{3}H-paroxetine binding sites in putamen. *Neurology.* 1986;36:556–560.

Radloff L. The CES-D Scale: a self-report depression scale for research in the general population. *Appl Psychol Measurement.* 1977;384–401.

Sandyk R. Locus coeruleus-pineal melatonin interactions and the pathogenesis of the "on-off" phenomenon associated with mood changes and sensory symptoms in Parkinson's disease. *Int J Neurosci.* 1989;49:95–101.

Sano M, Stanley M, Lawton L, et al. ^{3}H-Imipramine binding as a peripheral measure of serotonin in Parkinson's disease. *Neurology.* 1990;40:425.

Sano M, Stern Y, Williams JBW, et al. Coexisting dementia and depression in Parkinson's disease. *Arch Neurol.* 1989;46:1284–1286.

Schneider LS, Chui HC, Severson JA, Sloane RB. Decreased platelet binding in Parkinson's disease. *Biol Psychiatry.* 1988;24:348–351.

Spitzer R, Williams JBW, Gibbon M, First M. Structured clinical interview for DSM-HICR):1, history, rationale, and description. American Psychiatric Press Inc., Washington D.C., 1990.

Stanley M, Traskman-Bendz L, Dorovini-Zis K. Correlations between aminergic metabolites simultaneously obtained from human CSF and brain. *Life Sci.* 1985;37:1279–1286.

Stanley M, Virgilio J, Gershon S. Tritiated imipramine binding sites are decreased in the frontal cortex of suicides. *Science.* 1982;216:1337–1339.

Starkstein SE, Preziosi TJ, Berthier ML, et al. Depression and cognitive impairment in Parkinson's disease. *Brain.* 1989;112:1141–1153.

Van Praag HM. Depression. *Lancet.* 1982;2:1259–1264.

Van Praag HM, de Haan S. Central serotonin metabolism and frequency of depression. *Psychiatr Res.* 1979;1:219–224.

Williams JBW. A structured interview guide for the Hamilton depression rating scale. *Arch Gen Psychiatry.* 1988;45:742–747.

Wing JK, Eirley JLP, Cooper JE, et al. Reliability of a procedure for measuring and classifying "Present Psychiatric State" *Br J Psychiatry.* 1967;113:499–515.

Zweig RM, Jankel WR, Hedreen JC, Mayeux R. The pedunculopontine nucleus in Parkinson's disease. *Ann Neurol.* 1989;26:41–46.

18

Drug Treatment of Depression in Parkinson's Disease

JONATHAN M. SILVER AND STUART C. YUDOFSKY

Patients who suffer from Parkinson's disease (PD) may develop depressive symptoms that, in addition to being distressing to the individual, interfere with social, occupational, and cognitive functioning. This chapter deals with the psychopharmacological treatment of depression that occurs in patients with PD. Strategies to use antidepressant medications effectively and to minimize the side effects are discussed. Although the decision to start pharmacotherapy does not exclude other therapeutic modalities, such as psychotherapy and cognitive and behavioral therapies, these are not discussed in this chapter (Silver et al, 1990c). A discussion of electroconvulsive therapy in PD patients is found in Chapter 19.

PATHOPHYSIOLOGY OF PARKINSON'S DISEASE AND DEPRESSION

Similar neurotransmitter systems are involved in both depression and PD. Therefore, psychopharmacological treatment of depression may affect the motoric symptoms of PD, and likewise, those medications used to treat the movement disorder of PD, may affect mood. The neurotransmitters dopamine, norepinephrine, serotonin, and acetylcholine are decreased in PD patients (Chapter 2), and all have been hypothesized to play a role in the etiology of depressive disorders (Siever, 1987; Jimerson, 1987; Meltzer and Lowy, 1987; Janowsky and Risch, 1987). In patients with PD, a decrease in serotonin function is related to the severity of psychomotor retardation and loss of self-esteem (Mayeux et al, 1988). Slowing of mental processes (bradyphrenia) is correlated with decreased CSF levels of the norepinephrine metabolite 3-methoxy-4-hydroxyphenylene glycol (MHPG) (Mayeux et al, 1987). Wolfe and colleagues (1990) compared CSF levels of the dopamine metabolite homovanillic acid (HVA) in patients with PD, Alzheimer's disease, and major depression. They found that regardless of diagnosis, low HVA levels were associated with extrapyramidal motor symptoms, cognitive slowing, and more severe depression.

Treatment of the motoric symptoms of PD involves the use of medications that increase dopaminergic activity (i.e., dopamine agonists, such as L-dopa, bromocrip-

Table 18-1. Relative potencies of selected antidepressant drugs at receptors

Drug	Reuptake inhibition			Receptor Binding Affinity		
	Norepinephrine	Serotonin	Dopamine	Cholinergic	Histamine (H$_1$)	Adrenergic (alpha$_1$)
Imipramine	5[a]	3	10	5	3	7
Amitriptyline	6	2	4	1	2	2
Doxepin	7	8	6	4	1	1
Trimipramine	9	9	5	3	2	3
Desipramine	1	7	7	9	6	9
Nortriptyline	4	6	–	6	4	5
Protriptyline	2	6	3	2	5	10
Maprotiline	3	10	8	7	–	7
Amoxapine	3	4	1	8	–	4
Trazodone	11	5	11	12	7	6
Fluoxetine	8	1	9	10	–	11
Bupropion	10	11	2	11	–	12

[a]Numbers are relative ranking from most potent to least potent: 1 indicates most potent.
Adapted from Baldessarini. *Chemotherapy in Psychiatry: Principles and Practice.* Harvard University Press, 1985. Reproduced with permission from Silver and Yudofsky, 1988.

tine, amantadine) and decrease cholinergic activity (i.e., anticholinergic drugs, such as trihexyphenidyl). In addition, L-dopa increases noradrenergic activity but decreases serotonin turnover (Van Woert and Bowers, 1970). Antidepressant drugs acutely stimulate the serotonergic and catecholaminergic systems in the central nervous system and chronically increase receptor sensitivity of these systems. Antidepressants have weak inhibitory effects on the reuptake of dopamine. Bupropion, a novel nonheterocyclic antidepressant, has dopamine agonist properties. The relative affinities of the antidepressants in the inhibition of presynaptic reuptake of serotonin (5-HT) or norepinephrine (NE) are listed in Table 18-1. Because of the effects of these neurotransmitters on mood and motor function, it is likely that antiparkinsonian drugs may affect mood and that antidepressant drugs may affect the motoric and other symptoms of PD.

SUBTYPES OF DEPRESSION IN PARKINSON'S DISEASE

There are several subtypes of patients who have both PD and depressive symptoms (Table 18-2). The motoric symptoms of PD may or may not be under adequate control, and there may be a full or partial depressive syndrome. The partial depressive

Table 18-2. Subtypes of Parkinson's Disease and depression

Subtype	Parkinson's disease	Depressive syndrome
I	Treated and controlled	Partial syndrome
II	Treated and uncontrolled	Partial syndrome
III	Treated and controlled	Full syndrome
IV	Treated and uncontrolled	Full syndrome
V	Not treated and mild	Full syndrome

Table 18–3. Symptoms in full and partial depressive syndrome in patients with Parkinson's disease

Symptom	Full syndrome	Partial syndrome
Depressed mood	Present	Present
Lack of reactivity	Present	Absent
Diminished interest	Present	Can be motivated
Loss of appetite	Present	Absent
Sleep disorder	Present	Present
Fatigue	Present	Present, but patient can become involved
Guilt	Present	Absent
Decreased concentration	Present	Short-term memory intact
Suicidal thoughts	Present	Absent

syndrome in PD patients includes the symptoms of apathy and low arousal, but without anhedonia, guilt, or suicidal ideation, which frequently accompany major depression disorder (Table 18–3). Investigators have found no difference in the frequency of anergia, motor retardation, and early morning awakening in a group of PD patients with and without major depressive disorder (Sano et al, 1990; Starkstein et al, 1990a). If the depression is severe and incapacitating or there is suicidal ideation, immediate antidepressant treatment should be considered, including the use of electroconvulsive therapy (Chapter 19). The general steps in treating patients with depression and PD include reevaluation of antiparkinsonian medications, consideration of the effects of specific antidepressants on PD symptoms, and consideration of the side effects and dosing strategy for the chosen antidepressant.

EFFECT OF ANTIPARKINSONIAN MEDICATIONS ON MOOD

Because of the significant effects that antiparkinson drugs have on mood, a reevaluation of the prescribed antiparkinsonian drugs should be conducted before starting antidepressant medication. Psychotic symptoms may result from treatment with dopamine agonist medications, such as L-dopa, L-dopa/carbidopa (Sinemet), bromocriptine (Parlodel), and amantadine (Symmetrel), but they may result also from treatment with anticholinergic drugs. This latter category of drugs can cause disturbed sleep, hallucinations, mania, and delusions. The effects of antiparkinsonian drugs on memory, thought, and perception are covered elsewhere in Chapters 22 and 23.

L-Dopa may cause depression in patients with PD (Gangat et al, 1986; Damasio et al, 1971; Mindham et al, 1976). Patients with a previous history of affective disorders or other psychiatric illness are at higher risk of L-dopa causing additional mood problems (Damasio et al, 1971; Mindham et al, 1976). There is a correlation between depression in patients with early-onset left hemi-Parkinson's disease and higher doses of L-dopa (Starkstein et al, 1990a). Although L-dopa/carbidopa was effective in the treatment of depression in a small number of patients who did not have PD (Matussek et al, 1970; Goodwin et al, 1970), it was not as effective as tricyclic antidepressants (Goodwin et al, 1970). Andersen and colleagues (1980) have suggested that L-dopa may not be an effective antidepressant in patients with PD since L-dopa decreases serotonin turnover in addition to increasing norepinephrine turnover. Therefore, in depressed patients who require treatment with L-dopa, an antidepressant may reverse the effect of L-dopa on serotonin.

Bromocriptine (Parlodel) has been investigated as a treatment for several psychiatric disorders (Sitland-Marken et al, 1990). At low dosages, bromocriptine stimulates the presynaptic dopamine autoreceptor and inhibits the release of dopamine. At higher dosages, there is stimulation of the postsynaptic dopamine receptor and an increase in dopaminergic transmission. Preliminary data indicate that bromocriptine may have beneficial antidepressant effects (Sitland-Marken et al, 1990). Depressive and PD symptomatologies significantly improved in a group of 10 depressed PD patients who received high doses of bromocriptine (85 to 220 mg/day), although changes in motoric symptoms and depression were not correlated (Jouvent et al, 1983).

Amantadine, which is used as an initial treatment in mild PD in conjunction with L-dopa, has psychotropic activity. In a group of hospital workers who were taking amantadine for influenza prophylaxis and who reported emotional symptoms, 47 percent had elevation of mood, 41 percent had a worsening of mood, a decrease in energy, or hypersomnia, and 17 percent had fluctuations in mood (Flaherty and Bellur, 1981). A study examining elderly patients suffering from psychomotor deterioration found that amantadine treatment alleviated symptoms of depression, motor and intellectual impairment, and problems with short-term memory (Bavazzano et al, 1980).

Anticholinergic drugs that are administered to PD patients (e.g., biperiden, trihexylphenidyl) can be effective antidepressants (Kasper et al, 1981; Jimerson et al, 1982). Central cholinergic mechanisms may be involved in the pathophysiology of depression and are important in the overall modulation of the behavioral effects of stress (Dilsalver and Coffman, 1989; Janowsky and Risch, 1987).

Monoamine oxidase inhibitors (MAOI) intensify monoaminergic transmission by blocking the catabolism of several biogenic amines, including norepinephrine and serotonin (for MAO type A), and dopamine (for MAO type B). Deprenyl (Selegeline, Eldepryl) is a selective inhibitor of monoamine oxidase B that is used as an adjunct to L-dopa in the treatment of PD. At doses greater than 20 mg/day for the average size male, deprenyl is no longer a selective MAO B inhibitor but inhibits MAO A as well as MAO B. In addition, deprenyl is metabolized to amphetamine and methamphetamine, both of which may elevate mood (Karoum et al, 1982). Deprenyl is effective in the treatment of patients with depression (without PD) only when administered in dosages of 30 mg/day or greater (inhibition of both MAO A and MAO B). However, it is not effective when prescribed at 10 mg/day (inhibition of only MAO B) (Quitkin et al, 1984; Mann et al, 1989). Tariot and colleagues (1987) administered deprenyl to patients with dementia of the Alzheimer's type who were not depressed. They found that administration of 10 mg/day decreased anxiety, tension, and excitement and resulted in increased activity and social interactions. This effect was not seen when patients received 40 mg/day of deprenyl.

Deprenyl may have beneficial effects on mood in patients with PD. Eisler and colleagues (1981) found that 6 of 11 patients on deprenyl 10 mg and L-dopa/carbidopa had an elevation of mood. Although Tetrud and Langston (1989) found no change in depression scores when deprenyl 10 mg was given to PD patients, the results of the Parkinson Study Group (1989) showed that patients on deprenyl had an enhanced sense of well-being, as indicated by improved scores on the mental scale of the Unified Parkinson's Disease Rating Scale. These two studies treated PD patients who did not yet require L-dopa. Przuntek and colleagues (1989) treated 30 patients with deprenyl in addition to L-dopa/carbidopa. Deprenyl significantly improved both PD symptoms and depression. Interestingly, there was "more pronounced improvement of motor disability in depression patients" but no correlation between improvement in motor disability and depression.

These studies suggest that L-dopa may exacerbate depressive symptoms, and other antiparkinsonian medications may alleviate depression. Therefore, when a patient has depression coincident with PD, lowering the dosage of Sinemet (L-dopa/carbidopa) and using low dosages of several antiparkinsonian drugs (i.e., bromocriptine, aman-tadine, and deprenyl) may be effective in treating both depression and the motoric symptoms of PD.

PD PATIENT WITHOUT FULL DEPRESSIVE SYNDROME

PD patients may have diminished arousal and drive that are due to a deficiency of dopamine. They may, therefore, appear depressed but do not have the full depressive syndrome (Taylor and Saint-Cyr, 1990) (Table 18–3). A recent examination of the personality characteristics of PD patients revealed that they had the characteristics of low dopamine state, that is, low novelty seeking behavior (orderly, stoic, slow-tem-pered, rigid) (Cloninger, 1987; Menza et al, 1990). When the full depressive syndrome is present in PD patients, there can be prominent anhedonia, guilt, suicidal ideation, and loss of libido (Sano et al, 1990; Starkstein et al, 1990b). In the partial depressive syndrome, the patient has low arousal and apathy but is cooperative and responsive to the environment, maintains short-term memory, lacks feelings of guilt and negative self-worth, and exhibits motivated and socially sensitive behavior (Taylor and Saint-Cyr, 1990). For this group of patients (subtypes I and II in Table 18–2), the initial step in pharmacotherapy should be an optimization of the antiparkinsonian medications before the initiation of antidepressant medications.

Patients with early-onset PD develop depression that is correlated with cognitive impairment and duration of disease, whereas those patients with late-onset PD develop depression that is correlated with impairment in activities of daily living. This latter group has more severe motoric symptoms of PD (Starkstein et al, 1989, 1990a). This finding suggests that the initial treatment of patients with late-onset PD and depression should be focused on optimization of antiparkinsonian medications, since motoric symptoms and depressive symptoms may both result from a hypodopami-nergic state (Wolfe et al, 1990). In patients with early-onset PD, depression may result from a decrease in serotonergic transmission, and require antidepressant medications.

PD PATIENTS WITH FULL DEPRESSIVE SYNDROME

If the patient maintains a full depressive syndrome after adjustment of antiparkinso-nian medications (subtypes III and IV in Table 18–2) or if the patient has depression of sufficient severity that immediate psychiatric intervention is necessary, the addition of antidepressant medications may be effective. Several studies have examined the effect of antidepressants on mood and PD symptoms in patients concurrently treated with L-dopa. These are summarized as follows. Nortritptyline was administered in a double-blind, placebo-controlled crossover study to 19 PD patients with depression who were treated concomitantly with L-dopa (Andersen et al, 1980). The dosage of nortriptyline was increased to 150 mg/day, and a plasma level was obtained if side effects occurred to ensure that nortriptyline levels were within the therapeutic range. Although there was no change in motoric symptoms, depression scores significantly improved. The most frequent side effect was orthostatic hypotension.

Buproprion, a nonheterocyclic antidepressant that has indirect dopamine agonist effects, was administered at a maximum dosage of 450 mg/day for 9 weeks to 20 PD patients who were treated with L-dopa (19 patients) or trihexyphenidyl (1 patient) (Goetz et al, 1984). Ten patients had at least a 30 percent decrease in motoric symptoms. Although no diagnostic interviews or ratings were performed for the presence of depression, the authors stated that the mood of 5 of 12 patients with depression improved after buproprion administration. Four of these patients had a 30 percent decrease in motoric symptoms. In 2 patients, the antidepressant and antiparkinsonian effects occurred simultaneously, whereas in 3 patients, the antidepressant effects occurred earlier and was more dramatic than the antiparkinsonian effects. Side effects consistent with increased dopamine activity limited the use of buproprion, and these included nausea, vomiting, restlessness, postural tremor, hallucinations, confusion, and dyskinesias.

Buspirone is an anxiolytic drug that has mixed dopamine agonist and antagonist properties. It may have antidepressant effects when administered in dosages of 45 to 60 mg/day (Fabre, 1990). Ludwig and associates (1986) assessed the effects of buspirone in 16 PD patients in a double-blind placebo crossover study. Placebo was administered for 6 weeks, and buspirone, in doses ranging from 10 mg to 100 mg/day, was given for 12 weeks. Doses of buspirone between 10 and 60 mg had no effect on PD symptoms. The 100 mg dose decreased dyskinesias but increased ratings of PD disability, tension, insomnia, lightheadedness, and anxiety. Buspirone had no effect on depression at any dose administered.

Mayeux and colleagues (1988) administered the serotonin precursor, 5-hydroxy-tryptophan (5HTP) to seven patients with PD and major depression. All patients were treated concomitantly with L-dopa. An initial dose of 75 mg/day was increased by 25 mg every 3 days until the depression improved or the patient received 500 mg/day. The final dose of 5HTP was maintained for 4 months. Improvement in depression, as rated on the Hamilton Depression Scale, was documented in six patients. One patient who did not respond received electroconvulsive therapy with good results.

These studies indicate that antidepressants that modulate serotonergic activity are effective in treating depression in PD patients. Not only do PD patients with depression have low levels of the serotonin metabolite 5-hydroxyindole acetic acid (5HIAA) in the CSF (Mayeux et al, 1988), but L-dopa decreases serotonergic turnover (Van Woert and Bowers, 1970). However, antidepressants that predominantly affect the noradrenergic system still result in changes in the serotoninergic system. Therefore, it appears that most antidepressants should be effective in treating the full depressive syndrome that occurs in patients with PD.

TREATMENT OF PATIENTS WITH UNTREATED MILD PARKINSON'S DISEASE AND DEPRESSION

In many instances, the psychiatrist or geriatrician is asked to evaluate a patient who has depression and concurrent mild, untreated motoric symptoms of PD (subtype V, Table 18–2). For these patients, the clinician may be able to treat both the depressive and the mild motoric symptoms with a single medication. Studies have been performed on the effects of antidepressants on the symptoms of PD in patients who are not receiving L-dopa. Most of these reports were published before L-dopa was in accepted clinical use. Although focusing primarily on the response of motoric symptoms, comments and observations were made also about the response of emotional symptoms in those patients who are depressed. Strauss (1959) treated six depressed PD patients with imipramine 150 mg/day. Five patients "profited greatly from the use of the drug," although there was no change in tremor or akinesia in any patient. When Mandell and co-workers (1961) administered imipramine (doses up to 250 mg for 4 to 5 weeks) to 15 PD patients, 5 patients exhibited no improvement, 5 patients had mild improvement, and 5 patients had "dramatic" improvement in motoric symptoms of PD. This last group were all "quite depressed." The authors concluded that the "group of patients with predominately akinesias, rigidity, inertia, depression, irritability, and severe functional impairment" were the most responsive to imipramine. Definite improvement in motoric symptoms was observed in 63 percent of 68 patients with PD who were treated with imipramine (up to 150 mg for 4 weeks) (Gillhespy and Mustard, 1963). Fourteen patients had PD and depression, and 11 of these patients had improvement in both motoric and mood symptoms, although some patients had an amelioration of PD symptoms without exhibiting antidepressant effects.

In a 2-week double-blind crossover study of imipramine (150 mg) and placebo in eight nondepressed PD patients, two patients improved and three were greatly improved (Denmark et al, 1961). Two patients had mild mood elevation. Strang (1965) reported results of the treatment of 70 PD patients who received imipramine (up to 100 mg) or placebo. Fifty-three percent of patients had improvement in motoric symptoms. Of 20 patients with depression and PD, 12 improved. Three of 10 patients with moderate to good improvement of rigidity had no improvement of moderate to severe depression, and 4 of 12 patients who had improvement of depression had no improvement in motoric symptoms of PD. The clinical response of motoric symptoms was most often within 2 to 3 days. Laitinen (1969) administered desipramine (100 mg for 3 weeks) to 39 PD patients in a double-blind placebo-controlled study. One half of the patients on desipramine and 16 percent of the patients on placebo had a "good" (greater than 30 percent) response of the PD symptoms. Of the 10 patients who received desipramine and responded, 9 had improvements in depression or fatigue. In the placebo group, only 5 of 19 had improvement in depression.

These studies indicate that antidepressants may be of benefit in the treatment of PD if patients are not receiving L-dopa, possibly through the effect of the antidepressant on inhibition of the synaptic reuptake of dopamine (Andersen et al, 1980). Although it is possible that therapeutic effects were a result of the anticholinergic effects of the antidepressants, desipramine, which has relatively low anticholinergic properties, also was effective. Several medications may be initiated for the patient with mild untreated PD who is depressed. These include the tricyclic antidepressants, the selective MAO B inhibitor deprenyl that may increase dopaminergic activity, and the novel antidepressant buproprion that has dopamine agonist properties.

SIDE EFFECTS OF ANTIDEPRESSANTS

The choice of which antidepressant medication to use is most dependent on the side effect profile of the drug. For PD patients, the most important factors include orthostatic hypotension, anticholinergic effects, and extrapyramidal effects.

Orthostatic Hypotension

Patients with PD may have significant orthostatic hypotension—either from PD or as a side effect from medications such as L-dopa—that may be dangerously increased with the addition of antidepressant medication. Orthostatic hypotension is the cardiovascular side effect that most commonly results in serious morbidity, especially in the elderly and in patients with congestive heart failure (Glassman and Bigger, 1981; Glassman et al, 1983). The symptoms of orthostatic hypotension usually consist of dizziness or lightheadedness when the patient changes from a lying to sitting or sitting to standing position. Glassman and Bigger (1981) reported a physical injury rate of 4 percent in patients with an average age of 60 years who were treated with imipramine. These injuries included fractures and lacerations requiring sutures. Although orthostatic hypotension may occur from any heterocyclic antidepressant, nortriptyline has been found to cause less orthostatic hypotension than imipramine (Roose et al, 1981). Although this side effect usually correlates with the ability of these drugs to bind to the alpha$_1$-adrenergic receptor, trazodone can also cause orthostatic hypotension and dizziness (Glassman, 1984) (Table 18–1). No significant orthostatic hypotension occurred in 10 depressed patients with congestive heart failure who were treated with buproprion (average dose 445 mg/day) (Roose et al, 1987).

Anticholinergic Effects

Patients with PD have decreased cholinergic function, especially those patients with PD and dementia (Perry et al, 1983). When a group of patients with PD and dementia was treated with anticholinergic medications, 93 percent developed confusion, as compared with 46 percent who did not receive anticholinergic medications (De Smet et al, 1982). However, even nondemented PD patients had increased frontal lobe dysfunction when treated with anticholinergic medications (Dubois et al, 1990). Because PD patients frequently are treated with anticholinergic drugs, the addition of antidepressants with prominent anticholinergic properties will further impair cognition.

The antidepressant drugs vary greatly in their relative potential to produce anticholinergic side effects. The relative potency to which these drugs bind to the cholinergic receptor is listed in Table 18–1. Drugs, such as amitriptyline and protriptyline, have high affinities for the muscarinic receptors, whereas desipramine has approximately $\frac{1}{10}$ and trazodone has $\frac{1}{20,000}$ the muscarinic affinity of amitriptyline (Richelson, 1983). Therefore, antidepressants with low anticholinergic properties should be used.

Nortriptyline and desipramine are the heterocylcic drugs with the lowest anticholinergic activity. Of the novel antidepressants, fluoxetine, trazodone, and buproprion all have minimal or no anticholinergic action.

Extrapyramidal Effects of Antidepressants

Antidepressant medications have been reported to cause PD symptoms in depressed patients. The antidepressant that most frequently causes EPS is amoxapine, which is metabolized to the dopamine receptor blocking drug loxapine (Thornton and Stahl, 1984) and, therefore, should not be used to treat PD patients. Fluoxetine, a specific serotonin reuptake inhibitor, has been reported to cause PD symptoms, including tremor, akathisia, resting tremor, bradykinesia, rigidity, and dystonia Meltzer et al, 1979; (Bouchard et al, 1989). Bouchard and colleagues (1989) noted "unpublished observations of deterioration of parkinsonian patients receiving selective serotonin reuptake inhibitors that have been tried (Upstene) or are currently in use (Floxyfral) in France." The serotonin-specific antidepressants may produce enhanced serotonergic activity in the striatum that subsequently inhibits dopaminergic function and exacerbates PD symptoms (Waldmeier and Delini-Stula, 1979). Buproprion, through its mild dopaminergic agonist activity, may produce symptoms of increased dopaminergic function, that is, dyskinesias and psychosis. Lithium may produce extrapyramidal symptoms (Tyrer et al, 1980), including dyskinesias and hallucinations, when given in combination with L-dopa (Coffey et al, 1984). The nonselective MAO inhibitor phenelzine also has been reported to cause extrapyramidal symptoms, including bradykinesia, tremor, and rigidity (Teusink et al, 1984; Gillman and Sandyk, 1986). Nonselective MAO inhibitors should not be administered with L-dopa because of the risk of hypertensive crises.

Antidepressants, such as desipramine and imipramine, that affect predominantly the noradrenergic system, may produce a resting tremor and thereby exacerbate the tremor of PD. Dose reduction or changing the type of antidepressant ultimately may be required to alleviate the tremor, but treatment with a beta-adrenergic blocking drug (e.g., propranolol) usually provides symptomatic relief.

GUIDELINES FOR USE OF ANTIDEPRESSANTS FOR PD PATIENTS

The use of antidepressant medication in the treatment of the patient with PD and major depression must be guided by scientific principles tailored to the specific needs of individual patients (Silver and Yudofsky, 1988). Selected antidepressant drugs and dosages are listed in Table 18–4. A summary of the use of antidepressants in the treatment of PD patients is found in Table 18–5. Patients with neurological disease are more sensitive to the side effects of all medications, including antidepressants (Silver et al, 1990b,c). For this reason, antidepressant drugs are started at low dosages and slowly increased until clinical response or the recommended dosage is reached. Because of the frequent problems of PD patients with hypotension and dementia, those antidepressants with fewest effects on those systems should be prescribed, for example, nortriptyline or desipramine. Buproprion has few anticholinergic or cardiac effects and may improve PD symptoms, but there is the risk of increasing dyskinesia

Table 18–4. Selected antidepressant drugs and dosages

Class and generic name	Trade name	Usual daily maximum oral dose (mg)
Teritary amine tricyclics		
Imipramine	Tofranil	300
	Tofranil PM	
	SK-Pramine	
	Janimine	
Amitriptyline	Elavil	300
	Endep	
Doxepin	Adapin	300
	Sinequan	
Trimipramine	Surmontil	200
Secondary amine tricyclics		
Desipramine	Norpramin	300
	Pertofrane	
Nortriptyline	Aventyl	150
	Pamelor	
Protriptyline	Vivactyl	60
Tetracyclic		
Maprotiline	Ludiomil	200
Dibenzoxazepine		
Amoxapine	Asendin	400
Triazolopyridine		
Trazodone	Desyrel	600
Bicyclic		
Fluoxetine	Prozac	60
Unicyclic		
Buproprion	Wellbutrin	450

From Silver et al. In: Stoudemire, ed. *Clinical Psychiatry for Medical Students.* JB Lippincott Co, 1990.

Table 18–5. Guidelines for use of antidepressants in Parkinson's disease

1. Reevaluate antiparkinsonian medications
2. Categorize subtype of parkinson's disease and depression based on the severity and response of PD symptoms to treatment and the presence of a full or partial depressive syndrome (Table 18–2)
3. For subtypes I and II (and III and IV if depression is not severe), consider lowering the dosage of L-dopa/carbidopa (Sinemet) and using other dopamine agonists
4. For subtypes III and IV, use antidepressant medications with low anticholinergic effects and low incidence of orthostatic hypotension; preferred tricyclic antidepressants are nortriptyline and desipramine; if buproprion is used, watch for increased dopaminergic function; if fluoxetine is used, watch for increased PD symptoms; if trazodone is used, watch for orthostatic hypotension
5. For subtype V, consider the tricyclics nortriptyline and desipramine, buproprion, and deprenyl
6. Start at relatively low dosages (i.e., nortriptyline 10 mg bid) and increase slowly (i.e., by 10 mg every third day); the usual full therapeutic dosage ultimately may be required; monitor plasma levels when appropriate
7. Maintain the patient on antidepressants for at least 6 months after full therapeutic effect has been obtained

The authors express their appreciation to Barry Fogel, M.D., for his suggestions on categorization and treatment strategy.

and psychosis. Deprenyl, at dosages that maintain MAO B selectivity, may improve mood and prolong the time that a patient with mild PD may not need L-dopa. These two drugs (buproprion and deprenyl) may be particularly effective in the treatment of the depressed patient with mild untreated PD. Trazodone and fluoxetine have no anticholinergic effects and should, therefore, have little adverse effects on cognition. The full effectiveness of these two medications has yet to be explored adequately, and they may prove to be effective and safe antidepressants for PD patients. However, trazodone may produce hypotension, and fluoxetine may exacerbate PD symptoms in certain patients.

A complete trial of antidepressant medications consists of treatment with therapeutic doses of a drug for a total of 6 weeks, 3 of which should be at the maximum tolerated therapeutic dosage or the appropriate plasma level. No study has been performed as to whether PD patients with depression require long-term treatment with antidepressant medication. Therefore, in accordance with the usual therapeutic practice for patients with depression who do not have PD, antidepressant medications should be continued for at least 6 months after therapeutic response is obtained before tapering of the drug is attempted.

Although monitoring of plasma levels may not be necessary in the treatment of most patients, the clinician may prefer that an antidepressant with therapeutically meaningful levels be used. This may prove to be invaluable if a patient does not respond to a trial with standard doses of an antidepressant. The first-pass effect and hepatic metabolism of the heterocyclic antidepressants result in wide variation of plasma levels among patients. Because of this, clinicians must be concerned that the administered dosage may be sufficient to determine that an adequate therapeutic trial has occurred. Although many studies have been performed to assess the value of plasma level monitoring for the therapeutic use of the antidepressant drugs, plasma level studies have focused primarily on three antidepressants: imipramine, nortriptyline, and desipramine. The APA Task Force on the Use of Laboratory Tests in Psychiatry (1985) has developed guidelines for the use of plasma level monitoring. It should be noted, however, that these studies were conducted on patients with major depressive disorder that were not complicated by the presence of concomitant neurological disorders. We, therefore, have no recourse but to assume that many patients with depression and PD will require the usual therapeutic dosage of antidepressants. For an adequate therapeutic trial, plasma levels of imipramine and the desmethyl metabolite (desipramine) should be greater than 200 to 250 ng/ml, and desipramine levels should be greater than 125 ng/ml. A therapeutic window has been observed for nortriptyline, with optimal response between 50 and 150 ng/ml. Levels should be monitored after the drug has reached steady state (5 to 7 days) and approximately 10 to 14 hours after the last dose has been administered.

PD PATIENTS WITH DEPRESSION WITH ANXIETY

Many patients with PD and depression also have symptoms of anxiety and panic (Schiffer et al, 1988). Heterocyclic antidepressants, such as nortriptyline, desipramine, and imipramine, and the nonheterocyclic drug fluoxetine can all be effective in the treatment of panic disorder (Silver and Yudofsky, 1988). In the initial phases of treatment, patients with panic disorder also may be very sensitive to the uncomfortable stimulant effects of small doses of antidepressants. Therefore, we recommend initiating treatment with low doses of antidepressants (i.e., nortriptyline 10 mg or fluoxetine 5 mg). The use of benzodiazepines may mitigate these early stimulant effects and be used adjunctively until the reversal of panic symptoms has been established. Buspirone also may be used adjunctively with antidepressants to treat generalized anxiety. In addition, buspirone may have antidepressant properties when administered in dosages from 45 to 60 mg/day (Fabre, 1990). However, Ludwig and colleagues (1986) found no effect of buspirone when administered to PD patients in doses up to 60 mg/day on ratings of anxiety or depression. In comparison to benzodiazepines, buspirone appears to have no adverse effect on memory or alertness. However, unlike benzodiazepines, where antianxiety effects can be discerned after a single dose, the full therapeutic effect of buspirone may take 2 to 3 weeks to occur.

Nonselective monoamine oxidase inhibitors often are used to treat atypical depression and depression with anxiety and panic in patients who do not have PD. Because of the risk of a hypertensive reaction, these drugs (as well as deprenyl in nonselective dosages of 20 mg/day or greater) cannot be administered concomitantly with L-dopa.

CONCLUSION

Before treatment of the depressed PD patient is initiated, a review of currently prescribed medications and a careful documentation of depressive and cognitive symptomatologies are required. Depending on the clinical circumstances, the reduction or addition of the patient's antiparkinsonian medications may alleviate depressive symptoms. This is especially important if there are prominent motoric symptoms of PD or if the depressive picture features prominent withdrawal and apathy. For those patients with significant anhedonia, guilt, decreased libido, and suicidal ideation, antidepressant medication can be beneficial. A therapeutic trial of antidepressant medication includes prescribing an effective dosage for at least 6 weeks. For those patients who are severely depressed or suicidal and either cannot wait the required time for response or cannot tolerate antidepressant medications, electroconvulsive therapy can be a life-saving treatment.

REFERENCES

Andersen J, Aabro E, Gulmann N, et al. Anti-depressive treatment in Parkinson's disease: a controlled trial of the effect of nortriptyline in patients with Parkinson's disease treated with L-dopa. *Acta Neurol Scand.* 1980;62:210–219.

Baldessarini RJ. *Chemotherapy in Psychiatry: Principles and Practice.* Boston: Harvard University Press; 1985.

Bavazzano A, Guarducci R, Gestri G, et al. Clinical trial with amantadine and hydergine in elderly patients. *J Clin Exp Gerontol.* 1980;2:289–299.

Bouchard RH, Bourcher E, Vincent P. Fluoxetine and extrapyramidal side effects. *Am J Psychiatry.* 1989;146:1352–1353.

Cloninger CR. A systematic method for clinical description and classification of personality variants. *Arch Gen Psychiatry.* 1987;44:573–588.

Coffey CE, Ross ER, Massey EW, et al. Dyskinesias associated with lithium therapy in parkinsonism. *Clin Neuropharmacol.* 1984;7:223–229.

Damasio AR, Lobo-Antunes J, Macedo C. Psychiatric aspects in Parkinsonism treated with l-dopa. *J Neurol Neurosurg Psychiatry.* 1971;34:502–507.

De Smet Y, Ruberg M, Serdaru M, et al. Confusion, dementia, and anticholinergics in Parkinson's disease. *J Neurol Neurosurg Psychiatry.* 1982;45:1161–1164.

Denmark JC, Powell David JD, McComb SG. Imipramine hydrochloride (Tofranil) in parkinsonism: a preliminary report. *Br J Clin Practice.* 1961;15:523–524.

Dilsalver SC, Coffman JA. Cholinergic hypothesis of depression: a reappraisal. *J Clin Psychopharmacol.* 1989;9:173–179.

Dubois B, Pillon B, Lhermitte F, Agid Y. Cholinergic deficiency and frontal dysfunction in Parkinson's disease. *Ann Neurol.* 1990;28:117–121.

Eisler T, Teravainen H, Nelson R, et al. Deprenyl in Parkinson disease. *Neurology.* 1981;31:19–23.

Fabre LF. Buspirone in the management of major depression: a placebo-controlled comparison. *J Clin Psychiatry.* 1990;519(suppl):55–61.

Flaherty JA, Bellur SN. Mental side effects of amantadine therapy: its spectrum and characteristics in a normal population. *J Clin Psychiatry.* 1981;42:344–345.

Gangat AE, Simpson MA, Naidoo LR. Medication as a potential cause of depression. S Atr Med J 1986;70:224–226.

Gillhespy RO, Mustard DM. The evaluation of imipramine in the treatment of Parkinson's disease. *Br J Clin Pract.* 1963;17:205–208.

Gillman MA, Sandy KR. Parkinsonism induced by a monoamine oxidase inhibitor. Postgrad Med J 1986;62:235–236.

Glassman AH. The newer antidepressant drugs and their cardiovascular effects. *Psychopharmacol Bull.* 1984;20:272–279.

Glassman AH, Bigger JT. Cardiovascular effects of therapeutic doses of tricyclic antidepressants: a review. *Arch Gen Psychiatry.* 1981;39:815–820.

Glassman AH, Johnson LL, Giardina EGV, et al. The use of imipramine in depressed patients with congestive heart failure. *JAMA.* 1983;250:1997–2001.

Goetz CG, Tanner CM, Klawans HL. Buproprion in Parkinson's disease. *Neurology.* 1984;34:1092–1094.

Goodwin FK, Brodie HK, Murphy DL, Bunney WE. Administration of a peripheral decarboxylase inhibitor with l-dopa to depressed patients. Lancet 1970;653:908–911.

Janowsky DS, Risch SC. Role of acetylcholine mechanisms in the affective disorders. In: Meltzer HY, ed. *Psychopharmacology: The Third Generation of Progress.* New York; Raven Press; 1987:527–534.

Jimerson DC. Role of dopamine mechanisms in the affective disorders. In: Meltzer HY, ed. *Psychopharmacology: The Third Generation of Progress.* New York: Raven Press; 1987:505–512.

Jimerson DC, Nurnberger JI, Simmons S, et al. Anticholinergic treatment for depression. Presented at the 135th annual meeting of the American Psychiatric Association, Toronto, Canada, May 15–21, Syllabus, 1982:218–219.

Jouvent R, Abensour P, Bonnet AM. Antiparkinsonian and antidepressant effects of high doses of bromocriptine: an independent comparison. *J Affective Dis.* 1983;5:141–145.

Karoum F, Chuang L-W, Eisler TMS, et al. Metabolism of (−) deprenyl to amphetamine and methamphetamine may be responsible for deprenyl's therapeutic benefit: A biochemical assessment. *Neurology.* 1982;32:503–509.

Kasper S, Moises HW, Beckmann H. The anticholinergic biperiden in depressive disorders. *Pharmacopsychiatry.* 1981;14:195–198.

Laitinen L. Desipramine in treatment of Parkinson's disease: a placebo-controlled study. *Acta Neurol Scand.* 1969;45:109–113.

Ludwig CL, Weinberger DR, Bruno G, et al. Buspirone, Parkinson's disease, and the locus ceruleus. *Clin Neuropharmacology.* 1986;9:373–378.

Mandell AJ, Markham C, Fowler W. Parkinson's syndrome, depression and imipramine: a preliminary report. *Calif Med.* 1961;95:12–14.

Mann JJ, Aarons SF, Wilner PJ, et al. A controlled study of the antidepressant efficacy and side effects of (−)-deprenyl: a selective monoamine oxidase inhibitor. *Arch Gen Psychiatry.* 1989;46:45–50.

Mayeux R, Stern Y, Sano M, et al. Clinical and biochemical correlates of bradyphrenia in Parkinson's disease. Neurology. 1987;37:1130–1134.

Mayeux R, Stern Y, Sano M, et al. The relationship of serotonin to depression in Parkinson's disease. *Movement Disord.* 1988;3:237–244.

Meltzer HY, Lowy MT. The serotonin hypothesis of depression. In: Meltzer HJ, ed. *Psychopharmacology: The Third Generation of Progress.* New York: Raven Press; 1987:513–526.

Meltzer HY, Young M, Metz J, et al. Extrapyramidal side effects and increased serum prolactin following fluoxetine, a new antidepressant. *J Neural Transm.* 1979;45:165–175.

Menza MA, Forman NE, Goldstein HS, et al. Parkinson's disease, personality, and dopamine. *J Neuropsychiatry Clin Neurosci.* 1990;2:282–287.

Mindham RHS, Marsden CD, Parkes JD. Psychiatric symptoms during L-dopa therapy for Parkinson's disease and their relationship to physical disability. *Psychol Med.* 1976;6:23–33.

Parkinson Study Group. Effect of deprenyl on the progression of disability in early Parkinson's disease. *N Engl J Med.* 1989;321:1364–1371.

Perry RH, Tomlinson BE, Candy JM, et al. Cortical cholinergic deficit in mentally impaired parkinsonian patients. *Lancet.* 1983;1:789–790.

Przuntek H, Kuhn W, Draus P. The effect of *P*-(−)-deprenyl in de novo parkinsonian patients pretreated with levodopa and decarboxylase inhibitor correlated to depression and MHPG, HIAA, and HVA levels in the cerebrospinal fluid. *Acta Neurol Scand.* 1989;126:153–156.

Quitkin FM, Liebowitz MR, Stewart JW, et al. Deprenyl in atypical depressives. *Arch Gen Psychiatry.* 1984;41:777–781.

Richelson E. Antimuscarinic and other receptor-blocking properties of antidepressants. *Mayo Clin Proc.* 1983;58:40–46.

Roose SP, Glassman AH, Giardina EGV, et al. Cardiovascular effects of imipramine and buproprion in depressed patients with congestive heart failure. *J Clin Psychopharmacol.* 1987;7:247–251.

Roose SP, Glassman AH, Siris SG, et al. Comparison of imipramine- and nortriptyline-induced orthostatic hypotension. A meaningful difference. *J Clin Psychopharmacol.* 1981;1:316–319.

Sano M, Stern Y, Cote L, Williams JB, Mayeux R. Depression in Parkinson's disease: a biochemical model. *J Neuropsychiatry and Clin Neurosci* 1990;2:88–92.

Schiffer RB, Kurlan R, Rubin A, Boer S. Evidence for atypical depression in Parkinson's disease. *Am J Psychiatry.* 1988;145:1020–1022.

Siever LJ. Role of noradrenergic mechanisms in the etiology of the affective disorders. In: Meltzer HJ, ed. *Psychopharmacology: The Third Generation of Progress.* New York: Raven Press; 1987:505–512.

Silver JM, Yudofsky SC. Psychopharmacology and electroconvulsive therapy. In: Talbott JA, Hales RE, Yudofsky SC, eds. *American Psychiatric Press Textbook of Psychiatry.* Washington, DC: American Psychiatric Press; 1988:767–853.

Silver JM, Hales RE, Yudofsky SC. Biological Therapies for Mental Disorders In: Stoudemire A, ed. *Clinical Psychiatry for Medical Students.* Philadelphia: JB Lippincott Co; 1990a:459–496.

Silver JM, Hales RE, Yudofsky SC. Psychopharmacology of depression in neurologic disorders. *J Clin Psychiatry.* 1990b;51(1,suppl):33–39.

Silver JM, Hales RE, Yudofsky SC. Psychiatric consultation to neurology. In: Tasman A, ed. *American Psychiatric Press Review of Psychiatry,* vol 9. Edited by A. Washington, DC: American Psychiatric Press; 1990c:433–465.

Sitland-Marken PA, Wells BG, Froemming JH, et al. Psychiatric applications of bromocriptine therapy. *J Clin Psychiatry.* 1990;51:68–82.

Starkstein SE, Berthier ML, Bolduc PL, et al. Depression in patients with early versus late onset of Parkinson's disease. *Neurology.* 1989;39:1441–1445.

Starkstein SE, Preziosi TJ, Bolduc PL, Robinson RG. Depression in Parkinson's disease. *J Nerv Ment Dis.* 1990a;178:27–31.

Starkstein SE, Preziosi TJ, Forrester AW, Robinson RG. Specificity of affective and autonomic symptoms of depression in Parkinson's disease. *J Neurol Neurosurg Psychiatry.* 1990b;53:869–873.

Strang RR. Imipramine in treatment of Parkinsonism: a double-blind study. *Br Med J.* 1965;2:33–34.

Strauss H. Office treatment of depressive states with a new drug (imipramine). *NY State Med J.* 1959;59:2906–2910.

Tariot PN, Cohen RM, Sunderland T, et al. L-Deprenyl in Alzheimer's disease: preliminary evidence for behavioral change with monoamine oxidase B inhibition. *Arch Gen Psychiatry.* 1987;44:427–433.

Task Force on the Use of Laboratory Tests in Psychiatry. Tricyclic antidepressants: blood level measurements and clinical outcome: an APA Task Force Report. *Am J Psychiatry.* 1985;142:155–162.

Taylor AE, Saint-Cyr JA. Depression in Parkinson's disease: reconciling physiological and psychological perspectives. *J Neuropsychiatry Clin Neurosci.* 1990;2:92–98.

Tetrud JW, Langston JW. The effect of deprenyl (Selegiline) on the natural history of Parkinson's disease. *Science.* 1989;245:519–522.

Teusink JP, Alexopoulos GS, Shamoian CA. Parkinsonian side effects induced by a monoamine oxidase inhibitor. *Am J Psychiatry.* 1984;141:118–119.

Thornton JE, Stahl SM. Case report of tardive dyskinesia and parkinsonism associated with amoxapine therapy. *Am J Psychiatry.* 1984;141:704–705.

Tyrer P, Alexander MS, Regan A, Lee I. An extrapyramidal syndrome after lithium therapy. *Br J Psychiatry.* 1980;136:191–194.

Van Woert MH, Bowers MH. The effect of L-dopa on monamine metabolites in Parkinson's disease. *Experientia.* 1970;26:161–163.

Waldmeier PC, Delini-Stula AA. Serotonin–dopamine interactions in the nigrostriatal system. *Eur J Pharmacol.* 1979;55:363–373.

Wolfe N, Katz DI, Albert ML, et al. Neuropsychological profile linked to low dopamine in Alzheimer's disease, major depression, and Parkinson's disease. *J Neurol Neurosurg Psychiatry.* 1990;53:915–917.

19

The Role of Electroconvulsive Therapy in Parkinson's Disease

KEITH G. RASMUSSEN AND RICHARD ABRAMS

Electroconvulsive therapy (ECT), now over 50 years old, is a safe and technically sophisticated procedure that is used widely in psychiatry (Abrams, 1988; American Psychiatric Association, 1990). Less well known is the fact that ECT can also be effective in treating patients with Parkinson's disease (PD) or the parkinsonian syndrome even in the absence of psychopathology, especially those who are refractory to antiparkinsonian medications or who exhibit the on/off syndrome.

This chapter considers the various clinical indications for ECT in PD patients, describes potential neurobiological bases for its efficacy, details the risks and technical aspects of its administration in this population, provides a cost–benefit comparison with available neurosurgical procedures, and presents recommendations for current practice.

INDICATIONS FOR ECT IN PARKINSON'S DISEASE

Depression

The efficacy of ECT in treating major depression is well demonstrated in controlled comparisons against both placebo ECT and antidepressant drugs (Abrams, 1988). There are now five well-controlled studies demonstrating the superiority of genuine over sham ECT, in which anesthesia is administered without the subsequent electrical stimulus (Freeman et al, 1978; Johnstone et al, 1980; West, 1981; Brandon et al, 1984; Gregory et al, 1985). The single study failing to find such advantage (Lambourn and Gill, 1978) employed an ECT technique—unilateral electrode placement combined with low-dose electrical stimulation—that has been demonstrated subsequently to lack therapeutic value (Sackeim et al, 1987). Controlled comparisons of ECT and antidepressant medications document virtually without exception the greater efficacy of ECT (Greenblatt et al, 1964; Medical Research Council, 1965; Gangadhar et al, 1982; Abrams, 1988).

The prevalence of major depression in PD is estimated at 20 percent to 90 percent (Gotham et al, 1986). Differences in diagnostic criteria, patient selection, and depressive subtypes (e.g., melancholic, dysthymic) account for some of this wide variance. A further confounding factor is the overlap of extrapyramidal and depressive symptoms in PD. For example, apathy and psychomotor retardation, two cardinal manifestations of melancholia, are common subcortical symptoms of PD. Taylor and Saint-Cyr (1990) have described more subtle cognitive aspects of PD that may mimic depression, including inability to initiate and sustain action independent of external guidance. Despite this, Sano and colleagues (1990) argue that with careful attention to DSM III criteria (APA, 1980), a reliable diagnosis of depression can be made in over one third of PD patients.

Numerous case reports and small series attest to the efficacy of ECT in PD depression (Table 19–1). Although the main thrust of most of these reports is the serendipitous discovery of an antiparkinsonian effect of ECT, ECT appears to relieve the depression of PD without aggravating the course of the underlying disorder.

A recent American Psychiatric Association Task Force Report (APA, 1990) lists appropriate clinical circumstances for the psychiatric use of ECT, several of which are relevant to PD. Paramount among these are refractoriness to antidepressant medications or intolerance to their side effects, both phenomena frequently observed in PD patients, who tend to be elderly and, therefore, subject to a greater incidence of such problems (Blazer, 1989). Side effects include disorientation, dysmnesia, slurred speech, tremors, increased intraocular pressure, paralytic ileus, and urinary retention.

Medical conditions contraindicating antidepressants or other psychotropics can be an indication for the use of ECT in depressed PD patients. For example, narrow-angle glaucoma, heart block, urinary obstruction, and dementia all require avoiding medications with prominent anticholinergic effects, including many psychotropics and antiparkinsonian agents.

Psychiatric or medical urgency requiring a rapid, definitive treatment response provides a clinical indication for ECT. Suicidality, severe psychomotor retardation, and cachexia with poor food or fluid intake are typical features that may be encountered. The depressed PD patient, already plagued by motor immobility, may be particularly prone to such developments.

Mania

ECT was the sole antimanic therapy for decades before the introduction of psychopharmacological treatments (Kalinowsky and Hippius, 1969). Several retrospective chart reviews in large patient samples found ECT comparable to neuroleptics and superior to expectant treatment (McCabe, 1976; McCabe and Norris, 1977; Thomas and Reddy, 1982; Black et al, 1987), even in medication-resistant patients (Alexander et al, 1988). Prospective trials have confirmed these reports (Small et al, 1986; Mukherjee et al, 1988).

Although mania is rare in PD patients, some may have attacks induced by levodopa (Yager, 1989) or associated with the evolving dementia of PD. The usual antimanic agents create problems in management, since both lithium and neuroleptics can cause extrapyramidal symptoms. Moreover, neuroleptics enhance the risk of tardive dyskinesia in bipolar patients (Wolf et al, 1985; Mukherjee et al, 1986). In the two case reports of manic PD patients treated successfully with ECT (Atre-Vaidya and

Jampala, 1988; Roth et al, 1988), amelioration of the motor symptoms occurred as well as relief of the mood disturbance.

Psychosis

Psychotic depression occurs more often with advancing age (Blazer, 1989). Less responsive to pharmacotherapy than simple melancholia, it is nonetheless responsive to ECT (Abrams, 1988; Blazer, 1989). Nonaffective psychotic states also can respond to ECT, including schizophrenia (Gujavarty et al, 1987; Childers, 1964; Smith et al, 1967; Friedel, 1986; May et al, 1981; Taylor and Fleminger, 1980; Brandon et al, 1985; Janakiramaiah et al, 1982; Goswami et al, 1989; Bagadia et al, 1983) and a variety of organic psychoses and delirious states (Taylor, 1982; Dubovsky, 1986).

Secondary psychoses in PD patients can occur with virtually any of the antiparkinsonian medications (e.g., anticholinergic delirium, dopaminomimetic psychosis) or in association with dementia. The usefulness of neuroleptics in these states is limited by their exacerbation of extrapyramidal symptoms, often leading to further use of anticholinergic or dopaminergic agents and creating the unfortunate sequence that Yudofsky (1979) has dubbed the "pharmacologic seesaw." Judicious use of ECT in the psychotic PD patient can prevent this cycle (Hurwitz et al, 1988).

Parkinson's Disease Without Psychiatric Disorder

As early as 1953, Savitsky and Karliner commented on the antidepressant efficacy of ECT in 7 PD patients and mentioned that tremor improved in 3. Shapiro and Goldberg (1957) and Fromm (1959) also provided early reports of antiparkinsonian effects of ECT. Almost two decades passed, however, before Lebensohn and Jenkins (1975) systematically described the course of improvement of motor symptoms in PD patients receiving ECT for depression. Since then, over two dozen reports have appeared describing more than 60 patients in whom ECT has relieved the motor symptoms of PD or neuroleptic-induced parkinsonism (NIP). Table 19–1 enumerates these reports along with all others we could find describing the use and effects of ECT in PD patients. Table 19–2 presents similar data for NIP.

Some have questioned whether the antiparkinsonian effects of ECT are dependent on its antidepressant properties (Wilder, 1975). Jaeckle and Dilsaver (1986) report a patient with recurrent depressions whose PD occurred only during the depressions and remitted when they lifted. However, several reports clearly describe antiparkinsonian effects of ECT that precede any antidepressant effects or occur without them (Burke et al, 1988; Burkitt, 1988; Douyon et al, 1989; Young et al, 1985; Asnis, 1977). Burke and associates (1988) described a depressed PD patient who enjoyed remission of both sets of symptoms after ECT but whose PD later relapsed in the absence of depression, suggesting a dissociation of the two syndromes. Both reports on the efficacy of ECT in relieving the motor symptoms of manic PD patients (Atre-Vaidya and Jampala, 1988; Roth et al, 1988) describe improvement of the extrapyramidal symptoms before resolution of the mood disorder.

NIP also responds to ECT (Shapiro and Goldberg, 1957; Ananth et al, 1979; Gangadhar et al, 1983; Chacko and Root, 1983; Goswami et al, 1989), even in patients who remain on neuroleptics.

Table 19–1   Response of PD motor symptoms to ECT

Reference	Secondary diagnosis	Improvement
Savitsky and Karliner, 1953	Depression	3/7
Fromm, 1959	Unspecified	5/8
Lebensohn and Jenkins, 1975	Depression	2/2
Lebensohn, 1975	Depression	1/3
Rainey and Faust, 1975	Depression	1/1
Dysken et al, 1976	Depression	1/1
Asnis, 1977	Depression	1/1
Yudofsky, 1979	Depression	1/1
Balldin et al, 1980	None, depression	5/5
Ward et al, 1980	None, depression	1/6
Balldin et al, 1981	None	2/4
Levy et al, 1983	Depression	1/1
Holcomb et al, 1983	Depression	1/1
Raskin, 1984	Depression	1/1
Young et al, 1985	Depression	1/1
Jaeckle and Dilsaver, 1986	Depression	1/1
Andersen et al, 1987	Depression	9/11
Atre-Vaidya and Jampala, 1988	Mania	1/1
Roth et al, 1988	Mania	1/1
Burke et al, 1988	Depression	2/3
Birkett, 1988	Depression	4/5
Douyon et al, 1989	Depression	7/7
Lauterbach and Moore, 1990	Depression	1/1
Zervas and Fink, 1991	None, depression	4/4

A group of Swedish investigators (Balldin et al, 1980, 1981; Andersen et al, 1987) has described carefully a substantial number of nonpsychiatric, nondemented PD patients whose motor symptoms—characteristically the on/off syndrome—responded to ECT. Notably, Andersen and colleagues (1987) included a sham ECT control group that received anesthesia without an electrical stimulus. Several PD patients who received genuine ECT enjoyed relief of their motor symptoms, but none who received sham treatments improved. A few patients in the latter group then recovered when they were switched to genuine ECT.

There are two negative reports on the antiparkinsonian effects of ECT. Brown (1975) described an "unusually poor" response of PD motor symptoms to ECT in 7

Table 19–2.   Response of neuroleptic-induced parkinsonism to ECT

Reference	Diagnosis	Number
Ganghadar et al, 1983	Unspecified psychotic disorders	17/17
Chacko and Root, 1983	Schizophrenia	1/1
Goswami et al, 1989	Schizophrenia	9/9
Shapiro and Goldberg, 1957	Depression	1/1
Ananth et al, 1979	Schizophrenia	1/1

patients—although the data were retrospectively reviewed many years after treatment—and Ward and colleagues (1980) reported 5 nondepressed PD patients who received essentially no motor benefit from ECT and 1 who experienced only transient improvement.

Age correlates highly with the antiparkinsonian effects of ECT. The mean age of the Ward and colleagues (1980) sample of nonresponders was 57 years, similar to the nonresponders of Balldin and associates (1981), for whom the rank order correlation between age and improvement from ECT was 0.87. Douyon and colleagues (1989) report a similarly high correlation of 0.92. Balldin and associates (1981) found no correlation between response to ECT and either age at onset of PD or duration of illness. Duration of levodopa therapy correlated positively with outcome, suggesting that long-term levodopa might reduce dopamine receptor sensitivity, a phenomenon potentially reversed by ECT. A levodopa-induced dopamine receptor subsensitivity cannot explain all instances of antiparkinsonian benefits of ECT, however, since several patients without prior exposure to levodopa have responded to ECT (Jaeckle and Dilsaver, 1986; Burke et al, 1988; Holcombe et al, 1983).

Other factors found by Balldin and colleagues (1981) not to predict response were percent off time before treatment, initial improvement with levodopa, duration of on/ off symptoms, and pre-ECT basal and apomorphine-induced growth hormone and prolactin levels. Specifically, patients with the on/off syndrome responded well to ECT in both the Balldin and colleagues (1981) and Andersen and associates (1987) studies, regardless of duration or severity of illness.

Most of the reports in Table 19–1 used bilateral electrode placement and sine wave stimuli, although unilateral placements and brief pulse stimuli also have been reported effective (Burke et al, 1988; Roth et al, 1988).

Summary

Thus, an extensive literature spanning three decades and two continents attests to a beneficial effect of ECT on PD motor symptoms, whether primary or neuroleptic induced. Response failures are infrequent and tend to occur in younger patients. The beneficial effects are understandably temporary, lasting from a few hours to several months, with the modal remission lasting just a few weeks. This suggests a potential use for maintenance ECT, in which intermittent outpatient treatments are administered after a successful initial course of ECT (Abrams, 1988). Two reports support the efficacy of maintenance ECT for PD (Holcombe et al, 1983; Zervas and Fink, 1991), but more data are needed to support this approach.

NEUROBIOLOGICAL BASIS FOR THE EFFICACY OF ECT IN PARKINSON'S DISEASE

Motor Symptoms of Parkinson's Disease

Since the neuropathology of idiopathic PD includes loss of dopamine-containing neurons projecting to the striatum, it follows that interventions that enhance this deficit might be helpful. Both animal and human research support such an effect of ECT.

Animal Data

Electroconvulsive shock (ECS), the animal analogue of ECT in humans, affects brain dopamine (DA) content and synthesis and exhibits pre- and postsynaptic receptor and postreceptor effects (Lerer et al, 1984; Lerer, 1987). Several investigators found brain DA content and synthesis and striatal DA binding to be unaffected by daily ECS (Evans et al, 1976; Modigh, 1976; Bergstrom and Kellar, 1979; Atterwill, 1980; Deakin et al, 1981). Lerer and colleagues (1982), however, exploiting the fact that chronic haloperidol treatment reliably elevates striatal DA binding in the rat, found that although ECS alone did not change DA binding or apomorphine-induced behaviors, ECS combined with haloperidol attenuated the DA receptor supersensitivity caused by haloperidol alone, suggesting that ECS stabilized the DA receptor. Such a phenomenon would also provide a neurobiological basis for ECT's potential useful-ness in tardive dyskinesia, a syndrome thought to be partly caused by DA receptor supersensitivity (Lieberman, 1989).

In contrast to the apparent lack of increase in DA binding in the rat striatum after ECS, one group has found increased D1 binding in the substantia nigra after ECS (Fochtmann et al, 1987). There is evidence that D1 agonism in the substantia nigra increases nigrostriatal dopaminergic firing (Clark and White, 1987). Newman and Lerer (1989) have shown that a course of ECS may specifically enhance D1 receptor function in the rat striatum.

The differential behavioral responses to DA agonists after real vs sham ECS are well documented. Several studies have demonstrated that genuine, but not sham, ECS augments both generalized motor activity and motor stereotypes induced by the DA agonists apomorphine and methamphetamine or the combination of tranylcypro-mine and levodopa (Gangadhar et al, 1989; Modigh, 1975; Evans et al, 1976; Green et al, 1977, 1980; Grahame-Smith et al, 1978; Green and Deakin, 1980, Heal and Green, 1978; Deakin et al, 1981; Serra et al, 1981; Globus et al, 1981; Bhavsar et al, 1981). Only limited contradictory data exist (Wielosz, 1981). Peterson (1986) found that both ECS-pretreated rats and those given levodopa had greater reduction in head-turning behavior after electrical stimulation of the caudate than untreated controls, suggesting that ECS enhances dopaminergic activity, since DA is an inhibitory neu-rotransmitter in the caudate. Seizures induced chemically with flurothyl or bicuculline enhance DA functioning in similar behavioral paradigms (Green, 1978; Nutt et al, 1980). Using a different model, White and Barrett (1981) found that ECS-treated rats were more sensitive to the dopaminergic effects of D-amphetamine than their sham-ECS-treated littermates.

In doses well below those used in the preceding studies, apomorphine is a selective presynaptic autoreceptor agonist that attenuates nigrostriatal DA release (Clark and White, 1987), a phenomenon that is reduced by a course of ECS (Chiodo and Antel-man, 1980; Tepper et al, 1982; Creese et al, 1982). Thus, ECS may enhance nigrostri-atal firing by downregulating the nigrostriatal autoreceptor.

Other neurotransmitter changes postulated to play a role in mediating ECS enhancement of DA function include decreased GABA turnover and synthesis and increased GABA concentrations (presumably presynaptic) in the caudate and accumbens nuclei (Green et al, 1978). DA function is inhibited by GABA. Heal and colleagues (1978) provided support for this hypothesis by demonstrating that dibutyryl cAMP injections into rat caudate nucleus led to motor activity enhancement that was identical to that induced by DA injections. Pretreatment with the GABA transaminase inhibitor amino-oxyacetic acid, which promotes GABA function, prevented the dibutyryl cAMP-induced behavioral responses.

Green and colleagues (1978) also found that ECS increased caudate nucleus metenkephalin levels by 50 percent, suggesting decreased release and, therefore, decreased tone. Sandyk (1986) argued that a reduction in striatal opiate activity might directly—or indirectly via reduced inhibition of DA activity—alleviate the symptoms of PD.

Another putative mechanism for ECS-enhanced DA activity invokes neurochemical events distal to the postsynaptic receptor. After first demonstrating that cAMP worked distal to the postsynaptic receptor (Heal et al, 1978), Heal and Green (1978) found that dibutyryl cAMP injections into rat nucleus accumbens produced DA-mediated behaviors, an effect that was potentiated by ECS.

Human Data

With one exception (Jori et al, 1975), human ECT studies generally have found no evidence for increased synthesis or turnover of DA (Nordin et al, 1971; Abrams et al, 1976; Harnryd et al, 1979; Linnoila et al, 1983, 1984). Abrams and Swartz (1985a,b), however, found a progressive reduction in ECT-induced prolactin release across a course of treatment, suggesting enhanced sensitivity of the pituitary DA receptor.

More direct evidence for ECT-induced enhancement of pituitary DA receptors was provided by Balldin and colleagues (1982) in PD patients who exhibited significantly greater prolactin suppression by apomorphine before than after a course of ECT. Interestingly, in this study and another (Christie et al, 1982), ECT did not affect apomorphine-induced prolactin changes in depressed patients. Moreover, in neither PD nor depressed patients does ECT induce changes in the growth hormone response to apomorphine (Balldin et al, 1982; Christie et al, 1982).

The duration of ECS-enhanced DA functioning in animals may be relevant to the dopaminergic effects of ECT in humans. Most of the studies cited measured responses a day or so after the last ECS. Where measurements were repeated weeks later (Gangadhar et al, 1987; Bhavsar et al, 1981), the enhanced DA effects had subsided, demonstrating that the effects of ECS were similar in duration to the ameliorative effects of ECT on the parkinsonian syndrome and indirectly supporting the DA hypothesis.

Summary

Thus, substantial basic neuroscience research supports a rational basis for the efficacy of ECT in PD. A consensus among studies examining ECS effects on autoreceptors, postsynaptic receptors, postreceptor events, and modulatory neurotransmitters points to a dopamine-enhancing effect of electrically induced seizures, which is of obvious relevance in the management of PD.

PHYSIOLOGY AND RISKS OF ECT

Following induction of anesthesia with methohexital and succinylcholine, ECT is administered by passing an electric current through the brain via scalp electrodes placed either bitemporally or unilaterally over the right hemisphere. Stimulus intensity is adjusted to induce a grand mal seizure of 30 to 90 seconds duration, after which patients are monitored by recovery room personnel until orientation and alertness have returned, generally within 30 minutes.

Psychotropic agents are discontinued routinely before ECT, as are adjunctive antiparkinsonian medications whose anticholinergic properties might increase postictal confusion. Levodopa dosage should be reduced by 50 percent to prevent the development of emergent dyskinesias or delirium secondary to ECT-induced increases in dopamine receptor sensitivity (Douyon et al, 1989; Balldin et al, 1981; Zervas and Fink, 1991).

The cardiovascular and central nervous systems bear the brunt of the physiological impact of ECT (Abrams, 1988).

Cardiovascular Alterations with ECT

The electrical stimulus and resultant seizure elicit an initial intense parasympathomimetic response (e.g., bradycardia, hypotension) that electively may be blocked by an anticholinergic, such as atropine. An intense sympathoadrenal discharge rapidly ensues, characterized by sharp increases in blood pressure, heart rate, and rate–pressure product, all of which generally return to baseline shortly after seizure termination. Brief adrenergic dysrhythmias, such as premature ventricular contractions, are commonly observed during the immediate postictal phase and rarely require intervention.

Cardiovascular changes account for most of the mortality of ECT, although the great rarity of ECT-related deaths—1 per 50,000 treatments in the most recent estimate (Kramer, 1985)—makes identification of individual risk factors difficult. Serious or life-threatening morbidity (e.g., heart attack, stroke, ruptured aneurysm) is similarly rare, although it is more frequent in patients with preexisting cardiovascular disease. Correction or amelioration of the underlying condition before ECT, combined with appropriate use of selected cardioactive medications, improves the already high level of safety (Abrams, 1988; APA, 1990).

Neurological and Neuropsychological Alterations with ECT

EEG monitoring during ECT reveals characteristic hypersynchronous polyspikes followed by polyspike-and-slow-wave complexes, terminating in a period of electrical silence—a more or less flat line on the EEG—that is gradually and successively replaced by restoration of the baseline rhythms. After a course of ECT, the EEG may show diffuse slowing but generally returns to the pre-ECT pattern within a few weeks.

ECT is not reported to cause permanent EEG changes, and the rarely reported spontaneous seizures of the preanesthesia era no longer occur. In fact, ECT raises the seizure threshold and has been used to treat refractory seizure disorders (Post et al, 1986; Abrams, 1988; APA, 1990).

The immediate postictal period is often characterized by mild confusion that clears within half an hour or so. The occasional agitated postictal (emergence) delirium is rapidly responsive to intravenous diazepam.

ECT-induced cognitive dysfunction has been studied extensively (Abrams, 1988). In general, research confirms that bilateral electrode placement, especially with sine wave stimulation, can cause persistent autobiographical amnesia—6 months is the longest period studied so far—for some events occurring during the several months before ECT. However, Weiner and colleagues (1986) found that patients who received unilateral nondominant electrode placement with brief pulse stimulation exhibited no more memory disturbance than drug-treated control patients, yet improved just as much as those receiving sine wave bilateral ECT, the original method.

ECT is safe in demented patients (Tsuang et al, 1979; Demuth and Rand, 1980; Snow and Wells, 1981; McAllister and Price, 1982; Perry, 1983; Dubovsky et al, 1985), in whom it may help circumvent the need for psychotropic or antiparkinsonian medications that might otherwise exacerbate cognitive impairment. Moreover, depression-related cognitive dysfunction (depressive pseudodementia) often improves with antidepressant treatment, including ECT (Abrams, 1989; Stoudemire et al, 1989). For example, Jaeckle and Dilsaver (1986) reported substantial cognitive improvement in their parkinsonian patient treated with ECT, pari passu with improvements in depression and extrapyramidal symptoms.

RISKS AND BENEFITS OF ECT VS NEUROSURGERY FOR PARKINSON'S DISEASE

Despite initial enthusiasm for autologous adrenal medullary transplants into the striatum of PD patients (Madrazo et al, 1987), the results recently obtained tend to be more modest (Goetz et al, 1989; Ahlskog et al, 1990). The procedure involves abdominal as well as neurological surgery. Multiple specialty consultations, special nursing, and hospital costs can elevate total cost to over $20,000. Complications include stroke, pneumonia, depression, and possibly cognitive dysfunction (Ahlskog et al, 1990; Goetz et al, 1989). Fetal transplants also have been tried (Abrams, 1989), at a cost of about $10,000 per operation, with equivocal results.

In comparison, ECT is a noninvasive procedure that typically costs about $600 per treatment when administered in an outpatient setting. If both initial and maintenance ECT are used, the total first-year cost might range from $9000 to $12,000, falling to about $7000 to $9000 in subsequent years. Of course, if the initial course were ineffective, further treatments would not be given, and the cost of determining the efficacy of the method would be limited to $4000 or $5000. Considering the extremely low morbidity and mortality of ECT compared with neurosurgery and the generally far more favorable, although temporary, results reported with ECT, the latter appears to be a cost-effective alternative to surgery in the management of treatment-refractory PD.

We recommend a minimum course of six high-dose right unilateral ECTs for any PD patient who is being considered for neurosurgical amelioration of symptoms or who has received maximal tolerated dosages of levodopa and adjunctive antiparkinsonian therapy for at least 1 year without achieving satisfactory improvement in the quality of life. We further recommend that PD patients who improve significantly with an initial course of ECT be placed on an outpatient ECT schedule that is titrated to maintain the attained improvement with the minimum number of treatments. It is worth noting that with proper training, neurologists can and do routinely administer ECT in European countries (e.g., Germany).

REFERENCES

Abrams R. *Electroconvulsive Therapy.* New York: Oxford; 1988.

Abrams R. ECT for Parkinson's disease. *Am J Psychiatry.* 1989;146:1391–1393.

Abrams R, Swartz CM. ECT and prolactin release: Effects of stimulus parameters. *Convulsive Ther.* 1985a;1:115–119.

Abrams R, Swartz CM. ECT and prolactin release: Relation to treatment response in melancholia. *Convulsive Ther.* 1985b;1:38–42.

Abrams R, Essman WB, Taylor MA, Fink M. Concentration of 5-hydroxy-indoleacetic acid, homovanillic acid, and tryptophan in the cerebrospinal fluid of depressed patients before and after ECT. *Biol Psychiatry.* 1976;11:85–90.

Ahlskog JE, Kelly P, Van Heerden J, et al. Adrenal medullary transplantation into the brain for treatment of Parkinson's disease: clinical outcome and neurochemical studies. *Mayo Clin Proc.* 1990;65:305–328.

Alexander RC, et al. Convulsive therapy in the treatment of mania. *Convulsive Ther.* 1988;4:115–125.

American Psychiatric Association. *Diagnostic and Statistical Manual of Mental Disorders, 3rd ed.* Washington, DC: American Psychiatric Association, 1980.

American Psychiatric Association. *The Practice of Electroconvulsive Therapy: Recommendations for Treatment, Training, and Privileging.* Washington, DC: American Psychiatric Association; 1990.

Ananth J, Samra D, Kolivakis T. Amelioration of drug-induced parkinsonism by ECT. *Am J Psychiatry.* 1979;136:1094.

Andersen K, Balldin J, Gottfries C, et al. A double-blind evaluation of electroconvulsive therapy in Parkinson's disease with "on-off" phenomena. *Acta Neurol Scand.* 1987;76:191–199.

Asnis G. Parkinson's disease, depression and ECT: a review and case study. *Am J Psychiatry.* 1977;134:191–195.

Atre-Vaidya N, Jampala VC. Electroconvulsive therapy in parkinsonism with affective disorder. *Br J Psychiatry.* 1988;152:55–58.

Atterwill CK. Lack of effect of repeated electroconvulsive shock on [^{3}H] spiroperidol and [^{3}H] 5-hydroxy-tryptamine binding and cholinergic parameters in rat brain. *J Neurochem.* 1980;35:729–734.

Bagadia VN, Abhyankar RR, Doshi J, et al. A double blind controlled study of ECT vs. chlorpromazine in schizophrenia. *J Assoc Phys India.* 1983;31:637–640.

Balldin J, Eden S, Granerus A, et al. Electroconvulsive therapy in Parkinson's syndrome with "on-off" phenomenon. *J Neural Transm.* 1980;47:11–21.

Balldin J, Granerus A, Lindstedt G, et al. Predictors for improvement after electroconvulsive therapy in parkinsonian patients with on-off symptoms. *J Neural Transm.* 1981;52:199–211.

Balldin J, Granerus A, Lindstedt G, et al. Neuroendocrine evidence for increased responsiveness of dopamine receptors in humans following electroconvulsive therapy. *Psychopharmacology.* 1982;76:371–376.

Benson DF, Blumer D, eds. *Psychiatric Aspects of Neurologic Disease,* vol 2. New York: Grune & Stratton; 1982.

Bergstrom DA, Kellar KJ. Effect of electroconvulsive shock on mono-aminergic receptor binding sites in rat brain. *Nature.* 1979;278:464–466.

Bhavsar VH, Dhumal VR, Kelkar VV. The effect of some anti-epilepsy drugs on enhancement of the monoamine-mediated behavioral responses following the administration of electroconvulsive shocks to rats. *Eur J Pharmacol.* 1981;74:243–247.

Birkett DP. ECT in parkinsonism with affective disorder (letter). *British Journal of Psychiatry* 1988;152:712.

Black DW, Winokur G, Nasrallah H. Treatment of mania: A naturalistic study of electroconvulsive therapy versus lithium in 438 patients. *Journal of Clinical Psychiatry* 1987;48:132–139.

Blazer D. Depression in the elderly. *New England Journal of Medicine* 1989;320:164–166.

Brandon S, Cowley P, McDonald C, et al. Electroconvulsive therapy: Results in depressive illness from the Leicestershire trial. *British Medical Journal* 1984;288:22–25.

Brandon S, Cowley P, McDonald C, et al. Leicester ECT trial: Results in schizophrenia. *British Journal of Psychiatry* 1985;146:177–183.

Brown GL. Parkinsonism, depression, and ECT (letter to the editor). *Am J Psychiatry* 1975;132:1084.

Burke WJ, Peterson J, Rubin EH. Electroconvulsive therapy in the treatment of combined depression and Parkinson's disease. *Psychosomatics* 1988;29:341–346.

Chacko RC, Root L. ECT and tardive dyskinesia: Two cases and a review. *Journal of Clinical Psychiatry* 1983;44:265–266.

Childers RT. Comparison of four regimens in newly admitted female schizophrenics. *American Journal of Psychiatry* 1964;120:1010–1011.

Chiodo LA, Antelman SM. Electroconvulsive shock: Progressive dopamine autoreceptor subsensitivity independent of repeated treatment. *Science* 1980;210:799–801.

Christie JE, Whalley LJ, Brown NS, Dick H. Effect of ECT on the neuroendocrine response to apomorphine in severely depressed patients. *British Journal of Psychiatry* 1982;140:268–273.

Clark D, White FJ. Review: D1 dopamine receptors-the search for a function: A critical evaluation of the D1/D2 dopamine receptor classification and its functional implications. *Synapse* 1987;1:347–388.

Creese I, Kuczenski R, Segal D. Lack of behavioral evidence for dopaminergic autoreceptor subsensitivity after acute electroconvulsive shock. *Pharmacology, Biochemistry and Behavior* 1982;17:375–376.

Deakin JFW, Owen F, Cross AJ, Dashwood MJ. Studies on possible mechanisms of action of electroconvulsive therapy; Effects of repeated electrically induced seizures on rat brain receptors for monoamines and other neurotransmitters. *Psychopharmacology* 1981;73:345–349.

Demuth GW, Rand BS. Atypical major depression in a patient with severe primary degenerative dementia. *American Journal of Psychiatry* 1980;137:1609–1610.

Douyon R, Serby M, Klutchko B, Rotrosen J. ECT and Parkinson's disease revisited: A "naturalistic" study. *American Journal of Psychiatry* 1989;146:1451–1455.

Dubovsky SL. Using electroconvulsive therapy for patients with neurological disease. *Hospital and Community Psychiatry* 1986;37:819–825.

Dubovsky SL, Gay M, Franks R, Haddenhorst A. ECT in the presence of increased intracranial pressure and respiratory failure: Case report. *Journal of Clinical Psychiatry* 1985;46:489–491.

Dysken M, Evans HM, Chan CH, Davis JM. Improvement of depression and parkinsonism during ECT: A case study. *Neuropsychobiology* 1976;2:81–86.

Evans JPM, Grahame-Smith DG, Green AR, Tordoff FC. Electroconvulsive shock increases the behavioural responses of rats to brain 5-hydroxy tryptamine accumulation and central nervous system stimulant drugs. *British Journal of Pharmacology* 1976;56:193–199.

Fochtmann LJ, et al. Quantitative autoradiographic demonstration of increased D1 receptor binding in rat brain after repeated electroconvulsive shock. *Abstracts-Society for Neuroscience* 1987;13:1343.

Freeman CPL, Basson JV, Crighton A. Double-blind controlled trial of electroconvulsive therapy (ECT) and simulated ECT in depressive illness. *Lancet* 1978;1:738–740.

Friedel RO. The combined use of neuroleptics and ECT in drug resistant schizophrenic patients. *Psychopharmacology Bulletin* 1986;22:928–930.

Fromm GH. Observation on the effects of electroshock treatment in patients with parkinsonism. *Bulletin of Tulane University* 1959;18:71–73.

Gangadhar BN, Chowdhary JR, Channabasavanna SM. ECT and drug-induced parkinsonism. *Indian Journal of Psychiatry* 1983;25:212–213.

Gangadhar BN, Kapur RL, Kalyanasundaram S. Comparison of electroconvulsive therapy with imipramine in endogenous depression: A double blind study. *British Journal of Psychiatry* 1982;141:367–371.

Gangadhar BN, Pradhan N, Mayamil CSK. Dopamine autoreceptor down-regulation following repeated electroconvulsive shock. *Indian Journal of Medical Research* 1987;86:787–791.

Gangadhar BN, et al. Dopaminergic effects of repeated electroconvulsive shocks. *Convulsive Therapy* 1989;5:157–161.

Globus M, Lerer B, Hamburger R, Belmaker R. Chronic electroconvulsive shock and chronic haloperidol are not additive in effects on dopamine receptors. *Neuropharmacology* 1981;20:1125–1128.

Goetz CG, Olanow C, Koller W, et al. Multicenter study of autologous adrenal medullary transplantation to the corpus striatum in patients with advanced Parkinson's disease. *New England Journal of Medicine* 1989;320:337–341.

Goswami U, Dutta S, Kuruvilla K, et al. Electroconvulsive therapy in neuroleptic-induced parkinsonism. *Biological Psychiatry* 1989;26:234–238.

Gotham AM, Brown RG, Marsden CD. Depression in Parkinson's disease: A quantitative and qualitative analysis. *Journal of Neurology, Neurosurgery and Psychiatry* 1986;49:381–389.

Grahame-Smith DG, Green AR, Costain DW. Mechanism of the antidepressant action of electroconvulsive therapy. *Lancet* 1978;1:254–256.

Green AR. Repeated exposure of rats to the convulsant agent flurothyl enhances 5-hydroxytryptamine- and dopamine-mediated behavioural responses. *British Journal of Pharmacology* 1978;62:325–331.

Green AR, Costain DW, Deakin JWF. Enhanced 5-HTP and DA-mediated behavioural responses following convulsions. III: The effects of monoamine antagonists and synthesis inhibitors on the ability of ECS to enhance responses. *Neuropharmacology* 1980;19:907–914.

Green AR, Deakin JFW. Brain noradrenaline depletion prevents ECS-induced enhancement of serotonin and dopamine-mediated behavior. *Nature* 1980;285:232–233.

Green AR, Heal DJ, Grahame-Smith DG. Further observations on the effect of repeated electroconvulsive shock on the behavioural responses of rats produced by increases in the functional activity of brain 5-hydroxytryptamine and dopamine. *Psychopharmacology* 1977;52:195–200.

Green AR, Peralta E, Hong JS, et al. Alterations in GABA metabolism and metenkephalin content in rat brain following repeated electroconvulsive shocks. *Journal of Neurochemistry* 1978;31:607–611.

Greenblatt M, Grosser G, Wechster H. Differential response of hospitalized depressed patients in somatic therapy. *American Journal of Psychiatry* 1964;120:935–943.

Gregory S, Schawcross CR, Gill D. The Nottingham ECT study: A double blind comparison of bilateral, unilateral, and simulated ECT in depressive illness. *British Journal of Psychiatry* 1985;146:520–524.

Gujavarty K, Greenberg LB, Fink M. Electroconvulsive therapy and neuroleptic medication in therapy-resistant positive-symptom psychosis. *Convulsive Therapy* 1987;3:185–195.

Harnryd C, Bjerkenstedt L, Grimm V, Sedvall G. Reduction of MOPEG levels in cerebrospinal fluid of psychotic women after electroconvulsive treatment. *Psychopharmacology* 1979;64:131–134.

Heal DJ, Green AR. Repeated electroconvulsive shock increases the behavioural responses of rats to injection of both dopamine and dibutyryl cyclic amp into the nucleus accumbens. *Neuropharmacology* 1978;17:1085–1087.

Heal DJ, Phillips AG, Green AR. Studies on the locomotor activity produced by injection of dibutyryl cyclic 3^1 5^1 amp into the nucleus accumbens of rats. *Neuropharmacology* 1978;17:265–270.

Holcombe HH, Sternberg DE, Heninger GR. Effects of electroconvulsive therapy on mood, parkinsonism, and tardive dyskinesia in a depressed patient: ECT and dopamine systems. *Biological Psychiatry* 1983;18:865–873.

Hurwitz TA, Calne DB, Waterman K. Treatment of dopamino-mimetic psychosis in Parkinson's disease with electroconvulsive therapy. *Canadian Journal of Neurological Sciences* 1988;15:32–34.

Jaeckle RS, Dilsaver SC. Covariation of depressive symptoms, parkinsonism, and post-dexamethasone plasma cortisol levels in a bipolar patient: Simultaneous response to ECT and lithium carbonate. *Acta Psychiatrica Scandinavica* 1986;74:68–72.

Janakiramaiah N, Channabasavanna M, Narasimha Murthy NS. ECT/chlorpromazine combination versus chlorpromazine alone in acutely schizophrenic patients. *Acta Psychiatrica Scandinavica* 1982;66A:464–470.

Johnstone EC, Lawler P, Stevens M, et al. The Northwick Park electroconvulsive therapy trial. *Lancet* 1980;2:1317–1320.

Jori A, Dolfini E, Casati C, Argenta G. Effect of ECT and imipramine treatment on the concentration of 5-hydroxyindoleacetic acid (5-HIAA) and homovanillic acid (HVA) in the cerebrospinal fluid of depressed patients. *Psychopharmacologia* 1975;44:87–90.

Kalinowsky LB, Hippius H. *Pharmacological, convulsive, and other somatic treatments in psychiatry.* New York, Grune and Stratton, Inc., 1969.

Kramer BA. The use of ECT in California, 1977–1983. *American Journal of Psychiatry* 1985;142:1190–1192.

Lambourn A, Gill D. A controlled comparison of simulated and real ECT. *British Journal of Psychiatry* 1978;133:514–519.

Lauterbach EC, Moore NC. Parkinsonism-dystonia syndrome and ECT (letter). *American Journal of Psychiatry* 1990;147:1249–1250.

Lebensohn ZM. Parkinsonism, depression, and ECT (Letter to the Editor). *American Journal of Psychiatry* 1975;132:1084.

Lebensohn ZM, Jenkins RB. Improvement of parkinsonism in depressed patients treated with ECT. *American Journal of Psychiatry* 1975;132:283–285.

Lerer B. Neurochemical and other neurobiological consequences of ECT: Implications for the pathogenesis and treatment of affective disorders. In: *Psychopharmacology: The Third Generation of Progress.* Edited by H Meltzer. New York, Raven Press, 1987:577–588.

Lerer B, Jabotinsky-Rubin K, Bannet J, et al. Electroconvulsive shock prevents dopamine receptor supersensitivity. *European Journal of Pharmacology* 1982;80:131–134.

Lerer B, Weiner RD, Belmaker RH (editors). *ECT: Basic mechanisms.* Washington, DC, American Psychiatric Press, 1984.

Levy LA, Savit JM, Hodes M. Parkinsonism: Improvement by electroconvulsive therapy. *Archives of Physical Medicine and Rehabilitation* 1983;64:432–433.

Lieberman J. Dopamine pathophysiology in tardive dyskinesia. *Psychiatric Annals* 1989;19:289–296.

Linnoila M, Karoum F, Potter WZ. Effects of antidepressant treatments on dopamine turnover in depressed patients. *Archives of General Psychiatry* 1983;40:1015–1017.

Linnoila M, Litovitz G, Scheinin M, et al. Effects of electroconvulsive treatment on monoamine metabolites, growth hormone, and prolactin in plasma. *Biological Psychiatry* 1984;19:79–84.

Madrazo I, Drucker-Colin R, Diaz V, et al. Open microsurgical autograft of adrenal medulla to the right caudate nucleus in two patients with intractable Parkinson's disease. *New England Journal of Medicine* 1987;316:831–834.

May PRA, Tuma H, Dixon W, et al. Schizophrenia: A follow-up study of the results of five forms of treatment. *Archives of General Psychiatry* 1981;38:776–784.

McAllister TW, Price TRP. Severe depressive pseudodementia with and without dementia. *American Journal of Psychiatry* 1982;139:626–629.

McCabe MS. ECT in the treatment of mania: A controlled study. *American Journal of Psychiatry* 1976;133:688–691.

McCabe MS, Norris B. ECT vs. chlorpromazine in mania. *Biological Psychiatry* 1977;12:245–254.

Medical Research Council. Clinical trial of the treatment of depressive illness. *British Medical Journal* 1965;5439:881–886.

Modigh K. Electroconvulsive shock and post-synaptic catecholamine effects: increased psychomotor stimulant action of apomorphine and clonidine in reserpine-pretreated mice by repeated ECS. *Journal of Neural Transmission* 1975;36:19–32.

Modigh K. Long-term effects of electroconvulsive shock therapy on synthesis, turnover, and uptake of brain monoamines. *Psychopharmacology* 1976;49:179–185.

Mukherjee S, Rosen A, Caracci G, Shukla S. Persistent tardive dyskinesia in bipolar patients. *Archives of General Psychiatry* 1986;43:342–346.

Mukherjee S, Sackheim HA, Lee C. Unilateral ECT in the treatment of manic episodes. *Convulsive Therapy* 1988;4:74–80.

Newman ME, Lerer B. Effects of chronic electroconvulsive shock on D1 and D2 dopamine receptor-mediated activity of adenylate cyclase in homogenates of striatum and limbic forebrain of rat. *Neuropharmacology* 1989;28:787–790.

Nordin G, Ottosson TO, Roos BE. Influence of convulsive therapy on 5-hydroxyindoleacetic acid and homovanillic acid in cerebrospinal fluid in endogenous depression. *Psychopharmacologia* 1971;20:315–320.

Nutt DTR, Green AR, Grahame-Smith DG. Enhanced 5-hydroxytryptamine and dopamine-mediated behavioural responses following convulsions. I. The effects of single and repeated bicuculline-induced seizures. *Neuropharmacology* 1980;19:897–900.

Perry GF. ECT for dementia and catatonia. *Journal of Clinical Psychiatry* 1983;44:117.

Peterson SL. Electroconvulsive shock and L-dopa reduce head-turning induced by electrical stimulation of the caudate nucleus in the rat. *Experimental Neurology* 1986;91:463–470.

Post RM, Putnam F, Uhde TW, Weiss SR. Electroconvulsive therapy as an anticonvulsant: Implications for its mechanism of action in affective illness. In: *Electroconvulsive Therapy: Clinical and Basic Research Issues.* Edited by S. Malitz and HA Sackeim. New York, New York Academy of Sciences, 1986:376–388.

Rainey JM, Faust M. Parkinsonism masked by ECT and psychotropic medication (letter to the editor). *American Journal of Psychiatry* 1975;132:1084–1085.

Roth SD, Mukherjee S, Sackeim HA. Electroconvulsive therapy in a patient with mania, parkinsonism, and tardive dyskinesia. *Convulsive Therapy* 1988;4:92–97.

Sackeim HA, Decina P, Kanzler M, et al. Effects of electrode placement on the efficacy of titrated, low-dose ECT. *American Journal of Psychiatry* 1987;144:1449–1455.

Sandyk R. ECT, opioid system, and motor response in Parkinson's disease (letter to the editor). *Biological Psychiatry* 1986;21:235–236.

Sano M, Stern Y, Coté L, et al. Depression in Parkinson's disease: A biochemical model. *Journal of Neuropsychiatry and Clinical Neurosciences* 1990;2:88–92.

Savitsky N, Karliner W. Electroshock in the presence of organic disease of the central nervous system. *Journal of the Hillside Hospital* 1953;2:3–22.

Serra G, Argiolas A, Fadda F, et al. Repeated electroconvulsive shock prevents the sedative effect of small doses of apomorphine. *Psychopharmacology* 1981;73:194–196.

Shapiro MF, Goldberg HH. Electroconvulsive therapy in patients with structural disease of the nervous system. *American Journal of the Medical Sciences* 1957;233:186–195.

Small JG, Milstein V, Klapper MH, et al. Electroconvulsive therapy in the treatment of manic episodes. In: *Electroconvulsive therapy: clinical and basic research issues.* Edited by S Malitz and HA Sackeim. New York, New York Academy of Sciences, 1986:37–49.

Smith K, Surphilis WRP, Gynther MD. ECT-CPZ and chlorpromazine compared in the treatment of schizophrenia. *Journal of Nervous and Mental Disease* 1967;144:284–290.

Snow SS, Wells CE. Case studies in neuropsychiatry. Diagnosis and treatment of coexistent dementia and depression. *Journal of Clinical Psychiatry* 1981;42:439–441.

Stoudemire A, et al. Neuropsychological and biomedical assessment of depression-dementia syndromes. *Journal of Neuropsychiatry and Clinical Neurosciences* 1989;1:347–361.

Taylor AE, Saint-Cyr JA. Depression in Parkinson's disease: Reconciling physiological and psychological perspectives. *Journal of Neuropsychiatry and Clinical Neurosciences* 1990;2:92–98.

Taylor MA. Indications for electroconvulsive treatment. In: *Electroconvulsive Therapy: Biologic Foundations and Clinical Applications.* Edited by R Abrams and W Essman. New York, Spectrum Publications, 1982:7–39.

Taylor P, Fleminger JJ. ECT for schizophrenia. *Lancet* 1980;1:1380–1382.

Tepper JM, Nakamura S, Spanis C, et al. Subsensitivity of catecholaminergic neurons to direct acting agonists after single or repeated electroconvulsive shock. *Biological Psychiatry* 1982;17:1059–2070.

Thomas J, Reddy B. The treatment of mania: A retrospective evaluation of the effects of ECT, chlorpromazine, and lithium. *Journal of Affective Disorders* 1982;4:85–92.

Tsuang MT, Tidball JS, Geller D. ECT in a depressed patient with shunt in place for normal pressure hydrocephalus. *American Journal of Psychiatry* 1979;136:1205–1206.

Ward C, Stern G, Pratt R, McKenna P. Electroconvulsive therapy in parkinsonian patients with the "on-off" syndrome. *Journal of Neural Transmission* 1980;49:133–135.

Weiner RD, Rogers HJ, Davidson JR, Squire LR. Effects of stimulus parameters on cognitive side effects. In: *Electroconvulsive Therapy: Clinical and Basic Research Issues.* Edited by S Malitz and HA Sackeim. New York, New York Academy of Sciences, 1986:315–325.

West ED. Electric convulsion therapy in depression: A double-blind controlled trial. *British Medical Journal* 1981;282:355–357.

White DK, Barrett RJ. The effects of electroconvulsive shock on the discriminative stimulus properties of d-amphetamine and apomorphine: Evidence for dopamine receptor alteration subsequent to ECS. *Psychopharmacology* 1981;73:211–214.

Wielosz M. Increased sensitivity to dopaminergic agonists after repeated electroconvulsive shock (ECS) in rats. *Neuropharmacology* 1981;20:941–945.

Wilder J. Parkinsonism, depression, and ECT (letter to the editor). *American Journal of Psychiatry* 1975;132:1083–1084.

Wolf ME, DeWolfe A, Ryan J, et al. Vulnerability to tardive dyskinesia. *Journal of Clinical Psychiatry* 1985;46:367–368.

Yager J. Clinical manifestations of psychiatric disorders. In: *Comprehensive Textbook of Psychiatry: Volume One.* Edited by HI Kaplan and BJ Sadock. Baltimore, Williams and Wilkins, 1989:553–582.

Young RC, Alexopoulous GS, Shamoian CA. Dissociation of motor response from mood and cognition in a parkinsonian patient treated with ECT. *Biological Psychiatry* 1985;20:566–569.

Yudofsky SC. Parkinson's disease, depression, and electroconvulsive therapy: A clinical and neurobiologic synthesis. *Comprehensive Psychiatry* 1979;20:579–581.

Zervas IM, Fink M. ECT for refractory Parkinson's disease (letter to the editor). *Convulsive Therapy* 1991;7:222–223.

V
DRUG THERAPY
AND BEHAVIOR

20

Pharmacology of Parkinson's Disease

STEPHEN T. GANCHER

Several drugs are currently available for the treatment of Parkinson's disease (PD), including anticholinergics, amantadine, dopamine agonists, deprenyl, and levodopa. Some of these drugs, such as amantadine and anticholinergics, were empirically or serendipitously found to have antiparkinsonian action. In contrast, levodopa therapy emerged from several experimental observations: that parkinsonism was associated with a marked deficiency of striatal dopamine (Lloyd et al, 1975), that reserpine treatment in animals induced neurochemical and behavioral effects similar to parkinsonism, and that this reserpine syndrome was reversed with levodopa (Carlsson, 1971). These findings led to the development of levodopa as a specific pharmacological replacement therapy in PD that is still more effective than any other drug currently available.

However, chronic levodopa therapy is complicated by dyskinesias and diurnal motor fluctuations that affect most patients after several years of treatment (Fahn, 1974; Marsden and Parkes, 1977). A variety of treatments have been devised to delay or lessen levodopa-induced fluctuations, including the addition or substitution of dopamine agonists, deprenyl, and various dietary manipulations aimed at influencing the pharmacological profile of levodopa. Nonetheless, a better understanding of motor fluctuations remains a major challenge in the long-term treatment of PD.

LEVODOPA

Clinical Effects

Control of Specific Symptoms

Most patients improve with levodopa treatment, and a complete lack of response suggests an alternate diagnosis. However, not all symptoms improve to an equal degree. Bradykinesia and rigidity improve most consistently, whereas speech and gait abnormalities tend not to improve as much (Bonnet et al, 1987). The reason is not entirely clear, but some patients with prominent or selective gait abnormalities may have symptoms on a vascular basis (FitzGerald et al, 1989), a condition that responds less well to drugs.

Time Course of Drug Effects

Levodopa has both acute and chronic effects. The acute effect, termed the short-duration response (Muenter and Tyce, 1971), refers to improvement in PD symptoms within 1 or 2 hours after levodopa administration and may be recognized either by improvement after levodopa dosing or by reemergence of PD symptoms 3 to 6 hours later. Some patients exhibit a slower improvement days or weeks after initiating levodopa. This latter pattern, termed the long-duration response, occurs both with levodopa and dopamine agonists and may be sufficiently gradual to make it difficult for patients to describe when improvement in PD occurs. In some patients, the slow return of PD symptoms over days after discontinuing levodopa, which may take over 10 days to reach a nadir (Ogasahara et al, 1984), may be the only evidence of a beneficial effect of the drug. Both response patterns may occur in the same patient (Fig. 20–1).

Dyskinesia

A variety of involuntary movements may be induced by levodopa, most commonly choreoathetosis and dystonia. Levodopa-induced choreoathetosis may occur in a wide

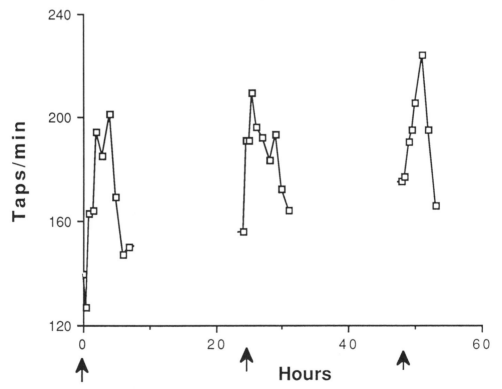

Figure 20–1.   This previously untreated patient received three doses of levodopa at the times indicated by the arrows. Improvement in bradykinesia within hours of levodopa administration (the short-duration effect, measured by tapping speed) and a slower improvement, seen by an increase in the baseline tapping rate (the long-duration response), are seen.

variety of muscle groups and may involve the face, neck, trunk, extremities, and occasionally the chest wall or diaphragm. Dystonia most commonly has a different distribution, mainly affecting the lower extremities, to produce extension, abduction, or flexion of the toes and inversion or eversion of the foot.

These movements occur in distinct temporal patterns. Most commonly, choreic movements appear at the same time as improvement in PD symptoms (peak-dose or on dyskinesia). Another pattern is for choreic or dystonic movements to appear at the start and the end of the period of improvement in PD. This pattern, termed diphasic dyskinesias or the D-I-D response (for dyskinesia-improvement-dyskinesia or dystonia-improvement-dystonia) (Muenter et al, 1977), occurs when plasma levodopa levels are rapidly rising or falling just above threshold levels and, in contrast to peak-dose dyskinesia, may improve if levodopa doses are raised.

Dystonic movements also occur in peak-dose or diphasic patterns. One type in particular, repetitive leg movements, seems to occur only in a diphasic pattern and is very distinctive (Obeso et al, 1989). Unlike choreoathetosis, dystonia also may occur during off periods (Poewe et al, 1988b), typically in the morning before levodopa administration, and may improve with levodopa or dopamine agonists. Paradoxically, the off dystonias are levodopa-induced, as they tend to disappear if levodopa is discontinued. Finally, fixed dystonias, not improving with levodopa or other drugs, also may occur in PD and may require bracing or surgical intervention.

Dose–Response Relationships

There are significant differences between patients in the timing and degree of response to levodopa. Some patients may be able to skip occasional doses of levodopa without noticing motor changes, whereas other patients experience large swings in mobility during the day and may be very dependent on the timing and amount of levodopa (on/off syndrome).

The reason for these differences between patients is unclear. The severity of the underlying PD may influence the response, since patients with severe disease before treatment, like those with MPTP-induced parkinsonism, tend to exhibit fluctuations and dyskinesias relatively soon after initiating levodopa (Langston and Ballard, 1984). However, chronic levodopa exposure may influence the response. Patients newly treated with levodopa show a longer duration of therapeutic response than do chronically treated patients, have a more gradual onset of effect and end of antiparkinsonian effect, and rarely experience dyskinesias (Barbeau and Roy, 1981; Gancher et al, 1988; Mouradian et al, 1988).

In contrast, patients with motor fluctuations have a shorter but more abrupt response to levodopa. These patients typically have an all-or-none response. Once levodopa doses are raised above threshold levels, further dose increases may produce a longer antiparkinsonian effect but one of no greater magnitude (Fig. 20–2) (Nutt and Woodward, 1986).

Dyskinesias appear only with chronic levodopa treatment and usually are minimal in patients without motor fluctuations. However, in patients who do have fluctuations, levodopa-induced dyskinesias tend to appear at the same doses needed for antiparkinsonian effect (Fahn, 1974). This latter feature makes it difficult to administer levodopa within a therapeutic window, that is, in doses sufficient to improve PD symptoms without inducing dyskinesias.

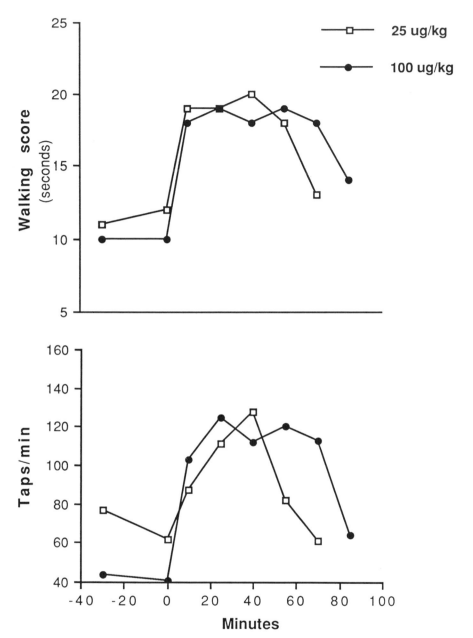

Figure 20–2. This patient with levodopa-induced fluctuations received 25 μg/kg and 100 μg/kg 10-minute infusions of apomorphine on separate days, with monitoring of tapping rate (bottom) and walking score (top, calculated by subtracting the time to arise from a chair, walk 15 feet, and return from 30 seconds). The duration, but not the magnitude of improvement, was dose dependent.

Levodopa Pharmacokinetics

Many factors that influence the pharmacokinetics of levodopa, including variable drug absorption, clearance, metabolism, and transport across the blood–brain barrier, may affect the response to the drug.

Absorption

Levodopa is a large, neutral amino acid preferentially absorbed in the proximal small bowel. One of the most important determinants of levodopa absorption is gastric emptying. Slowing of gastric emptying by high gastric acidity, food (in particular, fats) (Nutt et al, 1984), and drugs, particularly anticholinergics and antidepressants, retard levodopa absorption. Conversely, patients with gastrectomies may have very rapid levodopa absorption.

   In some patients (Fig. 20–3), a variable response to levodopa may result from variation in levodopa absorption due to erratic gastric emptying (Kurlan et al, 1988).

Clearance

Levodopa is cleared quickly from plasma. The elimination half-life is only 1 hour with standard levodopa preparations (Gancher et al, 1987). Because of this rapid clearance, levodopa does not accumulate in plasma with chronic administration and produces large fluctuations in plasma levodopa levels with oral administration. Controlled-release formulations slow absorption and retard the clearance of levodopa from plasma (Cederbaum et al, 1987) but do not eliminate oscillations in drug levels and usually are unable to fully reverse motor fluctuations.

Metabolism

Levodopa is a substrate for a variety of metabolic pathways (Fig. 20–4), including decarboxylation, methylation, and oxidation.

   The most quantitatively important metabolic pathway is decarboxylation to dopamine by aromatic amino acid decarboxylase (AAAD, also termed dopa decarboxylase). Without an AAAD inhibitor, such as carbidopa, over half of a dose of levodopa is metabolized in the small bowel mucosa before absorption, and the dose requirements for levodopa alone are up to five-fold higher than if administered with an AAAD inhibitor. It is estimated that between 75 mg and 100 mg of carbidopa is sufficient to maximally inhibit AAAD, but there is a large interpatient variation, and some patients may experience enhanced benefit or side effects with further supplemental carbidopa administration. In clinical practice, substitution of Sinemet 25/100 tablets for 10/100 tablets may result in a major change in clinical status.

   Catechol-O-methyltransferase (COMT) also metabolizes levodopa, producing 3-O-methyldopa (3OMD). Unlike levodopa, 3OMD has a long plasma half-life, approximately 15 hours, and accumulates in plasma to levels almost 5 to 10 times higher than levodopa. 3OMD is a large neutral amino acid and, like other amino acids, competitively inhibits transport of levodopa across the blood–brain barrier (Wade and Katzman, 1975b).

CNS Transport

To cross the blood–brain barrier, levodopa crosses brain capillaries by a saturable, carrier-dependent transport system that is shared by other large, neutral amino acids

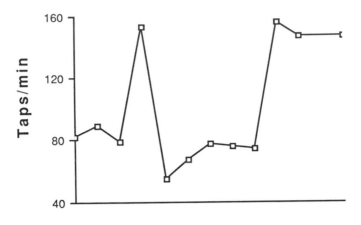

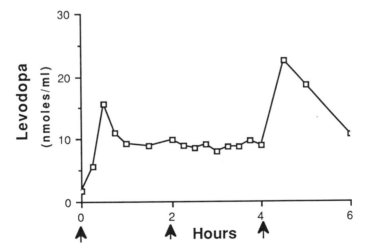

Figure 20–3. This patient with Parkinson's disease and levodopa-induced fluctuations received doses of levodopa/carbidopa at the times indicated by the arrows, with monitoring of plasma levodopa levels (bottom) and bradykinesia (tapping speed, top). The second levodopa dose was poorly absorbed and resulted in a failure of levodopa effect.

(LNAAs) (Wade and Katzman, 1975a). Since levodopa is quantitatively a small part of the total LNAA load in plasma, only a small amount of levodopa is transported into the brain, and an increase in plasma LNAA concentrations, including 3OMD, may interfere with levodopa's clinical effects (Fig. 20–5). Low-protein meals, which reduce plasma LNAA concentrations, may improve the response to levodopa in selected patients (Pincus et al, 1987; Riley et al, 1988).

CNS Metabolism

Levodopa is converted to dopamine by AAAD in the CNS, and this step may be partially deficient in PD. Rodents with a nigrostriatal lesion have much lower striatal dopamine levels after levodopa administration than do unlesioned animals (Spencer

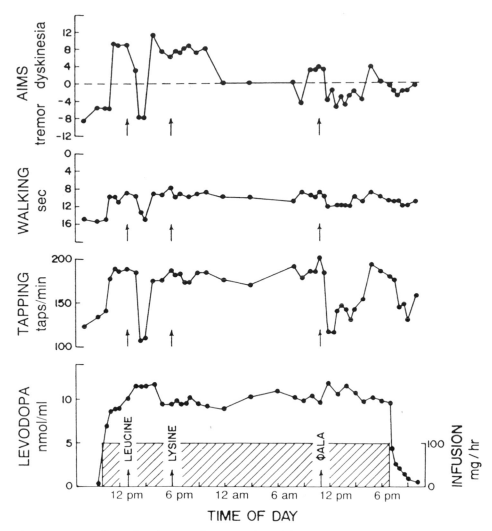

Figure 20-4. Effect of oral LNAA [leucine, phenylalanine (φALA)] and basic amino acid (lysine) challenges on response to levodopa. Plasma levodopa concentrations (bottom) and clinical effects (tapping and walking rate, middle; AIMS scale, top) were monitored during levodopa infusion. Worsening of Parkinson's disease was specific to LNAA challenges. (From Nutt et al., *N Engl J Med.* 1984;310:483–488.)

et al, 1984). Patients with PD imaged by PET after receiving F-18-labeled levodopa, have a decreased accumulation of radioactivity in the striatum (Leenders et al, 1986), suggesting a deficiency in dopamine synthesis, storage, or reuptake.

This decrease in the ability to store dopamine, presumably from loss of nigrostriatal nerve terminals, is thought by some investigators to represent the physiological abnormality that underlies the wearing-off effect and levodopa-induced fluctuations (Mouradian et al, 1988). However, not all studies are consistent with this hypothesis, and other pathophysiological alterations may exist in patients with fluctuations. Dopamine is also oxidized in the CNS by monoamine oxidase (MAO) to inactive, acidic

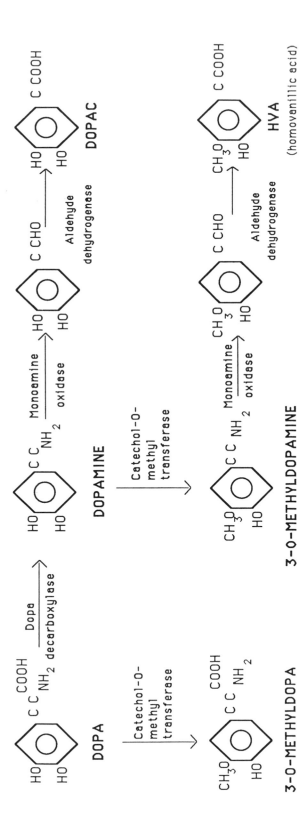

Figure 20–5. The most important metabolic pathways of levodopa are illustrated.

metabolites. A selective MAO B inhibitor, deprenyl, has been developed and is discussed later.

Finally, levodopa and dopamine in the CNS are both substrates for COMT, and COMT inhibitors enhance concentrations of levodopa and dopamine in the striatum after levodopa administration and are under investigation as adjunctive antiparkinsonian medications.

DEPRENYL

Deprenyl (seligiline) is a selective inhibitor of one of two isozymes of the enzyme monoamine oxidase (MAO) (Knoll, 1986), an enzyme that metabolizes dietary and endogenous monoamines, including dopamine, serotonin, norepinephrine, and epinephrine. It was discovered serendipitously that iproniazid, a drug for tuberculosis, had potent antidepressant effects and was discovered to be an MAO inhibitor. Other, nonselective MAO inhibitors were developed for treatment of depression but were prone to numerous dietary and drug interactions. The most notable interaction, the cheese effect, occurs with ingestion of foods containing tyramine. Tyramine acts pharmacologically as an indirect neurotransmitter, causing release of catecholamines from nerve terminals. Without MAO, tyramine and catecholamines accumulate in plasma and may precipitate life-threatening hypertensive crises.

MAO exists in two isozymes, A and B. Many tissues have both types. However, the striatum mainly contains MAO B, whereas intestinal MAO is type A. Unlike earlier MAO inhibitors, deprenyl is very selective for MAO B and lacks the dangerous cheese effect. Deprenyl is a lipophilic, long-acting drug and is an irreversible inhibitor of MAO B. Unlike other MAO inhibitors, which act by competitively binding MAO, deprenyl is a suicide inhibitor of MAO B, irreversibly binding and inhibiting the enzyme. Because new MAO B enzyme synthesis must occur to regain activity, it may take days or weeks for deprenyl's clinical effects to fully disappear. Deprenyl is metabolized to amphetamine and methamphetamine, which may cause a sense of well-being or mild insomnia but are not thought to account for deprenyl's pharmacological actions in PD.

Deprenyl has been studied in patients previously untreated with antiparkinsonian drugs and in patients with levodopa-induced fluctuations. By itself, deprenyl induces only minimal symptomatic benefit. In studies comparing deprenyl and placebo in otherwise untreated patients, only a very modest, statistically insignificant symptomatic effect was seen (Parkinson Study Group, 1989; Tetrud and Langston, 1989). However, in combination with levodopa, deprenyl is a useful adjunctive medication, decreasing the number of off hours per day and reducing off severity in patients with levodopa-induced fluctuations (Golbe et al, 1988).

It has been suggested that deprenyl may influence the natural history of PD. Animals or humans exposed to the drug MPTP develop irreversible parkinsonism. In humans, this disorder appears very similar to idiopathic PD (Langston and Ballard, 1984). This neurotoxic effect of MPTP results from conversion by brain MAO to MPP+ and is blocked by deprenyl. Since MPTP-induced parkinsonism appears clinically similar to idiopathic disease, it was reasoned that idiopathic PD also may result from chronic exposure to an endogenous or environmental toxin or precursor to a toxin. This hypothesis was tested by the DATATOP study, in which 800 patients with early PD received either deprenyl or placebo, and the time to needing symptomatic treatment (i.e., with levodopa) was measured. Deprenyl significantly delayed the need for symptomatic treatment with levodopa by an average of 13 months, even though the patients treated with deprenyl did not have any significant measurable symptomatic effect that could have accounted for the results (Parkinson Study Group, 1989). It was also reported in a retrospective analysis that patients treated with a combination of deprenyl and levodopa had less disability and a longer life expectancy than those treated with levodopa alone (Birkmayer, 1983). Taken together, these studies suggest that deprenyl may retard the progression of PD. However, further studies are needed to separate the small, insignificant symptomatic benefit of deprenyl from a possible prophylactic effect.

DOPAMINE AGONISTS

Several dopamine agonists are available for treatment of PD. It was discovered that some ergot alkaloids possessed dopaminergic activity, and a variety of dopamine agonists derived from ergot were developed, including bromocriptine, pergolide, and lisuride. The largest experience with these drugs in PD has been as adjunctive or replacement therapy in patients with levodopa-induced fluctuations. In these patients, these drugs may reduce the severity or frequency of off periods from levodopa. In general, these drugs have similar actions and adverse effects, though some patients with loss of benefit or intolerance to bromocriptine or pergolide may improve with substitution of another agonist (Goetz et al, 1989).

Apomorphine is a dopamine agonist that is chemically unrelated to the ergot alkaloids. A chemical breakdown product of morphine, apomorphine is a potent emetic and was used mainly as a treatment for poisoning. An early clinical trial, using orally administered apomorphine, produced nephrotoxicity (Cotzias et al, 1976), but more recent studies using parenteral routes have demonstrated that apomorphine is a safe, effective adjunctive medication in severe PD (Stibe et al, 1988; Poewe et al, 1988a). Apomorphine is a potent, lipophilic drug and may reverse PD within 5 minutes after subcutaneous injection. This rapid action facilitates its use as an emergency treatment for off periods that occur with oral antiparkinsonian drugs.

In the hopes of avoiding long-term difficulties with levodopa, dopamine agonists have been investigated as initial therapy in previously untreated patients. Most studies have noted improvement in all signs of PD roughly comparable to levodopa with both bromocriptine and pergolide (Jankovic, 1985), but recurrent symptoms develop frequently, requiring levodopa supplementation in most patients after 1 or 2 years of dopamine agonist treatment. Similar effects have been noted for lisuride and pergolide (Rinne, 1986).

The early combination of levodopa and a dopamine agonist before the appearance of fluctuations also has been suggested as a way to avoid some of the long-term complications observed with levodopa. In some studies, less levodopa-induced fluctuations are observed in patients receiving combination therapy compared with levodopa alone (Rinne, 1986). However, fluctuations also improve with the later addition of dopamine agonists, and it is still unclear to what extent early combination treatment is helpful.

One of the main difficulties in the use of dopamine agonists is frequent side effects. Most of the side effects that occur with bromocriptine, lisuride, pergolide, or apomorphine also occur with levodopa but are more prominent with these drugs. Side effects include nausea, vomiting, and postural hypotension. However, other more unusual adverse effects that are almost never seen with levodopa may occur with dopamine agonists. These include erythromelalgia, a painful, red edema of the lower extremities, and pleural fibrosis. These are of unclear cause, but the pleural reaction seen with pergolide and bromocriptine is similar to that described with the ergot alkaloid methysergide and may result from a structural similarity.

CNS side effects seen with levodopa also are common with dopamine agonists. They are wide ranging and vary from insomnia or other mild sleep disturbances to confusion and paranoia, benign visual hallucinosis with retained insight, delusions, or even a florid paranoid psychosis. These mental side effects also may occur with levodopa but may be more severe and persistent if induced by dopamine agonists.

ANTICHOLINERGICS AND AMANTADINE

Before levodopa, drug treatment of PD was limited to anticholinergic therapy. These drugs originally were derived from a variety of botanical sources, including *Atropa belladonna* (deadly nightshade) and *Datura stramonium* (jimson weed), containing scopolamine and atropine and were used for centuries in a variety of medical condition. These older drugs have been abandoned in favor of several synthetic compounds, including benztropine, trihexyphenidyl, biperidine, and ethopropazine. Despite their chemical differences, the clinical actions of all of these drugs are similar, and significant differences have not been described.

Anticholinergics are most useful for relief of rigidity and tremor and are only modestly effective otherwise. They may be used both as initial treatment in mildly affected patients and as an adjunct in patients chronically treated with levodopa with persistent tremor. They are especially useful for levodopa-induced dystonia.

Anticholinergics, in general, are poorly tolerated drugs with a narrow therapeutic margin, particularly in the elderly. Both peripheral side effects (dry mouth, constipation, accommodative paralysis, and urinary hesitancy) and CNS side effects (memory loss, confusion, disorientation, insomnia, or sedation) commonly occur with doses that improve PD symptoms. Some degree of tolerance develops to these adverse effects, and these drugs are most useful if very slowly increased over a period of weeks. Conversely, if side effects or lack of benefit necessitate discontinuation, drugs in this class should be tapered slowly, since sudden discontinuation may produce marked deterioration in PD.

Amantadine was developed as a prophylaxis against influenza A, and was discovered serendipitously to have antiparkinsonian effects (Schwab et al, 1969). By itself, amantadine may improve all symptoms of PD and acts quickly, but the improvement may wane over time. It is usually inadequate treatment for severe bradykinesia. Amantadine is usually well tolerated, but possible adverse effects include dry mouth, lower extremity edema, livedo reticularis, orthostatic hypotension, or worsening of congestive heart failure. CNS side effects, such as insomnia or agitation, also can occur but again are unusual. However, amantadine may have synergistic side effects with other antiparkinsonian drugs, and the addition of amantadine may worsen levodopa-induced dyskinesias, hallucinations, or orthostatic hypotension. Moreover, some patients, even without clear benefit, may have difficulty in reducing the dose due to withdrawal effects.

LATE-LEVODOPA COMPLICATIONS AND THE ON/OFF SYNDROME

Levodopa-induced fluctuations and dyskinesias are common in patients chronically treated with levodopa. The spectrum of fluctuations is large, varying from predictable, mild wearing-off effects to sudden, unpredictable swings between severe dyskinesia and immobility. The fluctuations may be classified in several ways, that is, by specific motor signs or symptoms that occur during on or off states or by the temporal pattern.

One useful approach is to divide fluctuations into predictable, in which the patient notices a relationship between levodopa dosing and signs or symptoms, and unpredictable, in which no pattern is obvious. Predictable fluctuations most commonly are manifest as wearing-off effects but also include peak-dose or diphasic dyskinesias, off dystonias, or a temporary flare in PD symptoms at the end of a levodopa dose cycle (Nutt et al, 1988). Less predictable fluctuations include failure of a levodopa dose to take effect and rapid, random changes in PD not clearly related to levodopa doses.

Nonmotor symptoms also may fluctuate during the day. Some patients experience pain, cramping, or dysesthesias when off, and these sensory symptoms may present a very difficult challenge in managing drug treatment (Snider et al, 1976). Autonomic symptoms also may fluctuate. These include urinary or bowel dysfunction, diaphoresis, dyspnea (either from off chest wall rigidity or respiratory dyskinesias when on), drooling, dysphagia, and particularly fluctuation in blood pressure. Levodopa or dopamine agonists have a hypotensive action and may cause peak-dose orthostatic dizziness or hypotension, or hypertension when off. Finally, mood and cognitive function may fluctuate with other symptoms and are discussed elsewhere.

Management

In approaching treatment for a patient with fluctuations, several historical features are useful in defining the problem. First, it is helpful to determine what specific symptom is fluctuating and if it occurs during episodes of PD symptoms or during periods of levodopa's action. To guide this, the history should include the amount, time, and frequency of levodopa administration, the usual latency to noting a benefit from levodopa, as well as its duration of effect, the effect of meals or exercise, and a description of typical on and off symptoms. Sometimes, the distinction between on and off symptoms is not clear by the history. For example, a complaint of intermittent, excessive "nervousness" with levodopa may be due to mild drug-induced dyskinesia, frequently a difficult sign or symptom for patients to recognize, or may represent akathisia during off periods. In these cases, examination of the patient during both on and off periods may prove fruitful.

A variety of treatments may help predictable off periods. Options include increasing the size of each levodopa dose, which would be expected to prolong the duration of action of each dose of levodopa, increasing the number of levodopa doses per day, or adding a dopamine agonist or deprenyl. Anticholinergics may be useful for control of tremor or off dystonia.

The first step in treatment of unpredictable off periods is to optimize levodopa absorption. Unless nausea is problematic, levodopa should be taken on an empty stomach, and the size of each levodopa dose should be increased as much as is feasible. With smaller doses, peak plasma levodopa may only rise to levels slightly above a minimally effective concentration, and any effect to retard or reduce levodopa absorption may cause a dose failure. Lowering plasma large, neutral amino acid concentrations by a protein-restricted diet may be helpful.

Treatment of adverse levodopa effects may include reduction in the size of each levodopa dose or reducing or eliminating adjunctive antiparkinsonian medications. Hallucinations or confusion, in particular, may require discontinuation of dopamine agonists but also may respond to discontinuation of anticholinergics or amantadine. Some adverse drug effects may benefit from the addition of specific, additional drug treatment. For example, levodopa-induced hypotension, if symptomatic, may benefit from the addition of flucortisone. Nausea may be treated by taking levodopa with food or reducing the dose, but domperidone, an antiemetic with little adverse effects on PD (Parkes, 1986) may be useful as well. In addition, some patients with nocturnal hallucinations may benefit from low-dose neuroleptic therapy without worsening of PD symptoms.

SUMMARY

Most patients with PD symptoms benefit to a significant extent from currently available drugs. In some patients, the improvement in symptoms after initiating levodopa therapy may be dramatic and may allow resumption of activities previously impossible due to bradykinesia. However, because of increasingly prevalent side effects in patients chronically treated with levodopa, the decision to start this potent drug should not be made lightly. Careful consideration of other treatment options should be made before initiating levodopa therapy, particularly in patients with mild symptoms that are not interfering with function.

The decision as to which of these options is the most beneficial for a given patient must be individualized, and financial considerations, peak-dose drug toxicity, other medical conditions, motivation and understanding of the patient, and spousal support are all important considerations in choosing the most beneficial treatment.

REFERENCES

Barbeau A, Roy M. Ten-year results of treatment with levodopa plus benzerazide in Parkinson's disease. In: *Research Progress in Parkinson's Disease.* Edited by FC Rose and R Capildeo. Kent, Pitman Medical, 1981:241–247.

Birkmayer W. Deprenyl (Selegiline) in the treatment of Parkinson's disease. *Acta Neurol Scand (suppl)* 1983;95:103–106.

Bonnet AM, Loria Y, Saint-Hilaire MH, et al. Does long-term aggravation of Parkinson's disease result from nondopaminergic lesions? *Neurology* 1987;37:1539–1542.

Carlsson A. Basic concepts underlying recent developments in the field of Parkinson's disease. In: *Recent Advances in Parkinson's Disease.* Edited by FH McDowell and CH Markham. Philadelphia, F. A. Davis, 1971:1–31.

Cederbaum JM, Breck L, Kutt H, McDowell FH. Controlled-release levodopa/carbidopa, II: Sinemet CR4 treatment of response fluctuations in Parkinson's disease. *Neurology* 1987;37:1607–1612.

Cotzias GC, Papavasilious PS, Tolosa ES, et al. Treatment of Parkinson's disease with aporphines. *N Engl J Med* 1976;294:567–572.

Fahn S. "On-off" phenomenon with levodopa therapy in parkinsonism. *Neurology* 1974;431–441.

FitzGerald PM, Jankovic J. Lower body parkinsonism: Evidence for vascular etiology. *Movement Disorders* 1989;4:249–260.

Gancher ST, Nutt JG, Woodward WR. Peripheral pharmacokinetics of levodopa in untreated, stable, and fluctuating parkinsonian patients. *Neurology* 1987;37:940–944.

Gancher ST, Nutt JG, Woodward W. Response to brief levodopa infusion in parkinsonian patients with and without motor fluctuations. *Neurology* 1988;38:712–716.

Goetz CG, Shannon KM, Tanner CM, et al. Agonist substitution in advanced Parkinson's disease. *Neurology* 1989;39:1121–1122.

Golbe LI, Lieberman AN, Muenter MD, et al. Deprenyl in the treatment of symptom fluctuations in advanced Parkinson's disease. *Clin Neuropharmacol* 1988;11:45–55.

Jankovic J. Long-term use of dopamine agonists in Parkinson's disease. *Clin Neuropharmacol* 1985;8:131–140.

Knoll J. The pharmacology of (−) deprenyl. *J Neural Transm (Suppl)* 1986;22:75–89.

Kurlan R, Rothfield KP, Woodward WR, et al. Erratic gastric emptying of levodopa may cause "random" fluctuations of parkinsonian mobility. *Neurology* 1988;38:419–421.

Langston JW, Ballard P. Parkinsonism induced by 1-methyl-4-phenyl-1,2,3,6-tetrahydropyridine (MPTP): Implications for treatment and the pathogenesis of Parkinson's disease. *Can J Neurol Sci* 1984;11:160–165.

Leenders KL, Palmer AJ, Quinn N, et al. Brain dopamine metabolism in patients with Parkinson's disease measured with positron emission tomography. *J Neurol Neurosurg Psychiatry* 1986;49:853–860.

Lloyd KG, Davidson L, Hornykiewicz O. The neurochemistry of Parkinson's disease: Effect of L-DOPA therapy. *J Pharmacol Exp Ther* 1975;195:453–464.

Marsden CD, Parkes JD. Success and problems of long-term levodopa therapy in Parkinson's disease. *Lancet* 1977;1:345–349.

Melamed E. Early-morning dystonia: a late side effect of long-term levodopa therapy in Parkinson's disease. *Arch Neurol* 1979;36:308–310.

Mouradian MM, Juncos JL, Fabbrini G, et al. Motor fluctuations in Parkinson's disease: Central pathophysiological mechanisms, part II. *Ann Neurol* 1988;24:372–378.

Muenter MD, Tyce GM. L-DOPA therapy of Parkinson's disease: Plasma L-DOPA concentration, therapeutic response, and side effects. *Mayo Clin Proc* 1971;46:231–239.

Muenter MD, Sharpless NS, Tyce GM, Darley FL. Patterns of dystonia ("I-D-I" and "D-I-D") in response to L-Dopa therapy for Parkinson's disease. *Mayo Clin Proc* 1977;52:163–174.

Nutt JG, Woodward WR. Levodopa pharmacokinetics and pharmacodynamics in fluctuating parkinsonian patients. *Neurology* 1986;36:739–744.

Nutt JG, Gancher ST, Woodward WR. Does an inhibitory action of levodopa contribute to motor fluctuations? *Neurology* 1988;38:1553–1557.

Nutt JG, Woodward WR, Hammerstad JP, et al. The "On-off" phenomenon in Parkinson's disease: Relation to levodopa absorption and transport. *N Engl J Med* 1984;310:483–488.

Obeso JA, Grandas F, Vaamonde J, et al. Motor complications associated with chronic levodopa therapy in Parkinson's disease. *Neurology Suppl 2)* 1989;39:11–19.

Ogasahara S, Nishikawa Y, Takahashi M, et al. Dopamine metabolism in the central nervous system after discontinuation of L-dopa therapy in patients with Parkinson's disease. *J Neurol Sci* 1984;66:151–163.

Parkes JD. Domperidone and Parkinson's disease. *Clin Neuropharmacol* 1986;9:511–532.

Parkinson Study Group. Effect of deprenyl on the progression of disability in early Parkinson's disease. *N Engl J Med* 1989;321:1364–1371.

Pincus JH, Barry K. Influence of diatary protein on motor fluctuations in Parkinson's disease. *Arch Neurol* 1987;44:270–272.

Poewe W, Kleedorfer B, Gersentbrand F, Oerterl W. Subcutaneous apomorphine in Parkinson's disease. *Lancet* 1988a;1:943.

Poewe WH, Lees AJ, Stern GM. Dystonia in Parkinson's disease: clinical and pharmacological features. *Ann Neurol* 1988b;23:73–78.

Riley D, Lang AE. Practical application of a low-protein diet for Parkinson's disease. *Neurology* 1988;38:1026–1031.

Rinne UK. Dopamine agonists as primary treatment in Parkinson's disease. *Adv Neurol* 1986;45:519–523.

Schwab RS, England AC, Poskanzer DC, Young RR. Amantadine in the treatment of Parkinson's disease. *JAMA* 1969;208:1168–1170.

Snider SR, Fahn S, Isgreen WP, Cote LJ. Primary sensory symptoms in parkinsonism. *Neurology* 1976;26:423–429.

Spencer SE, Wooten GF. Altered pharmacokinetics of L-dopa metabolism in rat stratium deprived of dopaminergic innervation. *Neurology* 1984;34:1105–1108.

Stibe CM, Kempster PA, Lees AJ, Stern GM. Subcutaneous apomorphine in parkinsonian on-off oscillations. *Lancet* 1988;1:403–406.

Tetrud JW, Langston JW. The effect of deprenyl (selegiline) on the natural history of Parkinson's disease. *Science* 1989;245:519–522.

Wade LA, Katzman R. Synthetic amino acids and the nature of L-DOPA transport at the blood-brain barrier. *J Neurochem* 1975a;25:837–842.

Wade LA, Katzman R. 3-0-methyldopa uptake and inhibition of L-DOPA at the blood-brain barrier. *Life Sci* 1975b;17:131–136.

21

The Effects of Dopamine Fluctuation on Cognition and Affect

DEAN C. DELIS AND PAUL J. MASSMAN

Fluctuations in the movement disorder of Parkinson's disease (PD) patients who are chronically treated with levodopa have been recognized and studied for over two decades (see review by Lees, 1989). However, possible fluctuations in cognition and affective state coinciding with the motor changes did not receive consideration until relatively recently, and the literature is still modest. This chapter aims to evaluate the nature and severity of these fluctuations in a variety of domains, including attention, learning and memory, visuospatial abilities, executive functions, and affect.

DIFFICULTIES IN EVALUATING AND COMPARING STUDIES

Most studies in this area refer to subjects who are tested when on (motor disability relatively mild) and when off (motor disability relatively severe). This terminology can be somewhat confusing because studies of motor fluctuations usually distinguish between on/off fluctuations (rapid, unpredictable changes between states of mobility and immobility) and wearing-off or end-of-dose deterioration (predictable decreases in mobility related to falling plasma dopa levels). Many of the cognitive studies actually involved wearing-off PD patients but used the on/off terminology.

Although controversy persists about the demarcation between the wearing-off and on/off phenomena and the mechanisms responsible for these fluctuations (Chapter 20) (Hardie et al, 1984; Lees, 1989; Wooten, 1988), the distinction between these types of fluctuations could be important. First, it appears that on/off fluctuations develop later in the disease course than do wearing-off effects (Mouradian et al, 1987). Second, when off, on/off patients have more severe motor deficits than do wearing-off patients (Fabbrini et al, 1988). Third, when on, on/off patients are more likely to display dyskinesia than are wearing-off patients (Wooten, 1988). Overall, it is likely that on/off patients suffer greater fluctuations in motor deficits (and presumably in dopaminergic functioning) than do wearing-off patients, and studies of on/off patients probably are more likely to detect cognitive and affective changes accompanying the motor changes than are studies of wearing-off patients.

A second potential problem for interpreting results of these studies concerns statistical power and the meaningfulness of statistically significant differences. In five of the nine studies reviewed in this chapter, 10 or fewer PD patients were tested. Even though the within-subjects design used in these investigations enhanced power markedly (assuming high correlations between measurements at the two time points), with sample sizes this small, Type II errors are still a concern. Meaningfulness of results is the other side of the question of power. In within-subjects studies that use relatively large samples and reliable measures, even small group differences will be statistically significant, but these effects might not be large enough to be of much importance. To address the power and meaningfulness issues, the sizes of effects (changes in mean scores relative to variability) are presented, in addition to their statistical significance. The calculation of effect size (ES) also is useful in comparing results across cognitive domains and across studies because ES is expressed in standard deviation units rather than the units of the particular measure. Unfortunately, because the number of studies in this area is small, a true meta-analysis cannot be performed, in which, for example, one could examine the association between subject characteristics (e.g., age, age of PD onset, duration of illness) and the magnitude of the ESs.

REVIEW OF THE LITERATURE

The first examination of cognitive fluctuation in PD patients did not appear in the research literature until 1982, with the publication of a case study by Delis and associates. The patient was a 51-year-old, college-educated man who suffered severe on/off motor fluctuations. Attention, immediate recall of verbal material, and immediate recognition of visual material were similar during on and off periods. Confrontation naming scores were also equivalent, but when off, the patient made more circumlocutory and perceptual errors before arriving at the correct response. On the FAS test of verbal fluency, he performed well when on and, remarkably, produced 30 more words when off. Over one fifth of his responses when off were perseverations however. Delayed recall of verbal information and delayed recognition of visual material decreased substantially from the on to the off state, and confabulation increased markedly when off.

A number of group studies were conducted after the Delis and associates (1982) case study. The characteristics and results of these studies are presented in Table 21–1. With the exception of the Starkstein and colleagues (1989) investigation, in which all subjects were evaluated first when off and later when on, all the studies were counterbalanced. It is difficult to compare the magnitude of subjects' motor changes in different studies because a variety of measures were used, which differed greatly in thoroughness and sensitivity. Thus, the ES estimates of the severity of change, listed in Table 21–1, provide only a crude means of comparing patients' fluctuations across studies.

The focus of this chapter is on the comparison of PD patients' performances in the on and off states, but a number of studies also included a normal control group. Thus, for the sake of completeness and perspective, on patients are contrasted also with normals. In the two ES columns of Table 21–1, positive values indicate that PD patients performed better when on than when off and that normals obtained better scores than on PD patients. Because there is a small-sample bias in the estimate of ES, all ESs in Table 21–1 were adjusted using Hedges' correction (1982), which mildly reduces the magnitude of ESs derived from small samples.

Table 21–1. A summary of studies comparing cognitive performance of patients with Parkinson's disease in on and off states

Study	n	Age	PD duration	Change in disability	Measure	On vs off		Normal vs on	
						p	ES	p	ES
On/off									
Brown et al, 1984	16	56.3 (9.8)	11.8 (4.3)	3.54	Accuracy on 79-item test of verbal and spatial reasoning	<0.01	0.46	<0.05	0.74
					Time to complete test of reasoning	NS	-0.32	NS	-0.02
Girotti et al, 1986	21	58.0 (8.1)	11.0 (4.8)	2.68	Symbol cancellation	NS	-0.01	<0.01	1.23
					Simple RT	NS	0.29	NS	0.72
					Choice RT	NS	0.24	NS	0.62
					Simple MT	<0.01	0.72	<0.01	1.24
					Choice MT	<0.05	0.69	<0.01	1.26
					Category fluency	NS	-0.16	<0.05	0.98
					Line orientation	NS	0.00	NS	0.57
					Story recall (immediate)	NS	-0.27	NS	0.76
Starkstein et al, 1989	7	64.7 (7.2)	11.6 (6.7)	2.99	Digits forward	NS	-0.66	—	—
					Digits backward	NS	-0.16	—	—
					P300 latency	<0.05	0.54	—	—
					P300 amplitude	NS	0.11	—	—
					Simple RT	NS	0.45	—	—
					Simple MT	<0.05	1.12	—	—
					FAS	NS	0.58	—	—
					Benton VRT	NS	0.07	—	—
					WCST categories	NS	-0.24	—	—
					WCST % perseverative error	NS	0.39	—	—

Study	N				Test				
Wearing-off									
Rafal et al, 1984	10	63.2 (11.5)	11.8 (5.2)	—	Simple RT	NS	—	—	—
					Choice RT	NS	—	—	—
					Covert orienting of attention	NS	—	—	—
					Short-term memory scanning speed	NS	—	—	—
Huber et al, 1987	32	—	—	—	List-learning–No. acquisition trials	<0.05	0.81	<0.05	0.81
					Delayed recall	NS	-0.10	NS	-0.19
					Delayed recognition	NS	-0.55	NS	0.24
Mohr et al, 1987	8	58.0 (13.3)	11.1 (5.9)	3.69	Category fluency	NS	-0.30	NS	0.98
					Embedded figures	NS	-0.09	<0.01	1.19
					Logical memory (immediate)	NS	0.23	<0.01	1.89
					Paired association (immediate)	NS	0.62	<0.01	1.39
					Visual form disc. (immediate)	NS	0.52	NS	0.14
					Logical memory (delayed)	<0.05	0.74	<0.01	2.04
					Paired association (delayed)	<0.05	0.57	<0.01	0.88
					Visual form disc. (delayed)	NS	0.12	NS	0.41
Pullman et al, 1988	5	49.2 (—)	—	2.04	Simple RT	NS	0.55	<0.01	1.25
					Choice RT	<0.01	1.55	NS	0.25
					Simple MT	<0.05	1.38	NS	0.48
					Choice MT	<0.05	1.43	NS	0.83
					PASAT-slow	NS	0.13	NS	0.45
					PASAT-fast	NS	0.27	NS	0.37
Gotham et al, 1988	16	64.4 (5.9)	9.9 (2.3)	—	Fluency measures[a]	—	—	—	—
					Category fluency	NS	0.26	NS	0.10
					Alternating fluency	NS	0.51	<0.01	1.05
					WCST categories	NS	-0.05	<0.05	0.91
					WCST % perseverance error	NS	-0.16	<0.05	0.78
					WCST nonperseverance error	NS	0.03	<0.01	0.80
					Associative learning	NS	0.27	<0.01	0.97
					Sub.-ordered point[b]	—	—	—	—
					Representative pictures	—	-0.14	—	0.63
					Abstract pictures	—	0.36	—	0.73
					Low-imagery words	—	-0.03	—	0.38

Table 21–1. A summary of studies comparing cognitive performance of patients with Parkinson's disease in on and off states (*Continued*)

Study	n	Age	PD duration	Change in disability	Measure	On vs off		Normal vs on	
						p	ES	p	ES
Mohr et al., 1989	10	59.0 (8.2)	12.0 (3.2)	3.15	Digits forward	NS	0.00	—	—
					Digits backward	NS	0.19	—	—
					Letter cancellation	NS	0.05	—	—
					FAS	NS	0.21	—	—
					Street map test	NS	−0.20	—	—
					Logical memory (immediate)	NS	0.28	—	—
					Paired association (immediate)	NS	0.30	—	—
					3 Words/shapes (immediate)	NS	0.08	—	—
					8-word list-learning	NS	−0.68	—	—
					Rey/Taylor figure (immediate)	NS	0.02	—	—
					Logical memory (delayed)	<0.05	0.52	—	—
					Paired association (delayed)	<0.05	0.84	—	—
					3 Words/shapes (delayed)	NS	0.60	—	—
					Delayed list recall	NS	0.16	—	—
					Rey/Taylor figure (delayed)	NS	0.24	—	—

[a]No significant group effects for the combined category and alternating fluency conditions, and no significant interactions between group and fluency condition.
[b]No significant group effects for the combined subject-ordered pointing tasks, and no significant interactions between group and task condition.

Attention

On forward digit-span, Starkstein and colleagues (1989) actually found that patients performed somewhat better when off than when on (this result was not statistically significant, however), but Mohr and associates (1989) found performance to be equivalent in the two states. Backward digit-span, which involves mental manipulation of numbers as well as attention, was similar in on and off periods (Mohr et al, 1989; Starkstein et al, 1989).

Digit-span performance requires only relatively brief periods of attention, so it is desirable to also use tests demanding sustained attention. One such test is the Paced Auditory Serial Addition Task (PASAT) (Gronwall and Wrightson, 1981). In this task, subjects listen to a series of 30 random single-digit numbers and are asked to add the most recent number to the number immediately preceding it and to report the total. PD patients' PASAT scores were found to be similar in the on and off states, whether the numbers were presented at the rate of 1 every 4 seconds or 1 every 2 seconds (Gotham et al, 1988). On patients did not differ significantly from normal subjects on either version of the PASAT, but the ESs were in the small to moderate range.

Other tests requiring sustained attention involve presenting subjects with a page of printed letters or symbols and asking them to make a pencil mark through as many of the designated target stimuli as possible in a set time limit. These tasks obviously also require visual scanning and a motor response, so they are not pure attentional measures. Somewhat surprisingly, although one might think that off patients' motor problems would interfere with their performances on these tests, it was found that their scores did not decline from those obtained when they were on (Girotti et al, 1986; Mohr et al, 1989). Normal subjects obtained substantially better scores than on patients (Girotti et al, 1986). Rafal and associates (1984) reported that covert orienting of attention in the visual field did not vary significantly with dopaminergic status. Overall, on the attentional measures on which on and off patients were compared, the mean ES was -0.02. This negligible change suggests that attentional abilities do not change significantly with fluctuations in dopamine levels. Starkstein and colleagues (1989) did find that the latency of the P300 component of the auditory event-related potential (thought to be related to attentional mechanisms) was longer when patients were off than when they were on. The ES was modest but significant. Amplitude of the P300 component was found to be similar in the two states.

Reaction Time

In three studies examining simple RT (Girotti et al, 1986; Pullman et al, 1988; Starkstein et al, 1989), patients performed somewhat faster when on than when off, but the mean ES was only 0.43, and in no case was the difference statistically significant. Rafal and associates (1984) also reported a nonsignificant difference in simple RT, but the ES could not be computed from the information provided in this study. The two studies comparing simple RT in normal subjects and on patients (Girotti et al, 1986; Pullman et al, 1988) yielded moderate to large ES estimates, with normal subjects responding more quickly.

Choice RT was found to be significantly faster when patients were on than when they were off in two of the studies (Pullman et al, 1988; Rafal et al, 1984) but did not differ between the on and off states in the investigation of Girotti and colleagues (1986). These results are inconclusive, but it appears possible that choice RT tasks (and their greater cognitive demands) are more affected by dopaminergic status than are simple RT tasks. Additionally, only small-to-moderate, nonsignificant differences between normal subjects' and on patients' choice RTs were found (Girotti et al, 1986; Pullman et al, 1988), and these effects appeared to be somewhat smaller than those reported for the simple RT tests. This pattern of results led Pullman and associates (1988) to speculate that simple and choice RT tasks could be mediated by relatively independent neural mechanisms, with choice RT tasks more dopamine-dependent than simple RT tests.

Not surprisingly, consistent with increased bradykinesia in the off state, patients' movement times (MTs), measured as the difference between the initiation of the response (i.e., RT) and the completion of the response, were much slower when off than when on during both simple and choice RT tests. The mean ES derived from five comparisons in three studies (Girotti et al, 1986; Pullman et al, 1988; Starkstein et al, 1989) was 1.08. Thus, it is clear that MT was more closely related to dopaminergic status than was RT. The optimally medicated on patients, however, had slower MTs than normal subjects, the mean ES from four comparisons in two studies (Girotti et al, 1986; Pullman et al, 1988) was 0.95.

Verbal Fluency

The only measures of language functions administered to fluctuating PD patients have been tests of verbal fluency. On the FAS test, differences between on and off periods were small to moderate in size and nonsignificant (Mohr et al, 1989; Starkstein et al, 1989). Similarly, on category fluency tests (e.g., generating animal names in a 1-minute time period), differences also were small and not statistically significant (Girotti et al, 1986; Gotham et al, 1988; Mohr et al, 1987). The mean ES derived from the five comparisons of verbal fluency performances was only 0.12. In two studies (Girotti et al, 1986; Mohr et al, 1987), normal subjects obtained markedly higher category fluency scores than on patients (mean ES of 0.98), but Gotham and colleagues (1986) reported only a negligible difference.

Visuospatial Functioning

Evaluation of on/off patients' visuospatial abilities has been sparse. It has been found that dopaminergic status is not significantly related to performance on the Line Orientation test (Girotti et al, 1986), the Street Map test (Mohr et al, 1989), or on a 5-item embedded figures test (Mohr et al, 1987). The mean ES derived from these three comparisons was only −0.10. Normal subjects obtained moderately higher scores than on patients on the Line Orientation and embedded figures tests, but the group difference was significant only for the latter measure (Girotti et al, 1986; Mohr et al, 1987).

Immediate Recall

Immediate recall of verbal material was evaluated in five studies (Table 21–1). There were six comparisons between PD patients when on and when off on tests of story recall or paired associate learning (Girotti et al, 1986; Mohr et al, 1987, 1989). All of these comparisons were nonsignificant, and the mean ES was only 0.21 (on patients had higher recall scores). Two studies (Huber et al, 1987; Mohr et al, 1989) employed list-learning tasks, but these tests were quite different. On a five-trial test using a short (eight-word) list, patients actually did somewhat better when off than when on, but this result was not statistically significant (Mohr et al, 1989). In the between-subjects study conducted by Huber and colleagues (1987) in which a group of on patients was compared with a separate group of off patients, the on group required significantly fewer acquisition trials than the off group to recall 12 words of a 24-word list composed of common four-letter words. As indicated in Table 21–1, this ES was moderately large—0.81. The investigation by Mohr and colleagues (1989) probably failed to demonstrate an advantage for on patients because the list length used did not sufficiently exceed the subjects' immediate recall spans. These immediate recall results suggest that free recall of structured verbal material is only mildly affected, at most, by dopamine depletion but that recall of unorganized information (requiring more effortful encoding and retrieval) might be more severely compromised. Four comparisons of normal subjects' and on patients' immediate recall performances revealed that normal subjects demonstrated clearly superior recall. The mean ES was 1.21 (Girotti et al, 1986; Huber et al, 1987; Mohr et al, 1987).

Regarding immediate recall of visuospatial material, nonsignificant differences between on and off periods were found on the Benton Visual Retention Test (BVRT) (Starkstein et al, 1989), on a 4-item version of the Benton Visual Form Discrimination Test—multiple choice recognition format (Mohr et al, 1987) and on the Rey-Osterrieth or Taylor Complex Figure Tests (Mohr et al, 1989). Even though the BVRT and Rey-Osterrieth tasks have substantial motor demands, dopaminergic status had little effect on performance. The mean ES for these two measures was only 0.05. On patients performed similarly to normal subjects on the Visual Form Discrimination Test (Mohr et al, 1987).

Finally, on a Sternberg-type memory scanning test, in which PD patients were shown a list of 1,2,4, or 6 digits and were then asked whether a target digit had been a member of the list, Rafal and colleagues (1984) found that memory scanning speed was not significantly different during on and off periods.

Delayed Recall and Recognition

In contrast to the findings of equivalent immediate recall of structured verbal material during on and off periods, it has been reported consistently that delayed recall of this material is poorer during the off state. In five comparisons from two studies (Mohr et al, 1987, 1989), the mean ES was 0.65, and four of these differences were statistically significant. It would have been informative to examine retention explicitly by computing savings scores (i.e., delayed recall score/immediate recall score), but this was not done. Group means for immediate and delayed recall can be compared to yield a rough estimate of savings. Using the data for Logical Memory reported in the two studies, the group savings scores during on periods were 81.6 percent and 96.3 percent, respectively, whereas the group savings scores during the off periods were 65.9 percent and 87.8 percent, respectively. It is not possible to ascertain whether off patients' delayed recall deficit was due to storage or retrieval problems. Storage difficulty would seem to be the more likely candidate, but it can be argued that delayed recall has higher retrieval demands than immediate recall, so a retrieval explanation cannot be ruled out. Recognition memory for the material could have shed some light on this issue, but this was not evaluated. Also, these studies did not tabulate intrusion errors in delayed recall, so it is unclear whether the increased confabulation reported in the Delis and colleagues (1982) case study can be generalized.

Normal subjects obtained substantially higher scores than on patients on tests involving delayed recall of structured verbal material (Mohr et al, 1987). However, these differences appeared to be attributable to differences in immediate recall. Group savings scores adjusting for level of immediate recall were very similar.

Delayed recall was assessed also in the two list-learning tasks described previously (Huber et al, 1987; Mohr et al, 1989). Interestingly, comparisons between the on and off states were small and nonsignificant. Delayed recognition of list words was also equivalent in on and off patients (Huber et al, 1987). It could be that when off patients are given multiple opportunities to encode and retrieve material during list-learning trials, their retention deficit subsides. However, their aforementioned delayed recall deficit on paired associate tests, which involved three learning trials, does not support this hypothesis. Normal subjects and on patients did not differ on either delayed recall or recognition of list items (Huber et al, 1987).

Regarding memory of nonverbal material, there were small, nonsignificant differences between on and off periods on tests involving 15-second delayed recognition of geometric figures (Mohr et al, 1987) and 30-minute recall of the Rey-Osterrieth or Taylor figures (Mohr et al, 1989). Additionally, group savings scores for the latter test appeared to be equivalent in the on and off states. These savings scores (38.0 percent and 42.4 percent) were relatively poor, but normal controls were not included in this study, so the degree of impairment cannot be ascertained. In any case, dopaminergic status did not appear to be related to retention of visuospatial information. On the four-item recognition test with a 15-second delay period, normal subjects and on patients did not differ significantly (Mohr et al, 1987).

State-Dependent Memory

In addition to evaluating retention of information within the on or off state, it is important to consider possible state-dependent memory effects. It has been well established that information learned in a particular physiological state is best recalled if the individual is in the same state when retrieval is attempted. Therefore, it could be that congruence of dopamine levels at the times of learning and delayed recall is a key variable in PD patients' retention abilities. Huber and associates (1987) conducted the first investigation in this area, employing a between-subjects design in which groups of PD patients learned and recalled verbal information (a 24-item word list) during dopamine-congruent periods (high–high or low–low) or dopamine-incongruent periods (high–low or low–high). Delayed recall occurred 24 hours after the learning session. It was found that the high–high and low–low groups' delayed recall performances did not differ from each other or from a normal control group. The high–high group recalled significantly more words than the high–low group, and the low–low group recalled more words than the low–high group, indicating that there was a state-dependent memory effect. On a delayed recognition memory test, the high–high, low–low, and control groups again did not differ. The low–low group performed significantly better than the low–high group, but the high–high and high–low groups did not differ significantly.

Huber and colleagues (1989) also conducted a within-subjects study of state dependency, testing PD subjects at eight different time points. Consistent with the between-subjects results, patients' delayed recall was better when dopamine levels were similar at learning and retrieval than when the levels were dissimilar. Delayed recognition did not display a state-dependent effect.

In an investigation by Mohr and co-workers (1989), patients learned information while on or off, were given a 30-minute delayed recall test in the same state, were medicated or allowed to wear off, then were given a 2-hour delayed recall test. It was reported that patients had a tendency to perform somewhat better when making the transition from off to on than when changing from on to off but that none of these differences were statistically significant. Because 2-hour delayed recall was not also assessed in a dopamine-congruent condition, no conclusions about a state-dependent effect could be drawn. However, the change scores from 30 minutes to 2 hours reported by Mohr and associates (1989) appeared to be quite small, which would suggest that there was minimal state dependency.

Executive Functions

On the Wisconsin Card Sorting Test, number of categories sorted and percent perseverative errors did not differ in the on and off states (Gotham et al, 1986; Starkstein et al, 1989). Similar numbers of nonperseverative errors were committed in the two states (Gotham et al, 1988). Compared with normal subjects, on patients performed significantly more poorly on all three of the measures, and the mean ES of 0.83 was moderately large.

On a conditional associative learning test, reported by Petrides (1985) to be sensitive to prefrontal lesions, in which subjects must learn associations between colors and nonmeaningful geometric designs, PD patients' performance did not vary significantly with dopaminergic status, but on patients' scores were poorer than normal subjects' scores (Gotham et al, 1986). Another test that has been reported to be sensitive to frontal lobe functioning is subject-ordered pointing (Petrides and Milner, 1982). PD subjects and normal subjects were presented with 12 cards in sequence, each bearing the same 12 stimuli arranged randomly on the card, and were asked to point to a different stimulus on each card (Gotham et al, 1988). Three different types of stimuli were used, including representational drawings, abstract designs, and low-imagery words. PD patients did not perform significantly differently during on and off states on these three pointing tasks, and the mean ES was only -0.18. On patients obtained significantly lower scores than normals, and the mean ES was 0.58. Patients' performance during on and off periods also did not differ significantly on a test of semantic shifting, in which they were instructed to alternately generate members from two categories (boys' names and fruit), but the ES of 0.51 was in the moderate range (Gotham et al, 1988). Normal subjects' performance was superior to that of the on patients, and this difference was large (ES = 1.05). Finally, on a test involving "general reasoning ability for verbal, numerical, and spatial material," patients obtained significantly higher scores when on than when off (ES = 0.46), and normal subjects obtained higher scores than on patients (Brown et al, 1984). Patients actually completed the test more quickly in the off state (ES = −0.32), suggesting that some of their errors in this state could have been due to impulsive responding.

Fluctuations in Affect

Most studies in this area have involved a cursory assessment of affect, and several were merely descriptive. Hardie and colleagues (1984) commented that 18 of 20 fluctuating PD patients "described significant depressive symptoms during 'off' periods." Nissenbaum and colleagues (1987) noted that 4 of 9 on/off patients who were clinically evaluated "had detectable mood changes characterized by depression and anxiety when 'off.'" Additionally, they conducted a survey of 31 fluctuating patients and found that 12 of these patients (38.7 percent) reported feeling "moderately more depressed" or "very much more depressed" when off than when on. Fourteen of the patients (45.2 percent) reported feeling "moderately more anxious" or "very much more anxious" when off than when on. Mohr and colleagues (1989) reported that Beck Depression Inventory scores did not differ significantly in on and off states but provided no descriptive statistics.

Girotti and associates (1986) found that patients obtained significantly higher (worse) scores when on than when off on seven items selected from the Brief Psychiatric Rating Scale. Two studies employed a 13-item scale of "subjective affect–arousal," in which subjects rated how they felt on a variety of dimensions defined by bipolar adjectives, such as "alert–drowsy" and "happy–sad" (Brown et al, 1984; Gotham et al, 1988). Patients' scores on this scale were significantly worse during off periods than during on periods. The mean ES for the on/off comparison found in these three studies was 0.98. The mean ES for the comparison between normals and on patients was 0.58.

Brown and colleagues (1984) reported that when the patients were on, the correlation between their affect–arousal score and their score on the test of reasoning accuracy described earlier was small (−0.24), but when they were off, the correlation was robust (−0.68). It was argued that this result indicated that alterations in affect–arousal mediated the cognitive changes associated with dopamine fluctuation. Obviously, however, correlation does not imply causation. Also, the variability in affect–arousal scores appeared to be markedly greater during the off period, and this expansion of range would permit a larger correlation to emerge. Finally, this finding was not replicated for the neuropsychological measures in the Gotham and associates (1988) study.

Interpretation of possible negative effects of dopamine depletion on affect–arousal is clouded by the possibility that the changes reflect merely a reaction to the increased motor disability of off periods. In an ingenious attempt to circumvent this difficulty, Cantello and colleagues (1986) compared fluctuating PD patients with rheumatoid arthritis patients, who exhibited a repetitive pattern of mobility and immobility, and levels of disability during "good" and "bad" periods similar to those of the PD patients. The rheumatoid arthritis patients displayed practically no change from mobile to immobile periods on the Beck Depression Inventory (excluding the "loss of weight" item) or on a six-item measure of "activation and euphoria" (e.g., rating on six-point scales how "alert," "excited," and "talkative" one feels). In contrast, there was a statistically significant (but small) difference between the Beck scores of PD patients during on and off periods, and these patients obtained markedly lower (worse) scores on the activation scale when they were off. This pattern of results suggests that the neurotransmitter changes associated with off periods are chiefly responsible for PD patients' changes in affect and arousal.

CONCLUSIONS

Summary of Research Findings

Similarities between PD patients' neuropsychological test performances when on and when off far outweighed the differences. Negligible differences were found on tests of attention, simple RT, verbal fluency, visuospatial abilities, executive functions, immediate recall of visuospatial stimuli, immediate recall of short stories or paired associates, delayed recall of visuospatial information, and delayed recall and recognition of verbal list items presented multiple times. Significant differences of moderate size were reported on tests of supraspan list learning, delayed recall of short stories or paired associates, and choice RT. Additionally, there was evidence of a state-dependent memory effect. Patients' delayed recall was optimal when dopaminergic status was congruent during learning and later retrieval. Finally, a substantial proportion of fluctuating PD patients experience increased symptoms of depression and anxiety during off periods, which do not appear to be reflective merely of negative reactions to increased motor disability (Cantello et al, 1986).

Theoretical and Pathophysiological Implications

The circumscribed, relatively minor nature of the changes in cognition found in fluctuating PD patients is strikingly dissimilar from the profound fluctuations in these patients' motor abilities. There are a number of possible explanations for this dissociation. Perhaps the neuropsychological functions evaluated in the studies are not significantly dopamine-dependent. Although this could be the case for some of these functions (e.g., visuospatial abilities), previous animal and human studies have indicated that dopaminergic input is important in learning and memory, motor activation, and executive functions (Brozoski et al, 1979; Newman et al, 1984; Stern and Langston, 1985; Quartermain et al, 1988; Berger et al, 1989; Wickens, 1989). The question thus arises: What could account for PD patients' failure to display marked deterioration on these tasks during their off periods? Based on a growing accumulation of anatomical and physiological data, it has been proposed that there are at least five distinct basal ganglia-thalmocortical circuits—motor, oculomotor, dorsolateral prefrontal, orbitofrontal, and anterior cingulate (Alexander et al, 1986). It appears that PD has a greater negative effect on the motor circuit than on the remaining circuits (Agid et al, 1987; Kish et al, 1988). In addition to the basal ganglia circuits, there are direct dopaminergic projections from the ventral tegmentum to cortical areas. In contrast to the almost complete annihilation of dopamine in the motor circuit, there are only 40 percent to 60 percent reductions of tegmental dopamine cells and of dopamine levels in their projection areas (e.g., frontal cortex, hippocampus, amygdala) (Agid et al, 1987). Overall, considering that dopamine loss in nonmotor circuits appears to be appreciably less than that in motor circuits and that residual neurons display substantial compensatory capacities (e.g., increased dopamine turnover), it is not surprising that dopamine-related cognitive functions would show less fluctuation than motor abilities.

The question that remains, however, is why are on PD patients impaired relative to normal subjects on many cognitive tests if the dopaminergic systems involved in these tasks are relatively intact and unaffected by dopamine fluctuations? This apparent inconsistency is not easily resolved, but there are several plausible explanations. First, neuropathological alterations in the noradrenergic locus ceruleus have been well documented in PD patients (Chan-Palay and Asan, 1989), and a substantial proportion of these patients also exhibit changes in the cholinergic system (Dubois et al, 1987). It has been proposed that these nondopaminergic abnormalities could be primarily responsible for PD patients' cognitive and affective disturbances (Pillon et al, 1989). If this were the case, an absence of cognitive fluctuations coinciding with dopaminergic changes would be expected. Clearly, much work needs to be done to elucidate the effects of deficits in multiple neurotransmitter systems and how interactions between these systems might vary with the levels of deficit within the individual systems. Regarding PD patients specifically, one important variable to consider is age because it is now well known that neurotransmitter changes accompany aging. Thus, the PD-related neurotransmitter deficits are superimposed on changes occurring naturally with aging, and different interactions could be evident in patients of different ages (and in the same patient across time).

Second, there could be a nonlinear, threshold effect, such that the relatively mild dopamine depletion occurring in nonmotor circuits does cause cognitive deficits (perhaps these higher-order functions are more vulnerable to the effects of neurotransmitter alterations than are motor functions, which are not affected until neurotransmitter changes are severe), but that further dopamine loss associated with motor fluctuations does not produce an additional decrement in cognitive functioning. It is possible that the cognitive effects of further dopamine depletion could vary with the initial dopamine level—perhaps a late-stage PD patient (with more severely compromised nonmotor dopaminergic circuits) would be more likely to display cognitive fluctuations than would an early-stage patient. Future research should address such possible individual differences.

REFERENCES

Agid Y, Javoy-Agid F, Ruberg M. Biochemistry of neurotransmitters in Parkinson's disease. In: *Movement Disorders 2.* Edited by CD Marsden and S Fahn. London, Butterworths, 1987:166–230.

Alexander GE, DeLong MR, Strick PL. Parallel organization of functionally segregated circuits linking basal ganglia and cortex. *Annual Review of Neuroscience* 1986;9:357–381.

Berger HJC, van Hoof JJM, van Spaendonck KPM, et al. Haloperidol and cognitive shifting. *Neuropsychologia* 1989;27:629–639.

Brown RG, Marsden CD, Quinn N, Wyke MA. Alterations in cognitive performance and affect-arousal state during fluctuations in motor function in Parkinson's disease. *Journal of Neurology, Neurosurgery, and Psychiatry* 1984;47:454–465.

Brozoski TJ, Brown RM, Rosvold HE, Goldman PS. Cognitive deficit caused by regional depletion of dopamine in prefrontal cortex of rhesus monkey. *Science* 1979;205:929–932.

Cantello R, Gilli M, Riccio A, Bergamasco B. Mood changes associated with "end-of-dose deterioration" in Parkinson's disease: A controlled study. *J Neurol Neurosurg Psychiatry* 1986;49:1182–1190.

Chan-Palay V, Asan E. Alterations in catecholamine neurons of the locus coeruleus in senile dementia of the Alzheimer type and in Parkinson's disease with and without dementia and depression. *Journal of Comparative Neurology* 1989;287:373–392.

Delis D, Direnfeld L, Alexander MP, Kaplan E. Cognitive fluctuations associated with on-off phenomenon in Parkinson's disease. *Neurology* 1982;32:1049–1052.

Dubois B, Danze F, Pillon B, et al. Cholinergic-dependent cognitive deficits in Parkinson's disease. *Ann Neurol* 1987;22:26–30.

Fabbrini G, Mouradian MM, Juncos JL, et al. Motor fluctuations in Parkinson's disease: Central pathophysiological mechanisms, Part I. *Ann Neurol* 1988;24:366–371.

Girotti F, Carella F, Pia Grassi M, et al. Motor and cognitive performances of Parkinsonian patients in the on and off phases of the disease. *J Neurol Neurosurg Psychiatry* 1986;49:657–660.

Gotham AM, Brown RG, Marsden CD. 'Frontal' cognitive function in patients with Parkinson's disease 'on' and 'off' levodopa. *Brain* 1988;111:299–321.

Gronwall D, Wrightson P. Memory and information processing capacity after closed head injury. *J Neurol Neurosurg Psychiatry* 1981;44:889–895.

Hardie RJ, Lees AJ, Stern GM. On-off fluctuations in Parkinson's disease. *Brain* 1984;107:487–506.

Hedges, LV. Estimation of effect size from a series of independent experiments. *Psychological Bulletin* 1982;92:490–499.

Huber SJ, Shulman HG, Paulson GW, Shuttleworth EC. Fluctuations in plasma dopamine level impair memory in Parkinson's disease. *Neurology* 1987;37:1371–1375.

Huber SJ, Shulman HG, Paulson GW, Shuttleworth EC. Dose-dependent memory impairment in Parkinson's disease. *Neurology* 1989;39:438–440.

Kish SJ, Shannak K, Hornykiewicz O. Uneven pattern of dopamine loss in the striatum of patients with idiopathic Parkinson's disease. *N Engl J Med.* 1988;318:876–880.

Lees AJ. The on-off phenomenon. *J Neurol Neurosurg Psychiatry.* 1989;(special suppl):29–37.

Mohr E, Fabbrini G, Ruggieri S, et al. Cognitive concomitants of dopamine system stimulation in Parkinsonian patients. *J Neurol Neurosurg Psychiatry.* 1987;50:1192–1196.

Mohr E, Fabbrini G, Williams J, et al. Dopamine and memory function in Parkinson's disease. *Movement Disorders* 1989;4:113–120.

Mouradian MM, Juncos JL, Fabbrini G, Chase TN. Motor fluctuations in Parkinson's disease: Pathogenic and therapeutic studies. *Ann Neurol* 1987;22:475–479.

Newman RP, Weingartner H, Smallberg SA, Calne DB. Effortful and automatic memory: Effects of dopamine. *Neurology* 1984;34:805–807.

Nissenbaum H, Quinn NP, Brown RG, et al. Mood swings associated with the 'on-off' phenomenon in Parkinson's disease. *Psychological Medicine* 1987;17:899–904.

Petrides M. Deficits on conditional associative-learning tasks after frontal- and temporal-lobe lesions in man. *Neuropsychologia* 1985;23:601–614.

Petrides M, Milner B. Deficits on subject-ordered tasks after frontal- and temporal-lobe lesions in man. *Neuropsychologia,* 1982;20:249–262.

Pillon B, Dubois B, Cusimano G, et al. Does cognitive impairment in Parkinson's disease result from non-dopaminergic lesions? *J Neurol Neurosurg Psychiatry.* 1989;52:201–206.

Pullman SL, Watts RL, Juncos JL, et al. Dopaminergic effects on simple and choice reaction time performance in Parkinson's disease. *Neurology.* 1988;38:249–254.

Quartermain D, Judge ME, Leo P. Attenuation of forgetting by pharmacological stimulation of aminergic neurotransmitter systems. *Pharmacol Biochem Behav.* 1988;30:77–81.

Rafal RD, Posner MI, Walker JA, Friedrich FJ. Cognition and the basal ganglia: separating mental and motor components of performance in Parkinson's disease. *Brain.* 1984;107:1083–1094.

Starkstein SE, Esteguy M, Berthier ML, et al. Evoked potentials, reaction time and cognitive performance in on and off phases of Parkinson's disease. *J Neurol Neurosurg Psychiatry.* 1989;52:338–340.

Stern Y, Langston JW. Intellectual changes in patients with MPTP-induced parkinsonism. *Neurology.* 1985;35:1506–1509.

Wickens J. Striatal dopamine in motor activation and reward-mediated learning: Steps towards a unifying model. *J Neural Transm.* 1990;80:9–31.

Wooten GF. Progress in understanding the pathophysiology of treatment-related fluctuations in Parkinson's disease. *Ann Neurol.* 1988;24:363–365.

22

Effect of Antiparkinsonian
Drugs on Memory

SANDER L. GLATT AND WILLIAM C. KOLLER

Advances in the drug therapy of Parkinson's disease (PD) over the last 20 years have led to dramatic clinical improvement of motor symptoms. The two most commonly used classes of agents are centrally active anticholinergic and dopaminergic medications. Anticholinergics have been used independently in patients with mild disease and as adjunctive therapy in advanced disease. They are most effective in the relatively young patient with a tremor-predominant PD syndrome. Dopaminergic agents are used when there has been sufficient motor deterioration to impair social, occupational, or ambulatory function. Dopaminergic drugs are effective for all symptoms, especially bradykinesia.

Pharmacological attempts to manipulate neurotransmitter systems related to motor function may have untoward effects on a variety of cognitive functions. This chapter deals with the effect of anticholinergic and dopaminergic drugs on memory. A better understanding of these effects may improve clinical management of the PD patient. In addition, PD may serve as an important model to examine the relationship of specific neurotransmitters and memory.

ANTICHOLINERGIC DRUGS

The efficacy of the belladonna alkaloids in PD has been known for over 100 years (Charcot, 1877). Duvoisin (1967) was the first to demonstrate the scientific basis for anticholinergic drug therapy in PD. He showed that the cholinesterase inhibitor physostigmine, an indirect cholinomimetic, exacerbates PD signs through blockade of the enzyme that breaks down acetylcholine. Anticholinergic agents that penetrate the blood–brain barrier into the central nervous system, such as scopolamine or benztrophine, reverse this effect. Anticholinergics block central cholinergic muscarinic receptors. Barbeau (1962) proposed that reduced dopaminergic input leads to cholinergic hyperactivity (Velasco et al, 1982) and that anticholinergics redress this imbalance between the cholinergic and dopaminergic circuits in the striatum.

Although a wide variety of anticholinergic agents have been used in PD, there are no significant differences in their efficacy or side effects (Comella and Tanner, 1990).

The most commonly used agents today are trihexyphenidyl (Artane) and benztrophine mesylate (Cogentin).

THE CHOLINERGIC HYPOTHESIS AND MEMORY

Administration of agents that affect neurotransmitter activity permits examination of their effect on cognitive function. Anticholinergic agents injected into the rat hippocampus inhibit the storage and retrieval of new memories (Deutsch et al, 1966; Deutsch, 1971). Drachman and Leavitt (1974) noted that scopolamine produced a loss of memory in humans. For example, women given scopolamine during delivery had no memory of the details of childbirth. This drug was shown also to interfere with memory storage and retrieval in normal controls. Physostigmine, a cholinomimetic, reversed much of the memory deficit caused by scopolamine. Amphetamine, which produces a nonspecific alerting effect, did not reverse the memory deficits produced by cholinergic blockade (Drachman, 1977). This was the first demonstration in humans of the role of the cholinergic system in memory.

Research with other cholinergic manipulations produced similar findings. Physostigmine facilitated the storage and retrieval of recently learned information in normal controls (Davis et al, 1978). Arecoline, a cholinergic agonist, improved serial learning. This effect was most prominent in controls with low pretreatment scores, suggesting that memory deficits related to cholinergic abnormalities might respond to drug therapy (Sitaram et al, 1978). Memory impairment of patients treated with psychotrophic medications correlated with serum anticholinergic levels (Tune et al, 1982).

The cholinergic hypothesis of memory dysfunction was also supported by research in Alzheimer's disease (AD) (Bartus et al, 1982; Coyle et al, 1983; Perry, 1986). Postmortem studies found a marked reduction (60 to 80 percent) of choline acetyltransferase (CAT), the enzyme responsible for acetylcholine synthesis, in the cerebral cortex (Davies and Maloney, 1976; Perry et al, 1977). The extent of the cortical cholinergic deficit correlated with cerebral histopathology findings as well as severity of mental status abnormalities (Perry et al, 1978; Wilcock et al, 1982).

The anatomy of cortical cholinergic inputs has been revealed by research. Studies using selective chemical lesions in the medial globus pallidus demonstrated that this was the principal source of cortical cholinergic input in animals (Johnston et al, 1979; Coyle et al, 1983). Neuropathological studies in AD showed that there was a corresponding loss of large neurons in the basal forebrain involving the basal nucleus of Meynert (Whitehouse et al, 1981). This structure is the primary source of cholinergic input to the cortex (Mesulam et al, 1983).

Rats with forebrain lesions and deficits in memory improved with cholinomimetic agents (Dunnett et al, 1987; Mandel and Thal, 1988), suggesting that attempts to treat the cholinergic deficit in AD were warranted. Trials of indirect cholinomimetic agents demonstrated mild improvement in AD. Intravenous physostigmine (Davis and Mohs, 1982) and a short-acting oral form of physostigmine (Thal et al, 1983) produced limited improvement of memory in AD patients. However, attempts to manipulate the cholinergic system via cholinergic precursors (cholinesterase inhibitors and receptor agonists) did not produce sufficient benefit to be of practical use (Galasko and Thal, 1990).

The cholinergic hypothesis has not provided a basis for significantly effective rational therapy in AD, but it has not been discarded. The large number of neurotransmitter deficits in AD may be one reason why exogenous therapy is of only limited benefit (Galasko and Thal, 1990).

ACETYLCHOLINE AND MEMORY IN PARKINSON'S DISEASE

Recently, research related to the cholinergic hypothesis of memory has focused on PD. One approach has been to examine the cognitive, pathological, and neurochemical abnormalities that may predispose PD patients to exacerbation of cognitive dysfunction when treated with anticholinergic agents.

Significant cognitive deficits are present in 30 to 40 percent of PD patients (Cummings, 1988). Subtle deficits in recent memory (Huber et al, 1986), visuospatial skills (Proctor et al, 1964), perceptual motor skills (Stern et al, 1983), and executive frontal lobe functions (Taylor et al, 1986) are common in PD patients. Demented PD patients have less difficulty with memory, language, and orientation but more severe problems with speed of information processing and mood compared with AD patients (Huber et al, 1989a).

The pathological basis of dementia in PD has not been clearly defined. Neuropathological studies have shown that cortical senile plaques and neurofibrillary tangles identical to those in AD are found in some patients with clinical and neuropathological evidence of PD (Boller et al, 1980; Hakim and Mathieson, 1979). This suggests that AD can cause dementia in some PD patients. Other investigators have demonstrated a subcortical dementia in PD that is not associated with cortical AD pathology (Chui et al, 1986), and most patients with PD and dementia do not have AD (Ball, 1984; Yoshimura, 1988). It seems likely that dementia in PD includes both patients with combined PD and AD and patients with a specific subcortical dementia syndrome (de La Monte et al, 1989).

Abnormalities in cortical cholinergic markers have been identified in PD (Ruberg et al, 1982), particularly in patients with dementia (Dubois et al, 1983). As in AD, cell loss in the nucleus basalis has been documented in PD dementia (Whitehouse et al, 1983), even in patients without accompanying cortical AD pathology (Nakano and Hirano, 1984). There was a positive correlation among severity of cholinergic deficit, dementia, and cell loss in the basal nucleus (Perry et al, 1985). Perry (1986) suggested that examination of PD dementia may provide a more straightforward model of the cholinergic hypothesis of memory because of the absence of cortical pathology.

MEMORY, COGNITION, AND ANTICHOLINERGICS IN PARKINSON'S DISEASE

The association between cholinergic deficits and dementia in PD raised concerns about clinical side effects of anticholinergics. De Smet and co-workers (1982) showed that the emergence of confusional states associated with anticholinergics is more common in PD patients with dementia. Sadeh and associates (1982) demonstrated a recent memory impairment in unselected PD patients given anticholinergics. Koller (1984) studied immediate and recent memory tasks in 12 nondemented patients with mild PD before and 1 month after treatment with trihexyphenidyl (6 mg/day). Declines were noted in a number of recent memory measures. All authors suggested caution when using anticholinergics in PD patients, particularly those who may be at risk for dementia.

PD patients without dementia were affected by subthreshold doses of subcutaneous scopolamine, although deficits were seen only in a more difficult drawing recognition memory task requiring effortful learning. Dubois and colleagues (1987) suggested that the memory deficit might be secondary to impaired selective attention and sequential planning indicative of frontal lobe dysfunction. These researchers have subsequently examined a variety of cognitive tasks in two matched groups of patients with PD with and without anticholinergic therapy (Dubois et al, 1990). Performance of the two groups differed on tests of frontal lobe function but not on memory tests.

This specific effect of anticholinergics on frontal lobe function may be peculiar to PD, where a frontal cholinergic deficit has been described (Dubois et al, 1983). Conversely, in AD, there is more marked involvement of the medial temporal structures: hippocampus, amygdala, and entorhinal cortex (Hyman et al, 1990). The underlying neuropathology in AD may cause memory to be most susceptible to anticholinergic blockade. In PD, the temporal lobes generally are spared.

Further investigations correlating specific cognitive abnormalities to regional neuropathology and neurochemistry are necessary to assess the precise risk involved in using anticholinergic agents in PD. At present, we suggest that they be restricted to either relatively young patients with mild disease or patients with advanced disease as a last resort when there is no evidence of dementia.

DOPAMINERGIC AGENTS

The scientific basis for dopaminergic therapy for PD was provided initially by Ehringer and Hornykiewicz (1960), who found a marked deficit of dopamine in the striatum of postmortem PD brains. More recently, the relationship of parkinsonism to dopamine deficiency was confirmed by investigators using the selective neurotoxin MPTP. This chemical was shown to produce a pure parkinsonian state in human and monkey by selectively destroying dopaminergic neurons in the substantia nigra and reducing striatal dopamine content (Burns et al, 1983).

Pathological changes in PD involve reduction of the pigmented neurons of the substantia nigra, which provide the dopaminergic innervation to the striatum. There is a greater than 80 percent depletion of dopamine in the striatum of PD patients studied at autopsy (Kish et al, 1988). Since a reduction of striatal dopamine appears sufficient to produce the motor manifestations of PD, the goal of therapy is to restore dopamine neurotransmission (Cotzias et al, 1969). Levodopa is the most effective drug for treatment of PD symptoms. Initiation of levodopa treatment usually is accompanied by a dramatic reduction in PD symptoms, and the lack of any response is inconsistent with the diagnosis of PD (Koller and Hubble, 1990). Since the advent of levodopa treatment, PD patients have normal life expectancies (Curtis et al, 1984). Levodopa has become the gold standard for the symptomatic treatment of PD and represents the best example of neurotransmitter replacement therapy (Koller and Hubble, 1990).

DOPAMINERGIC AGENTS AND MEMORY

The dramatic improvement in PD symptoms with levodopa is not accompanied by an equally robust recovery of cognitive function. Some early studies suggested improved cognitive function after dopaminergic therapy, but these reports have been criticized for faulty methodology (Riklan et al, 1976).

To adequately assess the effect of levodopa on memory, it is necessary to examine the contribution of the dopaminergic system to cognitive impairments of subcortical dementia. The syndrome of subcortical dementia has been described in progressive supranuclear palsy (Albert et al, 1974), Huntington's disease (McHugh and Folstein, 1975), and PD (Cummings and Benson, 1984; Huber et al, 1989b). The primary features include difficulties with cognitive processing speed, memory, and concept formation involving frontal lobe function (Bowen et al, 1975; Huber and Paulson, 1985).

The clearest evidence that such difficulties may be related to dopamine deficiency is derived from studies of patients exposed to MPTP. MPTP causes a relatively specific striatal dopaminergic lesion. Patients with MPTP-induced PD have deficits in construction, category naming, and tasks of frontal lobe executive functions (Stern and Langston, 1985). Even subjects with MPTP exposure and striatal dopaminergic deficits not sufficient to produce motor symptoms exhibit similar cognitive difficulties (Stern et al, 1990).

The observed correlation between severity of motor symptoms (particularly bradykinesia) in PD and intellectual deficits (Mortimer et al, 1982) also suggests a relationship between dopamine deficiency and cognitive symptoms. Patients with PD, AD, or depression with low levels of HVA (the principal dopamine metabolite) have impaired cognitive processing speed and frontal executive functions (Wolfe et al, 1990). Animal experiments have demonstrated that regional dopaminergic depletion can cause cognitive deficits that are responsive to levodopa (Brozoski et al, 1979; Zis et al, 1974). These findings support the hypothesis that dopaminergic deficiency contributes to the cognitive dysfunction of PD.

A putative anatomical locus for cognitive deficits in PD has been suggested. Dopaminergic cells in the ventral tegmental area project to the cingulate, entorhinal, and frontal regions (DeKeyser et al, 1990). The anatomical locus for the cognitive deficits of dopaminergic deficiency has been ascribed to the mesocortical dopaminergic system (Javoy-Agid and Agid, 1980). Histopathological mesocortical lesions have been reported in PD patients with dementia (Torack and Morris, 1988; Verity et al, 1990).

On/off effects are abrupt motor fluctuations while on stable doses of oral levodopa. Some investigations of PD patients have attempted to take advantage of the opportunity created by this complication of long-term dopaminergic therapy. These studies examined whether cognitive changes accompanied the motor fluctuations. Delis and colleagues (1982) reported a modest decline in cognitive performance while off in a PD patient undergoing erratic motor fluctuations. Huber and co-workers (1987) noted that the rate of memory acquisition improved in PD patients when plasma dopamine levels were higher. These researchers (Huber et al, 1989b) could not, however, replicate this finding using a more sensitive within-subjects design. Mohr and co-workers (1987, 1989) found modest improvement only in delayed recall of complex verbal material during on periods. Pillon and associates (1989) measured frontal executive function in PD patients and controls using a complex visual discrimination task. Levodopa had no effect on this task, whereas motor function improved significantly as the patients changed from off to on.

A state-specific impairment in memory has been noted in patients with on/off motor fluctuations. Huber and co-workers (1987, 1989a) demonstrated state-dependent memory impairments. If dopamine serum levels fluctuated between the time of memory acquisition and attempted retrieval, recall was impaired. The learned information was best remembered if retrieval was attempted in the same physiological state present during acquisition. As with the motor fluctuations, the state-dependent deficit was most likely to occur in patients on high doses of levodopa.

In most investigations, the effect of exogenous levodopa on cognitive function in PD has been minimal (Stern et al, 1990). However, as noted in the cholinergic system, there is a variety of potential pharmacological, biochemical, and histopathological explanations for the disappointing effects of dopaminergic therapy on cognition. Further investigation is required to adequately examine the role of dopaminergic deficiency in the subcortical dementia of PD.

COGNITIVE SIDE EFFECTS OF DOPAMINERGIC THERAPY

The cognitive side effects of levodopa were observed shortly after its introduction (Celesia and Barr, 1970), and patients with preexisting dementia were noted to be at greatest risk (Sacks et al, 1972). Although cognitive difficulties were not uncommon before levodopa, Sweet and co-workers (1976) noted that long-term dopaminergic therapy resulted in an agitated confusional state of varying severity in up to 60 percent of PD patients. Although recent efforts to limit total dopaminergic doses have decreased the incidence of behavioral side effects, they still represent a common clinical problem for patients on long-term therapy. Symptoms can include vivid dreams, nightmares, disturbed sleep patterns, visual illusions, confusion, and disorientation suggestive of toxic delirium (Moskovitz et al, 1978). Visual hallucinations are common and typically consist of formed objects, usually people or animals, and are usually nonthreatening. Insight is often lost as to their reality. Drug-induced behavioral alterations generally subside with drug reduction or withdrawal (Goetz et al, 1982). Although deficits in learning and memory may occur in PD patients with a hyperdopaminergic syndrome, they occur in the context of an attentional deficit due to toxic drug-induced delirium (Mayeux, 1987).

SUMMARY

Drug therapy of PD has resulted in a major improvement in motor function without a concomitant improvement in cognitive function. Lesions in the dopaminergic system may be responsible for the cognitive deficits associated with the syndrome of subcortical dementia, and cell loss in the nucleus basalis produces a cholinergic deficit in some PD patients. The cognitive response to dopaminergic therapy, however, has been disappointing. A dopaminergic state-dependent memory disorder has been identified in patients with motor fluctuations as a consequence of long-term therapy with levodopa. Anticholinergic agents appear to impair cognitive function, particularly in PD patients with dementia. The effect on PD patients without dementia is less clear-cut, but modest difficulties with frontal lobe tasks have been reported as a treatment effect.

REFERENCES

Albert ML, Feldman RG, Willis AL. The subcortical dementia of progressive supranuclear palsy. *J Neurol Neurosurg Psychiatry.* 1974;37:121–130.

Ball MJ. The morphological basis of dementia in Parkinson's disease. *Can J Neurol Sci.* 1984;11:180–184.

Barbeau A. The pathogenesis of Parkinson's disease: a new hypothesis. *Can Med Assoc J.* 1962;87:802–807.

Bartus RT, Dean RL III, Beer B, Lippa AS. The cholinergic hypothesis of geriatric memory dysfunction. *Science.* 1982;217:408–417.

Boller F, Mizutani T, Roessmann U, Gambetti P. Parkinson disease, dementia, and Alzheimer disease: clinicopathological correlations. *Ann Neurol.* 1980;7:329–335.

Bowen FP, Kamienny RS, Burns MM, Yahr MD. Parkinsonism: effects of levodopa treatment on concept formation. *Neurology.* 1975;25:701–704.

Brozoski TJ, Brown RM, Rosvold HE, Goldman PS. Cognitive deficits caused by regional depletion of dopamine in prefrontal cortex of rhesus monkey. *Science.* 1979;205:929–931.

Burns RS, Chiueh CC, Markey SP, et al. A primate model of parkinsonism: selective destruction of dopaminergic neurons in the pars compacta of the substantia nigra by N-methyl-4-phenyl-1,2,3,6-tetrahydropyridine. *Proc Natl Acad Sci USA.* 1983;80:4546–4550.

Celesia GG, Barr AN. Psychosis and other psychiatric manifestations of levodopa therapy. *Arch Neurol.* 1970;23:193–200.

Charcot JM. *Lectures on the Diseases of the Nervous System.* London: The Sydenham Society; 1877.

Chui HC, Mortimer JA, Slager U, et al. Pathological correlates of dementia in Parkinson's disease. *Arch Neurol.* 1986;43:991–995.

Comella CL, Tanner C. Anticholinergic drugs in the treatment of Parkinson's disease. In: Koller WC, Paulson G, eds. *Therapy of Parkinson's Disease.* New York: Marcel Dekker, Inc; 1990:123–141.

Cotzias GC, Papasiliou PS, Gellene R. Modification of parkinsonism. Chronic treatment with L-dopa. *N Engl J Med.* 1969;280:337–345.

Coyle JT, Price DL, DeLong MR. Alzheimer's disease: a disorder of cortical cholinergic innervation. *Science.* 1983;219:1184–1190.

Cummings JL. The dementias of Parkinson's disease: prevalence, characteristics, neurobiology, and comparison with dementia of the Alzheimer type. *Eur Neurol.* 1988;28(suppl):15–23.

Cummings JL, Benson DF. Subcortical dementia. Review of an emerging concept. *Arch Neurol.* 1984;41:874–879.

Curtis L, Lees AJ, Stern GM, Marmot MG. Effect of L-dopa on course of Parkinson's disease. *Lancet.* 1984;2:211–212.

Davies P, Malony AJF. Selective loss of central cholinergic neurons in Alzheimer's disease. *Lancet.* 1976;2:1403.

Davis KL, Mohs R. Enhancement of memory processes in Alzheimer's disease with multiple-dose intravenous physostigmine. *Am J Psychiatry.* 1982;139:1421–1424.

Davis KL, Mohs RC, Tinklenberg JR, et al. Physostigmine: improvement of long-term memory processes in normal humans. *Science.* 1978;201:272–274.

De Keyser J, Herregodts P, Ebinger G. The mesoneocortical dopamine neuron system. *Neurology.* 1990;40:1660–1662.

de la Monte SM, Wells SE, Hedley-Whyte ET, Growdon JH. Neurological distinction between Parkinson's dementia and Parkinson's plus Alzheimer's disease. *Ann Neurol.* 1989;26:309–320.

De Smet Y, Ruberg M, Serdaru M, et al. Confusion, dementia and anticholinergics in Parkinson's disease. *J Neurol Neurosurg Psychiatry.* 1982;45:1161–1164.

Delis D, Direnfeld L, Alexander MP, Kaplan E. Cognitive fluctuations associated with on-off phenomenon in Parkinson's disease. *Neurology.* 1982;32:1049–1052.

Deutsch JA. The cholinergic synapse and the site of memory. *Science.* 1971;174:788–794.

Deutsch JA, Hamburg MD, Dahl H. Anticholinesterase-induced amnesia and its temporal aspects. *Science.* 1966;151:221–223.

Drachman DA. Memory and cognitive function in man: does the cholinergic system have a specific role? *Neurology.* 1977;27:783–790.

Drachman DA, Leavitt J. Human memory and the cholinergic system. *Arch Neurol.* 1974;30:113–121.

Dubois B, Danzé F, Pillon B, et al. Cholinergic-dependent cognitive deficits in Parkinson's disease. *Ann Neurol.* 1987;22:26–30.

Dubois B, Pillon B, Lhermitte F, Agid Y. Cholinergic deficiency and frontal dysfunction in Parkinson's disease. *Ann Neurol.* 1990;28:117–121.

Dubois B, Ruberg M, Javoy-Agid F, et al. A subcortico-cortical cholinergic system is affected in Parkinson's disease. *Brain Res.* 1983;288:213–218.

Dunnett SB, Whishaw IQ, Jones GH, Bunch ST. Behavioral, biochemical and histochemical effects of different neurotoxic amino acids injected into nucleus basalis magnocellularis of rats. *Neuroscience.* 1987;20:653–669.

Duvoisin RC. Cholinergic-anticholinergic antagonism in parkinsonism. *Arch Neurol.* 1967;17:124–126.

Ehringer H, Hornykiewicz O. Verteilung von noradrenalin und dopamin (3-hydroxytyramin) im Gehirn des Menschen und ihr Verhalten bei Erkrankungen des extrapyramidalen systems. *Klin Wochenschr.* 1960;38:1236–1960.

Galasko DR, Thal LJ. Cholinomimetic agents. In: Cummings JL, Miller BL, eds. *Alzheimer's Disease. Treatment and Long-Term Management.* New York: Marcel Dekker, Inc; 1990:23–63.

Goetz C, Tanner C, Klawans HL. Pharmacology of hallucinations induced by long-term drug therapy. *Am J Psychiatry.* 1982;139:494–497.

Hakim AM, Mathieson G. Dementia in Parkinson disease: a neuropathologic study. *Neurology.* 1979;29:1209–1214.

Huber SJ, Paulson GW. The concept of subcortical dementia. *Am J Psychiatry.* 1985;142:1312–1317.

Huber SJ, Shulman HG, Paulson GW, Shuttleworth EC. Fluctuations in plasma dopamine level impairs memory in Parkinson's disease. *Neurology.* 1987;37:1371–1375.

Huber SJ, Shulman HG, Paulson GW, Shuttleworth EC. Dose-dependent memory impairment in Parkinson's disease. *Neurology.* 1989a;39:438–440.

Huber SJ, Shuttleworth EC, Freidenberg DL. Neuropsychological differences between the dementias of Alzheimer's and Parkinson's diseases. *Arch Neurol.* 1989b;46:1287–1291.

Huber SJ, Shuttleworth EC, Paulson GW. Dementia in Parkinson's disease. *Arch Neurol.* 1986;43:987–990.

Hyman BT, Van Hoesen GW, Damasio AR. Memory-related neural systems in Alzheimer's disease: an anatomic study. *Neurology.* 1990;40:1721–1730.

Javoy-Agid F, Agid Y. Is the mesocortical system involved in Parkinson's disease? *Neurology.* 1980;30:1326–1330.

Johnston MV, McKinney M, Coyle JT. Evidence for a cholinergic projection to neocortex from neurons in basal forebrain. *Proc Natl Acad Sci USA.* 1979;76:5392.

Kish SJ, Shannak K, Hornykiewicz O. Uneven pattern of dopamine loss in the striatum of patients with idiopathic Parkinson's disease. *N Engl J Med.* 1988;318:876–880.

Koller WC. Disturbance of recent memory function in parkinsonian patients on anticholinergic therapy. *Cortex.* 1984;20:307–311.

Koller WC, Hubble JP. Levodopa therapy in Parkinson's disease. *Neurology.* 1990;40(suppl 3):40–47.

Mandel RJ, Thal LJ. Physostigmine improves water maze performance following nucleus basalis magnocellularis lesions in rats. *Psychopharmacology.* 1988;96:421–425.

Mayeux R. Mental state. In: Koller WC, ed. *Handbook of Parkinson's Disease.* New York: Marcel Dekker, Inc; 1987:127–144.

McHugh PR, Folstein MP. Psychiatric syndromes of Huntington's chorea: a clinical and phenomenologic study. In: Benson DF, Blumer D, eds. *Psychiatric Aspects of Neurologic Disease.* New York: Grune & Stratton; 1975:267–285.

Mesulam MM, Mufson EJ, Levey AI, Wainer B. Cholinergic innervation of cortex by the basal forebrain. *J Comp Neurol.* 1983;11:264–267.

Mohr E, Fabbrini G, Ruggieri S, et al. Cognitive concomitants of dopamine system stimulation in parkinsonian patients. *J Neurol Neurosurg Psychiatry.* 1987;50:1192–1196.

Mohr E, Fabbrini G, Williams J, et al. Dopamine and memory function in Parkinson's disease. *Movement Disord.* 1989;4:113–120.

Mortimer JA, Pirozzolo FJ, Hansch EC, Webster DD. Relationship of motor symptoms to intellectual deficits in Parkinson disease. *Neurology.* 1982;32:133–137.

Moskovitz C, Moses H III, Klawans HL. Levodopa-induced psychosis: a kindling phenomenon. *Am J Psychiatry.* 1978;135:669–675.

Nakano I, Hirano A. Parkinson's disease: Neuron loss in the nucleus basalis without concomitant Alzheimer's disease. *Ann Neurol.* 1984;15:415–418.

Perry EK. The cholinergic hypothesis: 10 years on. *Br Med Bull.* 1986;42:63–69.

Perry EK, Curtis M, Dick DJ, et al. Cholinergic correlates of cognitive impairment in Parkinson's disease: comparisons with Alzheimer's disease. *J Neurol Neurosurg Psychiatry.* 1985;48:413–421.

Perry EK, Perry RH, Blessed G, Tomlinson BE. Necropsy evidence of central cholinergic deficits in senile dementia. *Lancet.* 1977;1:189.

Perry EK, Tomlinson BE, Blessed G, et al. Correlation of cholinergic abnormalities with senile plaques and mental test scores in senile dementia. *Br Med J.* 1978;2:1457–1459.

Pillon B, Dubois B, Bonnet A-M, et al. Cognitive slowing in Parkinson's disease fails to respond to levodopa treatment: the 15-objects test. *Neurology.* 1989;39:762–768.

Proctor F, Riklan M, Cooper IS, Teuber HL. Judgment of visual and postural vertical by parkinsonian patients. *Neurology.* 1964;14:287–293.

Riklan M, Whelihan W, Cullinan T. Levodopa and psychometric test performance in parkinsonism—5 years later. *Neurology.* 1976;26:173–179.

Ruberg M, Ploska A, Javoy-Agid F, Agid Y. Muscarinic binding and choline aceyltransferase activity in parkinsonian subjects with reference to dementia. *Brain Res.* 1982;232:129–139.

Sacks OW, Kohn MS, Messeloff CR, et al. Effects of levodopa in parkinsonian patients with dementia. *Neurology.* 1972;22:516–519.

Sadeh M, Braham J, Modan M. Effects of anticholinergic drugs on memory in Parkinson's disease. *Arch Neurol.* 1982;39:666–667.

Sitaram N, Weingartner H, Gillin JC. Human serial learning: enhancement with arecholine and choline and impairment with scopolamine. *Science.* 1978;210:274–276.

Stern Y, Langston W. Intellectual changes in patients with MPTP-induced parkinsonism. *Neurology.* 1985;35:1506–1509.

Stern Y, Mayeux R, Rosen J, Ilson J. Perceptual motor dysfunction in Parkinson's disease: a deficit in sequential and predictive voluntary movement. *J Neurol Neurosurg Psychiatry.* 1983;46:145–151.

Stern Y, Tetrud JW, Martin WRW, et al. Cognitive change following MPTP exposure. *Neurology.* 1990;40:261–264.

Sweet RD, McDowell FH, Feigenson JS, et al. Mental symptoms in Parkinson's disease during chronic treatment with levodopa. *Neurology.* 1976;26:305–310.

Taylor AE, Saint-Cyr JA, Lang AE. Frontal lobe dysfunction in Parkinson's disease. *Brain.* 1986;109:845–883.

Thal LJ, Fuld PA, Masur DM, Sharpless NS. Oral physostigmine and lecithin improve memory in Alzheimer disease. *Ann Neurol.* 1983;13:491–496.

Torack RM, Morris JC. The association of ventral tegmental area histopathology with adult dementia. *Arch Neurol.* 1988;45:497–501.

Tune LE, Strauss ME, Lew MF, et al. Serum levels of anticholinergic drugs and impaired recent memory in chronic schizophrenic patients. *Am J Psychiatry.* 1982;139:1460–1462.

Velasco F, Velasco M, Romo R. Effect of carbachol and atropine perfusions in the mesencephalic tegmentum and caudate nucleus of experimental tremor in monkeys. *Exp Neurol.* 1982;78:450–460.

Verity MA, Roitberg B, Kepes JJ. Mesolimbocortical dementia: clinico-pathological studies on two cases. *J Neurol Neurosurg Psychiatry.* 1990;53:492–495.

Whitehouse PJ, Hedreen JC, White CL III, Price DL. Basal forebrain neurons in the dementia of Parkinson's disease. *Ann Neurol.* 1983;13:243–248.

Whitehouse PJ, Price DL, Clark AW, et al. Alzheimer disease: evidence for selective loss of cholinergic neurons in the nucleus basalis. *Ann Neurol.* 1981;10:122–126.

Wilcock GK, Esiri MM, Bowen DM, Smith CT. Correlation of cortical choline acetyltransferase activity with the severity of dementia and histological abnormalities. *J Neurol Sci.* 1982;57:407–417.

Wolfe N, Katz DI, Albert ML, et al. Neuropsychological profile linked to low dopamine: in Alzheimer's disease, major depression, and Parkinson's disease. *J Neurol Neurosurg Psychiatry.* 1990;53:915–917.

Yoshimura M. Pathological basis for dementia in elderly patients with idiopathic Parkinson's disease. *Eur Neurol* 1988;28(suppl 1):29–35.

Zis AP, Fibiger HC, Phillips AG. Reversal by L-dopa of impaired learning due to destruction of the dopaminergic nigrostriatal projection. *Science.* 1974;185:960–962.

23

Neuropsychiatric Complications of Drug Treatment of Parkinson's Disease

JEFFREY L. CUMMINGS

Treatment of Parkinson's disease (PD), requires the use of powerful agents that affect the fundamental neurochemistry of the brain. It is not surprising that in addition to the alleviation of motor symptoms, these drugs frequently produce adverse side effects. These are sometimes dramatic and include delusions, visual hallucinations, and mania. Although undesirable, these psychotoxic symptoms may reveal important relationships between neurotransmitter function and neuropsychiatric disorders. In this chapter, the major types of behavioral alterations observed in the course of anti-parkinsonism therapy are discussed (Table 23-1). Behavioral disturbances were considered a consequence of therapy when they appeared for the first time soon after initiation of treatment or after an increase in drug dosage and improved when the drug was discontinued.

HALLUCINATIONS

Visual hallucinations are the most common neuropsychiatric side effect of antiparkinsonian treatment. They may result from treatment with all classes of drugs, including anticholinergic agents, amantadine, deprenyl, levodopa (with or without carbidopa), and dopamine receptor agonists (bromocriptine, pergolide, lisuride) (Parkes, 1981; Porteous and Ross, 1956; Postma and Van Tilburg, 1975). Table 23-2 presents representative studies reporting the prevalence of hallucinations arising in the course of treatment of PD. The frequency ranged from 6 percent to 38 percent, with most studies reporting the prevalence of hallucinations among patients treated with dopaminergic agents to be around 20 percent. There is a tendency for hallucinations to occur somewhat more frequently with levodopa than with other antiparkinsonian agents, and there is a trend for hallucinations to occur in patients treated with higher doses of drugs. The actual prevalence may be higher than suggested by the available reports because hallucinations may not have been sought systematically; they may be underreported by patients who believe them to be a sign of mental illness, and they may not have been properly distinguished from dreams, delusions, or delirium.

Hallucinations associated with dopaminergic agents typically occur in a normal state of consciousness without delirium. They are usually fully formed images of

Table 23-1.   Neuropsychiatric side effects reported with antiparkinsonian therapy

Hallucinations
  Visual
  Auditory
  Tactile
Psychosis
  Delusional syndrome
  Formal thought disorder
Mood disorders
  Mania, hypomania, euphoria
  Depression
Anxiety
Sexual alterations
  Hypersexuality
  Paraphilic behavior
Sleep disturbances
  Vivid dreams
  Nightmares
Delirium
Miscellaneous
  Rage
  Compulsive or ritualized behavior

humans or animals. Bizarre or exotic experiences sometimes are reported (Shaw et al, 1980). Moskovitz and colleagues (1978) reported that of 19 patients with visual hallucinations, 10 experienced images of people, 3 had images of animals and inanimate objects, 3 had unformed hallucinations, and 3 had combined formed and unformed hallucinations. The hallucinations were most common at night, recurred frequently (nearly every night), and were stereotyped for each patient. Seventy-two percent of the patients reported that the hallucinations were nonthreatening, whereas the others had frightening visions. The hallucinations are typically silent, although in rare cases, combined visual and auditory hallucinations occur. Vivid dreams and sleep disturbances commonly precede or accompany the visual hallucinosis. Nausieda and colleagues (1982) found that hallucinations were present in 39 percent of patients with and 4 percent of those without sleep complaints.

Hallucinations may occur in nonvisual modalities. Moskovitz and associates (1978) found that of 31 PD patients with hallucinations, 3 had pure auditory hallucinations, 1 had pure tactile hallucinations, and 8 had combined visual and auditory hallucinations. Lang and co-workers (1982) reported that 3 of 26 PD patients (11.5 percent) treated with pergolide experienced auditory hallucinations.

The determinants of visual hallucinations in the course of antiparkinsonian treatment are not completely known. In a review of 775 PD patients (257 with hallucinations), Tanner and colleagues (1983) found no associations between hallucinations and disease duration, duration of treatment, PD severity, or dyskinetic side effects. Patients with hallucinations, however, were older, had more often been treated with amantadine or anticholinergic agents, and had received these drugs for longer periods of time than nonhallucinating patients. These findings suggest that age, multiple-drug therapy, and anticholinergic treatment represent risk factors for hallucinosis. Glantz and colleagues (1986) found that PD patients with levodopa-induced hallucinations

Table 23-2. Representative studies reporting prevalence of visual hallucinations during antiparkinsonian treatment

Author	n	Drug	Dosage (mg/day) (mean or range)	Prevalence (%)
Mawdsley, 1970	32	Levodopa[a]	1500–9000	6.3
Moskovitz et al, 1978	88	Levodopa	NS[b]	32.3
Shaw et al, 1980	178	Levodopa	NS	8.4
Presthus, 1980	175	Levodopa	NS	11.4
Goetz et al, 1982	78	Levodopa	NS	32.1
Glantz et al, 1986	26	Levodopa	NS	35
Wilson and Smith, 1989	51	Levodopa	NS	38
Aaril and Gilhus, 1989	20	Levodopa CR[c]	200–2400	15
Bush et al, 1989	204	Levodopa CR	808	5
Birkmayer, 1983	1414	Levodopa + deprenyl	NS	5.2
Rinne, 1983	11	Levodopa + deprenyl	827 + 5–10	9
Gopinathan and Calne, 1981	118	Bromocriptine	72	15
Goetz et al, 1985	10	Bromocriptine	51	60
Burton et al, 1985	9	Bromocriptine	15–75	33.3
Rinne, 1985	76	Bromocriptine	28	7
Lang et al, 1982	26	Pergolide	0.4–15	19
Stern et al, 1984	19	Pergolide	NS	15.8
Quinn et al, 1984	43	Pergolide	0.2–10	6.9
Kurlan et al, 1985	9	Pergolide	2.2 ± 0.9	11
Tanner et al, 1982	23	Pergolide	2.8	17
Tanner et al, 1986	17	Pergolide	0.6–9	17.6
Olanow and Alberts, 1986a	22	Pergolide	1.5–4.25	18.2
LeWitt et al, 1982	28	Lisuride	4.5	25
Burton et al, 1985	11	Mesulergine	8–68	36.3
Jankovic et al, 1985	20	Mesulergine + levodopa	6.7	30
Frankel et al, 1990	57	Subcutaneous apomorphine + levodopa	10.2 + 815	5
Parkes et al, 1975	22	Levoamphetamine	50	9
Goetz et al, 1984	20	Buproprion	400	15
Birkmayer and Riederer, 1984	380	Deprenyl	10	2.8

[a] 17% on non-levodopa drug regimens.
[b] NS, unspecified; levodopa administered with carbidopa.
[c] CR, continuous release.

scored higher on the hypochondriasis, psychasthenia, and schizophrenia subscales of psychiatric rating instruments. Abnormalities were considered to be indicative of impairment in life-functioning, heightened concern with bodily functioning, anxiety, self-doubt, self-devaluation, social alienation, bizarre feelings, and general dissatisfaction. Moreover, these abnormalities were present in PD patients with ongoing hallucinations as well as in those who progressed to hallucinatory states later in their clinical course. Thus, these behavioral findings appeared to have predictive value for which patients were in prodromal phases of hallucinosis or were vulnerable to the hallucinatory effects of levodopa.

Hallucinatory syndromes produced by dopaminergic agents may be distinguishable from those caused by anticholinergic therapy (Goetz et al, 1982). Hallucinations associated with anticholinergic toxicity tend to be threatening, occur in conjunction with delirium, are less well formed, and are more likely to be accompanied by hallucinations in other modalities.

Hallucinations nearly always respond to reduction of drug dosage, although the response may not be immediate. Reduction of either anticholinergic or dopaminergic therapy usually is efficacious (Goetz et al, 1982). Management of hallucinations co-occurring with delusions is discussed below.

DELUSIONS

Delusions are false beliefs that are based on incorrect inference, are held despite evidence to the contrary, and are not ordinarily accepted by other members of the person's culture or subculture (American Psychiatric Association, 1987). The occurrence of delusions in untreated PD is notably rare, and the occurrence of psychosis in PD usually is indicative of an adverse treatment response (Crow et al, 1976). Delusions have been described in conjunction with all types of antiparkinsonian therapy, including anticholinergic agents, amantadine, levodopa, bromocriptine, pergolide, and deprenyl (Parkes, 1981; Porteous and Ross, 1956; Postma and Van Tilburg, 1975). In comparative studies, amantadine, levodopa, and lisuride had approximately equal psychotogenic potency (Fischer et al, 1990). Table 23-3 lists representative studies reporting the frequency of delusions in PD patients treated with a variety of antiparkinsonian drugs. The range of prevalence of delusions was 3 percent to 30 percent, and

Table 23-3. Representative studies reporting delusions in response to antiparkinsonian treatment

Authors	n	Drug	Dosage (mg/day) (mean or range)	Prevalence (%)
Jenkins and Groh, 1970	90	Levodopa	NS[a]	7
Celesia and Barr, 1970	45	Levodopa	<8000	17.7
Goodwin, 1971[b]	180	Levodopa	NS	3.6
O'Brien et al, 1971	16	Levodopa	4000–12,000	6.2
Moskovitz et al, 1978	88	Levodopa[c]	NS	12.5
Shaw et al, 1980	178	Levodopa	NS	3.3
Presthus, 1980	175	Levodopa	NS	9.7
Serby et al, 1978	66	Bromocriptine	15–80	3.0
Lang et al, 1982	26	Pergolide	0.4–15	3.8
Quinn et al, 1984	43	Pergolide	NS	4.6
Lieberman et al, 1981[a]	10	Lisuride	3.6	30
Lieberman et al, 1981[b]	20	Lisuride + levodopa	5 + 1030	10
Obeso et al, 1986	30	Lisuride infusion	2.7	30
Critchley et al, 1986	12	Lisuride infusion	1.4	83
Moses et al, 1986	20	Mesulergine	NS	5
Serby et al, 1978	53	Lergotrile	15–85	5.6

[a]NS, unspecified; levodopa administered with carbidopa.
[b]Review.
[c]17% on non-levodopa drug regimens.

delusions were more common among patients treated with higher doses of drugs. These figures probably underestimate the true frequency of delusions in treated PD patients, since they have rarely been specifically sought, the investigators were frequently unfamiliar with psychiatric interviewing techniques, and patients and families may underreport these disturbing and embarrassing phenomena. In addition, some authors failed to distinguish among delusions, delirium, and hallucinations when reporting psychiatric side effects of treatment.

The frequency of delusions is similar for all agents except lisuride infusions. The delivery of lisuride through a pump, providing continuous intravenous therapy, is associated with a markedly elevated prevalence rate (Critchley et al, 1986; Obeso et al, 1986).

Levodopa-related delusions frequently are antedated by two other behavioral changes: dreams and visual hallucinations (Klawans, 1978; Moskovitz et al, 1978; Nausieda et al, 1982). Their occurrence is evidence of emerging toxicity and should lead to dosage modifications. Delusions are uncommon before at least 2 years of levodopa therapy has elapsed (Klawans, 1978). The delusional–hallucinatory syndrome may occur in conjunction with overt delirium or in a clear sensorium as the sole evidence of psychotoxicity (Celesia and Barr, 1970; Moskovitz et al, 1978). The delusions, particularly those occurring in the absence of delirium, are usually complex, well-formed belief systems buttressed by supporting observations. They are typically persecutory in nature, involving fears of being injured, influenced, poisoned, filmed, or tape recorded (Jenkins and Groh, 1970; Moskovitz et al, 1978; Serby et al, 1978). In some cases, the delusions have specific themes, such as the Capgras syndrome (the belief that a spouse, family member, or acquaintance has been replaced by an identical appearing imposter) (Lipper, 1976). A few of the delusional patients reported in the literature have been aggressive, vociferous, and behaviorally disturbed (Celesia and Barr, 1970). Older patients and those with dementia syndromes may be particularly vulnerable to the development of delusions (Celesia and Barr, 1970; Fischer et al, 1990; Pederzoli et al, 1983; Sacks et al, 1972).

Pharmacotoxic delusions in PD usually occur in the absence of a formal thought disorder (loosening of associations, tangentiality, incoherence, neologisms, blocking, clanging), but there is modest evidence suggesting that levodopa may occasionally produce a characteristic thought disorder syndrome. Beardsley and Puletti (1971), using the MMPI, found that PD patients treated with levodopa had elevations on the schizophrenia subscale, whereas patients treated with anticholinergic agents or thalamotomies did not. No firm conclusion regarding the possible effect of dopaminergic agents on thought form is currently possible, but these agents are much more likely to induce delusions and abnormal thought content than to affect thought structure.

Neuropathological investigations specifically addressing psychosis in PD have been rare. In one of the few studies exploring this issue, Birkmayer and Riederer (1975) found elevated levels of 5-hydroxytryptamine and noradrenalin in the caudal substantia nigra, raphe, red nucleus, and globus pallidus of delusional patients. Striatal levels of dopamine, noradrenaline, and 5-hydroxytryptamine were the same in those with and without delusions. The authors suggested that transmitter alterations at extrastriatal sites are responsible for the psychosis. Dopamine receptor hypersensitivity also has been invoked as the neurophysiological basis of delusions in PD (Moskovitz et al,

1978), and the production of a psychotogenic endotoxin from dopamine also has been postulated (Clark, 1970).

The first step in the management of delusions is withdrawal of anticholinergic agents and amantadine. If delusions persist, the dosage of levodopa–carbidopa or other dopaminergic agents should be reduced to the minimal level compatible with acceptable patient mobility. Patients with drug-induced psychoses that remit with dosage reduction may later tolerate higher doses without recurrence of the psychotic symptoms (Teychenne et al, 1986). If delusions continue despite dose modifications, pharmacotherapy of the delusional syndrome may be undertaken. L-Tryptophan has successfully reduced paranoid delusions in a few patients (Miller and Nieburg, 1974). Low dosages of neuroleptic medications—molindone, thioridazine, pherphenazine, haloperidol—may be administered, although considerable caution should be exercised to avoid exacerbating the extrapyramidal disorder (Hale and Bellizzi, 1980). Clozapine, an antipsychotic agent with few extrapyramidal side effects, also has been used successfully to treated delusions in PD (Friedman and Lannon, 1989; Roberts et al, 1989). Sedation, confusion, and increased PD symptoms may occur with clozapine therapy, however, and patients usually will be intolerant of doses larger than 100 mg daily (Pfeiffer et al, 1990; Wolters et al, 1990). Clozapine may cause agranulocytosis, and hematological monitoring is mandatory. Electroconvulsive therapy occasionally has been successfully used to alleviate levodopa-induced delusions (Hurwitz et al, 1988).

MANIA, HYPOMANIA, AND EUPHORIA

Levodopa has definite mood-elevating properties in some patients. The behavioral changes vary from simple euphoria with feelings of well-being to fully developed manic episodes with elation, grandiosity, pressured speech, racing thoughts, hyperactivity, diminished need for sleep, increased libido, and risk-taking behaviors (O'Brien et al, 1971; Ryback and Schwab, 1971). Celesia and Barr (1970) observed euphoria in 10 percent of levodopa-treated patients. In all cases, the elevated mood occurred in conjunction with drug-induced dyskinesias and subsided when the total levodopa dose was reduced. In a review of 908 patients treated with levodopa, Goodwin (1971) reported that hypomania had occurred in 8 (1.5 percent). He also noted that hypomania occurred in essentially all patients who had histories of mania before PD onset. Jouvent and colleagues (1983) reported hypomania in 2 of 10 patients treated with bromocriptine. Neither patient had a previous history of manic behavior. Lang and associates (1982) reported 1 case of euphoria among 26 PD patients given pergolide. Feelings of elation and even manic behavior may accompany the on period in patients with the on/off phenomenon (Keshavan et al, 1986; Nissenbaum et al, 1987). The elation and sense of energy and well-being experienced with dopaminergic agent ingestion probably account for the development of a pattern of abuse, dependency, and drug-seeking behavior observed in a few PD patients (Nausieda, 1985).

Mania typically subsides when the drug dosage is reduced. Lithium administration has benefited some patients but not others (Ryback and Schwab, 1971; Van Woert et al, 1971).

DEPRESSION

Levodopa has sometimes been impugned as a depressogenic agent. Several studies have noted an apparent increase in the number of depressed patients after initiation of levodopa therapy (Barbeau, 1969; Celesia and Barr, 1970; Cherington, 1970; Damasio et al, 1971; Shaw et al, 1980; Wagshul and Daroff, 1969; Wilson and Smith, 1989). Raft and Spencer (1972) reported the suicide of a depressed PD patient who had recently begun levodopa treatment. Maskin and colleagues (1973) assessed depression in PD using the depression scale of the MMPI and found a significantly higher depression score in patients treated for more than 18 months compared to those treated for shorter periods of time. Likewise, Huber and associates (1988) found that depressed PD patients had significantly higher levodopa dosages and had been taking the drug for a longer period of time than nondepressed patients. Mindham and co-workers (1976) found that patients treated with levodopa evidenced more depression than those treated with anticholinergics or amantadine. The percentage of patients receiving levodopa and manifesting depressive symptoms varies from 2 to 50 percent, approximately the same range as the reported prevalence in PD regardless of treatment status and similar to the prevalence among untreated PD patients. Thus, levodopa may precipitate depression or may make depressive mood changes more evident but does not appear to alter the overall frequency of depression.

When long-term levodopa therapy leads to the on/off phenomenon, depression frequently accompanies the abrupt onset of PD symptoms and abates when motility returns (Nissenbaum et al, 1987).

PD depression is treated with conventional antidepressant agents or electroconvulsive therapy (Chapters 18 and 19).

ANXIETY

Celesia and Barr (1970) described anxiety in 4 of 45 (8.8 percent) PD patients treated with levodopa. The syndrome was characterized by apprehension, nervousness, irritability, and feelings of impending disaster, as well as palpitations, hyperventilation, and insomnia. Most of the patients had not experienced these symptoms before treatment. Rondot and colleagues (1984) found a high prevalence of anxiety among PD patients before therapy but also observed exacerbation of anxiety syndromes after levodopa treatment.

Lang and associates (1982) noted an unusually high frequency (19 percent) of anxiety symptoms among patients given pergolide. None of the patients had experienced anxiety on other drug regimens. Markham and Diamond (1986) reported anxiety in 9 percent of patients treated with pergolide, and Olanow and Alberts (1986b) observed anxiety in 13 percent of patients receiving this agent. Yahr and colleagues (1983) noted a 20 percent incidence of anxiety when deprenyl was added to levodopa therapy in 69 patients with long-duration disease and on/off episodes. These observations are preliminary but suggest that pergolide and deprenyl may be more likely to induce anxiety than are other antiparkinsonian agents.

Anxiety occurs in approximately two thirds of patients experiencing on/off episodes, with anxious symptoms increasing during the off state (Nissenbaum et al, 1987). In addition, the depression syndrome manifested in PD is often characterized by prominent anxiety symptoms (Schiffer et al, 1988).

Anxiety improves with reduction in drug dosage or treatment with an antianxiety agent (Celesia and Barr, 1970).

ALTERED SEXUAL BEHAVIOR

PD patients may experience a remarkable resurrection of sexual interest and potency in conjunction with antiparkinsonian therapy. In some cases, increased libido reaches pathological proportions, with hypersexuality. Exaggerated libido may represent one aspect of a manic syndrome as discussed or may occur without other symptoms of mania. This section summarizes observations regarding increased or aberrant sexual behavior in the absence of other evidence of mania.

Case series generally have reported increased libido in 1 to 10 percent of PD patients treated with levodopa. Goodwin (1971) described hypersexual behavior in 8 of 908 patients (0.9 percent). Bowers and co-workers (1971) carefully assessed sexual function in 19 patients receiving levodopa and found that one third had an activation of sexual interests. O'Brien and colleagues (1971) found that of 20 patients treated with levodopa, 2 developed spontaneous erections and 4 had increased libido. In 1 patient, hypersexuality occurred. Wodak and colleagues (1972) observed pathologically increased libido in 2 of 16 (13 percent) patients treated with levodopa, and Lesser and associates (1979) noted hypersexuality in 4 of 131 levodopa-treated patients (3 percent). Case reports of hypersexual responses in individual patients treated with levodopa (Harvey, 1988; Shapiro, 1973; Vogel and Schifter, 1983) document increased masturbation, more numerous attempts at intercourse with the patient's spouse, and initiation of extramarital affairs for sexual gratification. The reports concern males more frequently than females. Most cases of hypersexuality have involved PD patients treated with levodopa, but pergolide also has been observed to produce hypersexual behavior (Quinn et al, 1984).

Paraphilic (i.e., sexually deviant) behavior also may be induced or exaggerated by levodopa. Miller and colleagues (1986) reported a PD patient with no history of paraphilic tendencies who developed sexual masochistic behavior while being treated with levodopa, injuring his penis by inserting a pencil into the urethra. A patient reported by Harvey (1988) acknowledged deviant sexual interests throughout life, but he had not acted on them before receiving levodopa. After reaching maximal doses, he engaged in pedophilia, voyeurism, and scatologic letter writing and described pederastic and rape fantasies. Quinn and colleagues (1983) reported 2 patients who had had sadomasochistic fantasies before treatment with levodopa but had engaged in little or no paraphilic behavior. Once treatment was initiated, the masochism was no longer contained, and they engaged in flagellation and bondage. Both patients also had exhibitionistic thoughts, and one exposed himself in public lavatories. In one patient, the sexual deviations did not recur when treatment was changed to a dopaminergic receptor agonist (bromocriptine), but in the other, the behavior occurred both with levodopa and the receptor agonist pergolide.

These reports indicate that dopaminergic therapy regularly results in increased libido, produces hypersexuality in a minority of PD patients, and may lead to paraphilic behavior, particularly in predisposed individuals.

SLEEP DISTURBANCES

Sleep in PD patients treated with levodopa is characterized by diminished deep (stage III and IV) sleep, decreased rapid eye movement (REM) sleep, and increased sleep fragmentation with multiple arousals and awakenings (Emser et al, 1988). Jenkins and Groh (1970) reported that 19 of 90 patients (21 percent) treated with levodopa reported insomnia, and 3 complained of hypersomnia; 17 (19 percent) described vivid dreams or nightmares. Lesser and colleagues (1979) recorded complaints of insomnia in 11 of 131 patients (8 percent) treated chronically with levodopa. Wilson and Smith (1989) described nightmares in 4 percent of elderly PD patients treated with levodopa. Vivid dreams have occurred with pergolide treatment (Lang et al, 1982) as well as levodopa. Dreams and nightmares frequently precede the occurrence of waking hallucinations and delusions and may serve as an early warning for these more dire effects.

Sleep disturbances are particularly common among PD patients with treatment-related psychiatric disorders. Nausida and co-workers (1982) found that 39 percent of patients with sleep complaints had benign hallucinations, whereas only 4 percent of patients without sleep complaints had hallucinations. Nineteen percent of those with sleep complaints had confusional states, and none of those without sleep disturbances were confused

CONFUSION

Confusion and delirium are loosely used words, and the exact syndrome described when the terms are applied in conjunction with drug therapy in PD rarely has been carefully defined. Nevertheless, it is evident that a portion of patients treated with antiparkinsonian agents develop delirious states, with fluctuating arousal, impaired attention, and incoherent verbal output. Table 23–4 summarizes the results of representative studies in which this syndrome was recorded. Mild confusion may well have gone unobserved, and the reported figures probably underestimate the actual prevalence of the syndrome. The frequency ranges from 5 percent to 25 percent in most studies, with prevalence rates noted to be higher in investigations using the higher potency ergot agents, such as bromocriptine, pergolide, and mesulergine.

MISCELLANEOUS DRUG-INDUCED BEHAVIOR CHANGES

In addition to the behaviors described, there are a few behavioral alterations that have been observed only rarely but seemed to have been precipitated by drug treatment of PD patients. Stern and co-workers (1984) described a patient who manifested depression, irritability, insomnia, and rage attacks while being treated with pergolide. All psychiatric symptoms abated within 7 days of stopping the drug. Sacks and colleagues

Table 23-4. Representative studies reporting frequency of confusional states in course of antiparkinsonian therapy

Authors	n	Drug	Dosage (mg/day)	Prevalence (%)
Goodwin, 1971	908	Levodopa	NS[a]	4.4
Shaw et al, 1980	178	Levodopa	NS	14
Bush et al, 1989	204	Sinemet CR[b]	814	4
Birkmayer, 1983	1414	Levodopa + deprenyl	NS	15.5
Rinne, 1983	11	Levodopa + deprenyl	827 + 5–10	9
Gopinathan and Calne, 1981	48	Bromocriptine	68	12
Lieberman et al, 1982	56	Pergolide	2.5	10.7
Kurlan et al, 1985	9	Pergolide	2.2 ± 0.9	33
Markham and Diamond, 1986	11	Pergolide	3.14	9
Pfeiffer et al, 1986	20	Mesulergine	20	25
Goetz et al, 1984	20	Buproprion	400	15
Porteous and Ross, 1956	52	Benzhexol HCl	NS	19

[a]NS, not specified.
[b]Sinemet CR, continuous release.

(1972) reported that a few patients with postencephalitic PD manifested either unusual hyperkinetic syndromes with tics, stereotyped movements, banging, and moaning, or peculiar cataleptic trancelike states. Similarly, Hardie and colleagues (1984) noted that PD patients occasionally exhibit complex mannerisms and organized rituals in conjunction with on/off fluctuations.

CONCLUSIONS

Antiparkinsonian therapy results in a remarkable array of neuropsychiatric alterations, including hallucinations, delusions, mania, anxiety, sexual behavior changes, vivid dreams and nightmares, and confusion. In most cases of levodopa-induced behavioral changes, delirium is not present, and the neuropsychiatric alterations occur in a clear sensorium. Behavioral alterations associated with anticholinergic agents, in contrast, usually occur as part of a delirium. Delusions and hallucinations, the two most common side effects of dopaminergic therapy, are not uncommon, occurring in at least 10 to 25 percent of patients. Behavioral complications are dose-related, occurring most frequently in patients treated with high-dose regimens. Levodopa is the only naturally occurring substance, playing a vital role in normal human neurophysiology, known to have these dramatic psychotogenic and hallucinogenic properties. The behavioral properties of levodopa appear to be shared by the dopamine receptor agonists, including bromocriptine, pergolide, lisuride, and mesulergine.

Levodopa rarely is given to nonparkinsonian patients, so it is not known if this substance would have the same behavioral impact if given to normal individuals. Bromocriptine, however, occasionally is administered to otherwise healthy patients for amenorrhea and galactorrhea. In these circumstances, it has had behavioral effects similar to those observed in PD. It has produced schizophrenia-like psychoses with delusions and auditory and visual hallucinations and has caused mania with grandiosity, elation, motor hyperactivity, and flight of ideas (Brook and Cookson, 1978; Shukla et al, 1985; Taneli et al, 1986; Vlissides et al, 1978). The behavioral changes have been observed in patients with no known history of psychiatric illness. On rare occasions, levodopa has been given to patients with a history of manic-depressive illness, and in that setting, it regularly precipitates manic episodes (Ko et al, 1981; Murphy et al, 1971). When administered to patients with schizophrenia, levodopa produces a worsening of paranoid ideation, hallucinations, and behavioral dyscontrol (Angrist et al, 1973; Yaryura-Tobias et al, 1972). These observations suggest that behavioral alterations with dopaminergic agents are not limited to PD patients but also occur in normal individuals. When administered to patients with preexisting bipolar or schizophrenic illnesses, dopaminergic agents regularly precipitate or worsen the underlying psychiatric disorder.

There is considerable pharmacological heterogeneity among dopaminergic agents. They all exert D2 agonist effects, but pergolide also has potent D1 agonist properties, lisuride is a serotonin agonist, and bromocriptine has noradrenergic agonist effects (Karobath, 1986; Lieberman et al, 1987). The shared behavioral effects are most likely mediated by the common pharmacological property of D2 stimulation.

The emergence of neuropsychiatric complications in the course of antiparkinsonian therapy cannot be predicted in every case, but factors that increase the likelihood of such effects include older age, dementia, higher drug dosage, mixed anticholinergic–dopaminergic treatment regimens, and a history of a psychiatric illness before PD onset (Celesia and Barr, 1970; Pederzoli et al, 1983; Tanner et al, 1983).

More comprehensive study of the behavioral complications of antiparkinsonian therapy will improve the management of PD and may provide important insights into the neurochemical mediation of neuropsychiatric syndromes.

ACKNOWLEDGMENTS

This project was supported by the Department of Veterans Affairs.

REFERENCES

Aarli JA, Gilhus NE. Sinemet CR in the treatment of patients with Parkinson's disease already on long-term treatment with levodopa. *Neurology.* 1989;39(suppl 2):82–85.

American Psychiatric Association. *Diagnostic and Statistical Manual of Mental Disorders,* 3rd ed rev. Washington, DC: American Psychiatric Press; 1987.

Angrist B, Sathananthan G, Gershon S. Behavioral effects of L-dopa in schizophrenic patients. *Psychopharmacologia.* 1973;31:1–12.

Barbeau A. L-Dopa therapy in Parkinson's disease: a critical review of nine years' experience. *Can Med Assoc J.* 1969;101:791–800.

Barr GC, Barr AN. Psychosis and other psychiatric manifestations of levodopa therapy. *Arch Neurol.* 1970;23:193–200.

Beardsley JV, Puletti F. Personality (MMPI) and cognitive (WAIS) changes after levodopa treatment. *Arch Neurol.* 1971;25:145–150.

Birkmayer W. Deprenyl (selegiline) in the treatment of Parkinson's disease. *Acta Neurol Scand* 1983;(suppl 95):103–106.

Birkmayer W, Riederer P. Deprenyl prolongs the therapeutic efficacy of combined L-dopa in Parkinson's disease. In: Hassler RG, Christ JF, eds. *Advances in Neurology,* vol 40. *Parkinson-Specific Motor and Mental Disorders.* New York: Raven Press; 1984:475–481.

Birkmayer W, Riederer P. Responsibility of extrastriatal areas for the appearance of psychotic symptoms (clinical and biochemical human post-mortem findings). *J Neural Transm.* 1975;37:175–182.

Bowers MB Jr, Van Woert M, Davis L. Sexual behavior during L-dopa treatment for parkinsonism. *Am J Psychiatry.* 1971;127:1691–1693.

Brook NM, Cookson IB. Bromocriptine-induced mania? *Br Med J.* 1978;1:790 (letter).

Burton K, Larsen A, Robinson RG, et al. Parkinson's disease: a comparison of mesulergine and bromocriptine. *Neurology.* 1985;35:1205–1208.

Bush DF, Liss CL, Morton A. Sinemet CR multicenter study group. An open multicenter long-term treatment evaluation of Sinemet CR. *Neurology.* 1989;39(suppl 2):101–104.

Celesia GG, Barr AN. Psychosis and other psychiatric manifestations of levodopa therapy. *Arch Neurol.* 1970;23:193–200.

Cherington M. Parkinsonism, L-dopa and mental depression. *J Am Geriatr Soc.* 1970;43:513–516.

Clark WG. Some aspects of the pharmacology of the psychic and behavioral effects of L-3-4-dihydoxyphenylalanine (L-dopa). In: Barbeau A, McDowell FA, eds. *L-Dopa and Parkinsonism.* Philadelphia: F. A. Davis; 1970:349–359.

Critchley P, Perez FG, Quinn N, et al. Psychosis and the lisuride pump. *Lancet* 1986;2:239 (letter).

Crow TJ, Johnstone EC, McClelland HA. The coincidence of schizophrenia and parkinsonism: some neurochemical implications. *Psychol Med.* 1976;6:227–233.

Damasio AR, Lobo-Antunes J, Macedo C. Psychiatric aspects in parkinsonism treated with L-dopa. *J Neurol Neurosurg Psychiatry.* 1971;34:502–507.

Emser W, Brenner M, Stober T, Schimrigk K. Changes in nocturnal sleep in Huntington's and Parkinson's disease. *J Neurol.* 1988;235:177–179.

Fischer P, Danielczyk W, Simanyi M, Streifler MB. Dopaminergic psychosis in advanced Parkinson's disease. In: Streifler MB, Korczyn AD, Melamed E, Youdin MBH, eds. *Advances in Neurology,* vol 53. *Parkinson's Disease: Anatomy, Pathology, and Therapy.* New York: Raven Press; 1990:391–397.

Frankel JP, Lees AJ, Kempster PA, Stern GM. Subcutaneous apomorphine in the treatment of Parkinson's disease. *J Neurol Neurosurg Psychiatry.* 1990;53:96–101.

Friedman JH, Lannon MC. Clozapine in the treatment of psychosis in Parkinson's disease. *Neurology.* 1989;39:1219–1221.

Glantz RH, Bieliauskuas L, Paleologos N. Behavioral indicators of hallucinosis in levodopa-treated Parkinson's disease. In: Yahr MD, Bergmann KJ, eds. *Advances in Neurology,* vol 45. *Parkinson's Disease.* New York: Raven Press; 1986:417–420.

Goetz CG, Tanner CM, Glantz RH, Klawans HL. Chronic agonist therapy for Parkinson's disease: a 5-year study of bromocriptine and pergolide. *Neurology.* 1985;35:749–751.

Goetz CG, Tanner CM, Klawans HL. Bupropion in Parkinson's disease. *Neurology.* 1984;34:1092–1094.

Goetz CG, Tanner CM, Klawans HL. Pharmacology of hallucinations induced by long-term drug therapy. *Am J Psychiatry.* 1982;139:494–497.

Goodwin FK. Psychiatric side effects of levodopa in man. *JAMA.* 1971;218:1915–1920.

Gopinathan G, Calne DB. Actions of ergot derivatives in parkinsonism. In: Rose FC, Capilideo R, eds. *Research Progress in Parkinson's Disease.* Turnbridge Wells, Kent: Pitman Medical; 1981:324–332.

Hale MS, Bellizzi J. Low-dose perphenazine and levodopa/carbidopa therapy in a patient with parkinsonism and a psychotic illness. *J Nerv Ment Dis.* 1980;168:312–314.

Hardie RJ, Lees AJ, Stern GM. On-off fluctuations in Parkinson's disease. *Brain.* 1984;107:487–506.

Harvey NS. Serial cognitive profiles in levodopa-induced hypersexuality. *Br J Psychiatry.* 1988;153:833–836.

Huber SJ, Paulson GW, Shuttleworth EC. Depression in Parkinson's disease. *Neuropsychiatry Neuropsychol Behav Neurol.* 1988;1:47–51.

Hurwitz TA, Calne DB, Waterman K. Treatment of dopaminomimetic psychosis in Parkinson's disease with electroconvulsive therapy. *Can J Neurol Sci.* 1988;15:32–34.

Jankovic J, Orman J, Jansson B. Placebo-controlled study of mesulergine in Parkinson's disease. *Neurology.* 1985;35:161–165.

Jenkins RB, Groh RH. Mental symptoms in parkinsonian patients treated with L-dopa. *Lancet.* 1970;2:177–180.

Jouvent R, Abensour P, Bonnet AM, et al. Antiparkinsonian and antidepressant effects of high doses of bromocriptine. *Biol Psychiatry.* 1983;5:141–145.

Karobath M. Dopamine agonists: new vistas. In: Fahn S, Marsden CD, Jenner P, Teychenne P, eds. *Recent Developments in Parkinson's Disease.* New York: Raven Press; 1986:175–182.

Keshavan MS, David AS, Narayanen HS, Satish P. "On-off" phenomena and manic-depressive mood shifts: case report. *J Clin Psychiatry.* 1986;47:93–94.

Klawans HL. Levodopa-induced psychosis. *Psychiatr Annu.* 1978;8:447–451.

Ko GN, Leckman JF, Heninger GR. Induction of rapid mood cycling during L-dopa treatment in a bipolar patient. *Am J Psychiatry.* 1981;138:1624–1625.

Kurlan R, Miller C, Levy R, et al. Long-term experience with pergolide therapy of advanced parkinsonism. *Neurology.* 1985;35:738–742.

Lang AE, Quinn N, Brincat S, et al. Pergolide in late-stage Parkinson disease. *Ann Neurol.* 1982;12:243–247.

Lesser RP, Fahn S, Snider SR, et al. Analysis of the clinical problems in parkinsonism and the complications of long-term levodopa therapy. *Neurology.* 1979;29:1253–1260.

LeWitt PA, Gopinathan G, Ward CD, et al. Lisuride versus bromocriptine treatment in Parkinson's disease: a double-blind study. *Neurology.* 1982;32:69–72.

Lieberman AN, Goldstein M, Gopinathan G, Neophytides A. D-1 and D-1 agonists in Parkinson's disease. *Can J Neurol Sci.* 1987;14:466–473.

Lieberman AN, Goldstein M, Gopinathan G, et al. Further studies with pergolide in Parkinson disease. *Neurology.* 1982;32:1181–1184.

Lieberman A, Goldstein M, Neophytides A, et al. Lisuride in Parkinson disease: efficacy of lisuride compared to levodopa. *Neurology.* 1981a;31:961–965.

Lieberman AN, Goldstein M, Leibowitz M, et al. Lisuride combined with levodopa in advanced Parkinson disease. *Neurology.* 1981b;31:1466–1469.

Lipper S. Psychosis in patients on bromocriptine and levodopa with carbidopa. *Lancet.* 1976;2:571–572.

Markham CH, Diamond SG. Pergolide: a double-blind trial as adjunct therapy in Parkinson's disease. In: Fahn S, Marsden CD, Jenner P, Teychenne P, eds. *Recent Developments in Parkinson's Disease.* New York: Raven Press; 1986:331–337.

Maskin MB, Riklan M, Chabot D. Emotional function in short-term vs long-term L-dopa therapy in parkinsonism. *J Clin Psychol.* 1973;29:493–495.

Mawdsley C. Treatment of parkinsonism with levo-dopa. *Br Med J.* 1970;1:331–337.

Miller BL, Cummings JL, McIntyre H, et al. Hypersexuality or altered sexual preference following brain injury. *J Neurol Neurosurg Psychiatry.* 1986;49:867–873.

Miller EM, Nieburg HA. L-Tryptophan in the treatment of levodopa-induced psychiatric disorders. *Dis Nerv Syst.* 1974;35:20–23.

Mindham RHS, Marsden CD, Parkes JD. Psychiatric symptoms during L-dopa therapy for Parkinson's disease and their relationship to physical disability. *Psychol Med.* 1976;6:23–33.

Moses H III, Uhl G, Preziosi T, et al. Mesulergine (CU 32-085) in idiopathic parkinsonism. In: Fahn S, Marsden CD, Jenner P, Teychenne P, eds. *Recent Developments in Parkinson's Disease.* New York: Raven Press; 1986:363–368.

Moskovitz C, Moses H III, Klawans HL. Levodopa-induced psychosis: a kindling phenomenon. *Am J Psychiatry.* 1978;135:669–675.

Murphy DL, Brodie HKH, Goodwin FK, Bunney WE Jr. Regular induction of hypomania by L-dopa in "bipolar" manic-depressive patients. *Nature.* 1971;229:135–136.

Nausieda PA. Sinemet "abusers." *Clin Neuropharmacol.* 1985;8:318–327.

Nausieda PA, Weiner WJ, Kaplan LR, et al. Sleep disruption in the course of chronic levodopa therapy: an early feature of the levodopa psychosis. *Clin Neuropharmacol.* 1982;5:183–194.

Nissenbaum H, Quinn NP, Brown RG, et al. Mood swings associated with the "on-off" phenomenon in Parkinson's disease. *Psychol Med.* 1987;17:899–904.

O'Brien CP, DiGiacomo JN, Fahn S, Schwarz GA. Mental effects of high-dosage levodopa. *Arch Gen Psychiatry.* 1971;24:61–64.

Obeso JA, Liquin MR, Martinez-Lage JM. Lisuride infusions pump: a device for the treatment of motor fluctuations in Parkinson's disease. *Lancet.* 1986;1:467–470.

Olanow CW, Alberts MJ. Double-blind controlled study of pergolide mesylate as an adjunct to sinemet in the treatment of Parkinson's disease. In: Yahr MD, Bergmann KJ, eds. *Advances in Neurology,* vol 45. *Parkinson's disease.* New York: Raven Press; 1986a:555–560.

Olanow CW, Alberts MJ. Double-blind controlled study of pergolide mesylate in the treatment of Parkinson's disease. In: Fahn S, Marsden CD, Jenner P, Teychenne P, eds. *Recent Developments in Parkinson's Disease.* New York: Raven Press; 1986b:315–321.

Parkes JD. Adverse effects of antiparkinsonian drugs. *Drugs.* 1981;21:341–353.

Parkes JD, Tarsy D, Marsden CD, et al. Amphetamines in the treatment of Parkinson's disease. *J Neurol Neurosurg Psychiatry.* 1975;38:232–237.

Pederzoli M, Girotti F, Scigliano G, et al. L-Dopa long-term treatment in Parkinson's disease: age-related side effects. *Neurology.* 1983;33:1518–1522.

Pfeiffer RF, Kang J, Granber B, et al. Clozapine for psychosis in Parkinson's disease. *Movement Disord.* 1990;5:239–242.

Pfeiffer RF, Wilken KE, Glaeske CS. Mesulergine: 18 months experience. In: Fahn S, Marsden CD, Jenner P, Teychenne P, eds. *Recent Developments in Parkinson's Disease.* New York: Raven Press; 1986:355–361.

Porteous HB, Ross DN. Mental symptoms in parkinsonism following benzhexol hydrochloride therapy. *Br Med J.* 1956;2:138–140.

Postma JU, Van Tilburg W. Visual hallucinations and delirium during treatment with amantadine (symmetrel). *J Am Geriatr Soc.* 1975;23:212–215.

Presthus J. Psychiatric side effects occurring in parkinsonism during long-term treatment with levodopa alone and in combination with other drugs. In: Rinne UK, Klinger M, Stamm G, eds. Parkinson's Disease—Current Progress, Problems, and Management. New York: Elsevier/North-Holland Biomedical Press; 1980:255–270.

Quinn NP, Lang AE, Thompson C, et al. Pergolide in the treatment of Parkinson's disease. In: Hassler RG, Christ JF, eds. *Advances in Neurology,* vol 40. *Parkinson-Specific Motor and Mental Disorders.* New York: Raven Press; 1984:509–513.

Quinn NP, Toone B, Lang AE, et al. Dopa dose-dependent sexual deviation. *Br J Psychiatry.* 1983;142:296–298.

Raft D, Spencer R. Suicide on L-dopa. *South Med J.* 1972;65:312–313.

Rinne UK. Combined bromocriptine-levodopa therapy early in Parkinson's disease. *Neurology.* 1985;35:1196–1198.

Rinne UK. Deprenyl (selegiline) in the treatment of Parkinson's disease. *Acta Neurol Scand.* 1983;(suppl 95):107–111.

Roberts HE, Dean RC, Stoudemire A. Clozapine treatment of psychosis in Parkinson's disease. *J Neuropsychiatry Clin Neurosci.* 1989;1:190–192.

Rondot P, de Recondo J, Coignet A, Ziegler M. Mental disorders in Parkinson's disease after treatment with L-dopa. In: Hassler RG, Christ JF, eds. *Advances in Neurology,* vol 40. *Parkinson-Specific Motor and Mental Disorders.* New York: Raven Press; 1984:259–269.

Ryback RS, Schwab RS. Manic response to levodopa therapy. Report of a case. *N Engl J Med.* 1971;285:788–789.

Sacks O, Kohl MS, Messeloff CR, Schwartz WF. Effects of levodopa in parkinsonian patients with dementia. *Neurology.* 1972;22:516–519.

Schiffer RB, Kurlan R, Rubin A, Boer S. Evidence for atypical depression in Parkinson's disease. *Am J Psychiatry.* 1988;145:1020–1022.

Serby M, Angrist B, Lieberman A. Mental disturbances during bromociptine and lergotrile treatment of Parkinson's disease. *Am J Psychiatry.* 1978;135:1227–1229.

Shapiro SK. Hypersexual behavior complicating levodopa (L-dopa) therapy. *Minn Med.* 1973;56:58–59.

Shaw KM, Lees AJ, Stern GM. The impact of treatment with levodopa on Parkinson's disease. *Q J Med.* 1980;49:283–293.

Shukla S, Turner WJ, Newman G. Bromocriptine-related psychosis and treatment. *Biol Psychiatry.* 1985;20:326–328.

Stern Y, Mayeux R, Ilson J, et al. Pergolide therapy for Parkinson's disease: neurobehavioral changes. *Neurology.* 1984;34:201–204.

Taneli B, Ozaskinli S, Kirli G, Bora I. Bromocriptine-induced schizophrenic syndrome. *Am J Psychiatry.* 1986;143:935 (letter).

Tanner CM, Goetz CG, Glantz RH, et al. Pergolide mesylate and idiopathic Parkinson disease. *Neurology.* 1982;32:1175–1179.

Tanner CM, Goetz CG, Glantz RH, Klawans HL. Pergolide mesylate: four years experience in Parkinson's disease. In: Yahr MD, Bergmann KJ, eds. *Advances in Neurology,* vol 45. *Parkinson's Disease.* New York: Raven Press; 1986:547–549.

Tanner CM, Vogel C, Goetz CG, Klawans HL. Hallucinations in Parkinson's disease: a population study. *Ann Neurol.* 1983;14:136 (abstract).

Teychenne PF, Bergsrud D, Racy A. Subcategories of Parkinson patients treated with bromocriptine. In: Fahn S, Marsden CD, Jenner P, Teychenne P, eds. *Recent Developments in Parkinson's Disease.* New York: Raven Press; 1986:303–313.

Van Woert MH, Ambani LM, Weintraub MI. Manic behavior and levodopa. *N Engl J Med.* 1971;285:1326 (letter).

Vlissides DN, Gill D, Castelow J. Bromocriptine-induced mania? *Br Med J.* 1978;1:510 (letter).

Vogel HP, Schifter R. Hypersexuality—a complication of dopaminergic therapy in Parkinson's disease. *Pharmacopsychiatry.* 1983;16:107–110.

Wagshul AM, Daroff RB. Depression during L-dopa treatment. *Lancet.* 1969;2:592 (letter).

Wilson JA, Smith RG. The prevalence and aetiology of long-term L-dopa side effects in elderly parkinsonian patients. *Age Ageing.* 1989;18:11–16.

Wodak J, Gilligan BS, Veale JL, Dowty BJ. Review of 12 month's treatment with L-dopa in Parkinson's disease, with remarks on unusual side effects. *Med J Australia.* 1972;2:1277–1282.

Wolters ECh, Hurwitz TA, Mak E, et al. Clozapine in the treatment of parkinsonian patients with dopaminomimetic psychosis. *Neurology.* 1990;40:832–834.

Yahr MD, Mendoza MR, Moros D, Bergmann KJ. Treatment of Parkinson's disease in early and late phases. Use of pharmacological agents with special reference to deprenyl (selegiline). *Acta Neurol Scand.* 1983;(suppl 95):95–102.

Yaryura-Tobias JA, Diamond B, Merlis S. Psychiatric manifestations of levodopa. *Can Psychiatr Assoc J.* 1972;17(suppl):SS123–SS128.

24

Behavioral Effects of Intrastriatal Adrenal Medullary Surgery in Parkinson's Disease

GLENN T. STEBBINS AND CAROLINE M. TANNER

Since the first attempt to transplant analogous adrenal medullary cells into the striatum of patients with Parkinson's disease (PD) (Backlund et al, 1985), transient behavioral disturbances have been noted. From this initial report and subsequent replication and extension of the technique, it has been evident that these disturbances appear soon after surgery and are typically short-lived. The mechanisms responsible for the behavioral changes are not known at the present time but may include neurochemical changes after transplantation or the effects of trauma associated with the surgery. The occurrence of psychological disturbances associated with surgical interventions in PD is not new. From the first attempts to control the movement disorder with cortical ablation to the current use of thalamotomy, changes in behavior following brain surgery in PD have been noted.

This chapter reviews the history of surgical treatments of PD, then summarizes the development of recent implantation techniques. The specific behavioral syndromes accompanying adrenal medullary implantation are reviewed.

SURGICAL TREATMENT OF PARKINSONISM

In the early twentieth century, Horsley (1909) noted that removal of the precentral cortex could control abnormal movements in parkinsonism. Putman (1938) found that lesioning the pyramidal tract was beneficial in unilateral parkinsonism, and Bucy (1942) and Klemme (1940) noted that disruption of the motor and premotor cortex alleviated tremor and rigidity in PD patients. These procedures led to marked changes in behavior in some patients, including hemiparesis, speech disturbances, and visuospatial impairment.

Advances in knowledge of the neuroanatomy of movement disorders enabled surgeons to select better targets for lesioning (Browder, 1948; Guiot and Pecker, 1949; Meyers, 1951). In addition, improvements in surgical techniques (Schaltenbrand and Bailey, 1959; Hassler and Riechert, 1955; Spiegel and Wycis, 1952) allowed for finer control of the site of lesion. Current surgical approaches to the treatment of movement disorders include stereotactic lesions to the ventral lateral, central median, and ventral intermedius nuclei of the thalamus and the medial globus pallidus.

The effects of subcortical surgery on abnormal movements include a major reduction in tremor and rigidity, with a concomitant mild decrease in bradykinesia. The morbidity associated with thalamotomy is high in the short term, but the procedure appears to be of lasting benefit in the treatment of PD, essential tremor, intentional tremor, dystonia, and hemiballismus (Grossman, 1988).

In a sample of patients with PD, postencephalitic parkinsonism, and multisystem degeneration, the mortality associated with stereotactic surgery was approximately 1 percent, hemorrhage at the lesion site being the most common cause of death (Markham and Rand, 1963). The morbidity associated with the procedure was divided into short-term and long-term effects in this study. The most common causes of long-term morbidity were hemiparesis (3.4 percent) (mostly after unilateral surgery) and dysarthria (2 percent) (mostly after bilateral surgery). The most frequent short-term adverse effect was the occurrence of psychological dysfunction. This was characterized by "lethargy, disturbance of recent memory, disorientation to place and time, difficulty in simple calculations, and disturbed judgment and labile emotions" (Markham and Rand, 1963, p 628). It occurred in 27.4 percent of the series. These behavioral disturbances tended to clear within a short time after surgery (1 to 2 weeks), with only 1.4 percent of patients manifesting psychological disturbances a year after the operation.

In a report of 1000 PD patients who had undergone basal ganglia surgery, Cooper (1960) also noted transient behavioral disturbances. He found that within the first week, 8 percent of the patients experienced episodes of somnolence, confusion, or changes in level of consciousness. These abnormal behaviors cleared in the short term in all but a few of the older patients. Nagaseki and colleagues (1986), however, reported no psychological disturbances in a sample of 27 PD patients and 16 patients with essential tremor who underwent stereotactic lesioning of the ventral intermedius nucleus.

The similarity between these behavioral disturbances and those seen in adrenal medullary implant surgery in PD is striking. Sleep disturbances, confusion, and emotional changes are frequently reported adverse effects in neural implant procedures in PD. In addition, other psychological disturbances, such as delusions and hallucinations, that have not been reported in thalamotomy patients, appear to be common findings in adrenal medulla implant series (Goetz et al, 1990b).

NEURAL TRANSPLANTATION IN PARKINSON'S DISEASE

With the advent of dopaminergic therapy, the use of thalamotomy for PD treatment has waned, although the procedure may still be used in patients with severe tremor (Tasker, 1987). Dopaminergic medications combat PD through replacement of dopamine lost to the striatum due to death of the dopamine-producing cells in the pars compacta of the substantia nigra (Hornykiewicz, 1966) (Fig. 24–1). This loss of nigral dopamine is offset by the use of centrally acting dopaminergic preparations, such as L-dopa, a dopamine precursor that can cross the blood–brain barrier and be converted to dopamine within the central nervous system.

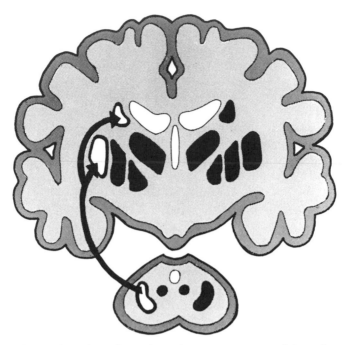

Figure 24-1. Dopaminergic pathway from the pars compacta of the substantia nigra to the striatum.

The pioneering work in neural transplantation of Olson (1970), showing that dopamine-producing adrenal medulla cells could be successfully transplanted into the anterior eye chamber of the rat, led to a renewed interest in surgical treatment for PD. The medullary cells of the adrenal gland are derived from the neural crest in embryogenesis and are known to produce many neural active substances, including catecholamines. Implantation of catecholamine-producing adrenal tissue into the striatum was postulated to be an alternative source of dopamine. Adrenal medullary cells and fetal mesocortical neuronal tissue, known to produce dopamine, have shown promise in animal preparations as potential grafting material (Bjorklund and Stenevi, 1985). Both autografted adrenal medullary cells and transplanted fetal mesocortical neuronal tissue have been used in humans with PD.

A full discussion of neural transplant surgery in PD is beyond the scope of this chapter (see the excellent reviews by Perlow, 1987; Dunnett and Richards, 1990). In 1982, implantation of adrenal medullary cells to the striatum was performed in two PD patients. One adrenal gland from the patient was removed, and the chromaffin medullary cells were dissected away from the adrenal cortical tissue. These medullary cells were then placed in a steel holder and implanted deep within the head of the right caudate via a closed stereotactic technique. Each patient showed mild improvement in functioning immediately after the grafting procedure. However, the only lasting improvement was a mild change in motor functioning in one patient (Backlund et al, 1985).

In 1985, a similar procedure, this time using the putamen as target for the grafted tissue, was performed in two patients (Lindvall et al, 1987). This change in host target was made because the putamen is more affected by the loss of substantia nigral dopamine than is the caudate (Nyberg et al, 1983). Therefore, if production of dopamine by the grafted tissue were to replace lost dopaminergic effects, the putamen would be the ideal target. These changes in procedure did not improve the outcome of the grafting, however. The two patients again showed mild short-term improvement of motor deficits but no long-lasting amelioration of parkinsonian symptoms.

Madrazo and colleagues (1987a) modified this technique by using an open craniotomy approach. In addition, instead of placing the implant deep within the nuclear structure, they placed the adrenal medulla graft on the surface of the right caudate (Fig. 24–2), exposing the graft to the CSF. After the implant procedure, PD symptoms were dramatically reduced at 3 and 10 months in the two patients with the best therapeutic response. In a later report on 10 patients, Madrazo and colleagues (1987b), continued to note dramatic improvements in almost all areas of the patients' functioning, including a decreased need for antiparkinsonian medications. The authors attributed their success to the placement of the graft on the surface of the caudate, where it was in contact with CSF, which theoretically promoted the diffusion of dopamine produced by the grafted adrenal tissue.

Stimulated by these results, movement disorder specialists began attempts to replicate Madrazo's findings. In the United States and Canada, it has been estimated that over 150 adrenal medulla implant procedures have been conducted (Goetz et al, 1990a). However, only one center in China (Jiao et al, 1989) reported a similar level of amelioration of PD symptoms as those reported by Madrazo and colleagues (Lewin, 1988). Whether the procedures closely resemble Madrazo's technique (Tulipan, 1988; Lieberman et al, 1988; Penn et al, 1988; Allen et al, 1989; Goetz et al, 1989, 1990b; Jankovic et al, 1989) or use stereotactic procedures (Hitchcock et al, 1988; Kelly et al, 1989; Lindvall et al, 1990), only moderate improvements in PD symptoms have been reported. Moreover, the mechanism underlying postsurgical improvement is uncertain. The initial concept that implanted adrenal cells would produce dopamine clearly is incorrect. The implanted tissue may supply trophic factors that stimulate sprouting of dopaminergic fibers (Gage et al, 1987; Fiandaca et al, 1988).

In addition to the mild improvements in motor functioning reported after adrenal medulla implant surgery in PD, most studies have noted the occurrence of specific behavioral disturbances. These disturbances typically include somnolence, changes in pain perception, delusions, hallucinations, and depression. In most studies, the alteration in behavior occurs in the period immediately after surgery and tends to clear quickly, although in some patients, symptoms may persist for as long as 1 year postsurgery (Goetz et al, 1990a).

BEHAVIORAL DISTURBANCES ASSOCIATED WITH IMPLANT SURGERY IN PARKINSON'S DISEASE

The literature on behavioral disturbances in neural implant surgery in PD patients presents several problems. First, not all reports contain information on the postoperative period most frequently associated with the occurrence of behavioral disturbances, or if data from this time period is presented, no discussion of behavior is included. Second, most reports do not provide definitions of the psychological distur-

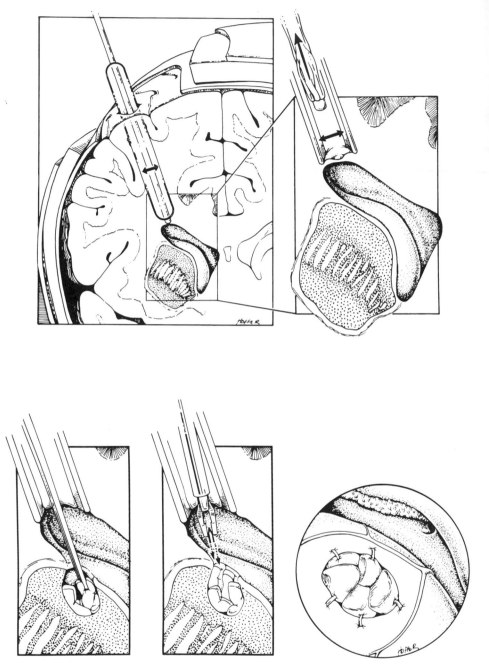

Figure 24–2. **A**. Coronal view of the catheter being expanded to a diameter of 2 cm. **B**. Deflation of the balloon, its removal, and placement of the self-retaining retractors. **C**. Small caudate nucleus biopsy and creation of a cavity for implantation and placement of the medullary tissue into the cavity. **D**. Clipping of the superficial pieces to the surface of the caudate nucleus. **E**. View through the microscope showing the small hemoclips holding the medullary tissue in the cavity. (From Penn et al., *Neurosurgery.* 1988;22:999–1004.)

bances. Some authors follow standard diagnostic schemata (Tanner et al, 1988), and others only mention the behavioral phenomena without specifying how the diagnoses were made (Ostrosky-Solis et al, 1988). Third, behavioral disturbances may occur in PD patients not undergoing surgery and must be distinguished from surgery-related changes.

We use the American Psychiatric Association (1987) definitions for behavioral disturbances, as presented in DSM IIIR. To date, only one report has used standard diagnostic criteria in detailing the behavioral changes after surgery (Tanner et al, 1988).

Most reports describing behavioral changes in implanted patients do not discuss the patients' preoperative psychiatric functioning. This information is vital because behavioral abnormalities have been associated with PD regardless of treatment status. Even before the use of dopaminergic medications, which have been associated with the development of changes in dream quality, visual hallucinations, and acute paranoid reactions (Weiner and Lang, 1989), specific behavioral changes have been noted, including sleep disturbances, confusion, agitation, and hallucinations (Ball, 1882; Schwab et al, 1950). If preoperative psychiatric functioning is not carefully assessed, preexisting behavioral changes may be considered erroneously to be the result of surgery.

Despite these limitations, some information about specific changes in patients' psychiatric state after adrenal medullary implant is available. In the first report to discuss behavioral disturbances after adrenal implantation, Backlund and colleagues (1985) found that one of the two patients developed a short period of paranoia 2 weeks after surgery. This disturbance was attributed to a synergistic effect between the dopamine produced by the graft and renewed treatment with dopamine replacement medication. In the two patients receiving putamen implantations (Lindvall et al, 1987), no psychological disturbances were reported.

Madrazo and colleagues (1987a) did not mention behavioral disturbances in their original report. However, later they reported (Ostrosky-Solis et al, 1988) a series of seven patients with dramatic decreases in pain perception after surgery despite both cranial and abdominal incisions. In addition, five of the seven patients had visual hallucinations during the first 3 days postimplant. Although the patients were not receiving dopaminergic therapy, the hallucinations were similar to those accompanying levodopa treatment, that is, visual hallucinations of people familiar to the patients, or small insects, which did not evoke anxiety in the patients. Perioperative depression, delusions, and somnolence were not mentioned (although Madrazo is cited in Penn et al, 1988, as noting increased somnolence in his patients). The visual hallucinations were attributed to dopamine released by the grafted tissue, and the increased pain threshold to release of metenkephalins.

Subsequent neural implant studies have noted similar, as well as additional, disturbances in patients (Table 24–1). Currently there are two published reports of multicenter registries for neural transplantation in PD. The first is a registry compiled by the American Association of Neurological Surgeons (Bakay et al, 1990), which discusses safety in surgical procedures in 118 patients. The second registry is compiled by the United Parkinson Foundation (Goetz et al, 1990a) and details the efficacy of the procedure in 61 patients.

Bakay and colleagues (1990) present data on 118 patients from 22 centers in the Americas and in Europe. They note that a majority of patients experienced transient

Table 24-1. Behavioral disturbances in reports of adrenal medullary implant and fetal transplant studies in PD patients

Authors	n	Procedure[a]	Tissue type	Symptoms	Character of disturbance
Backlund et al, 1985	2	S	Adrenal	+	Short-term paranoia in 1 patient
Backlund et al, 1987	2	S	Adrenal	−	No disturbances reported
Ostrosky-Solis et al, 1988	7	C	Adrenal	+	Visual hallucinations, decreased pain
Penn et al, 1988	5	C	Adrenal	+	Increased somnolence, decreased pain, delusions, depression
Madrazo et al, 1988	2	C	Fetal	−	No disturbances reported
Lieberman et al, 1988	6	C	Adrenal	+	Increased somnolence, depression
Allen et al, 1989	18	C	Adrenal	+	Disorientation, delusions, paranoia, disturbed sleep
Kelly et al, 1989	8	S	Adrenal	+	Increased somnolence, depression, confusion, hallucinations
Goetz et al, 1989	19	C	Adrenal	+	Increased somnolence, depression, hallucinations, delusions
Jankovic et al, 1989	3	C	Adrenal	+	Increased somnolence, hallucinations, delusions
Bakay et al, 1990	118	C+S	Adrenal	+	Psychoses, confusion
Freed et al, 1990	1	S	Fetal	−	No disturbances reported
Goetz et al, 1990b	7	C	Adrenal	+	Increased somnolence, depression, hallucinations, delusions
Goetz et al, 1990a	61	C+S	Adrenal	+	Sleep disburbances, hallucinations, delusions, confusion, depression
Hitchcock et al, 1990	12	S	Fetal	−	No disturbances reported
Lindvall et al, 1990	1	S	Fetal	−	No disturbances reported
Madrazo et al, 1990	7	C	Fetal	−	No disturbances reported

[a]C, craniotomy; S, stereotactic.

changes in mental status and that the occurrence of these behavioral disturbances was dependent on the age of the patients (Table 24–2), with older patients having more behavioral disturbances. No detailed description of the behavioral abnormalities is provided other than the terms "psychoses" and "confusion."

In the United Parkinson Foundation report of the efficacy of adrenal medulla/caudate implant surgery in PD, Goetz and colleagues (1990a) present results of 61 patients

Table 24-2. Frequency of transient postoperative confusion or delusions related to age as reported from all centers ($n = 88$)

Age range (years)	Number	Percent
26–30	0	0
31–35	0	0
36–40	0	0
41–45	1	8
46–50	2	12
51–55	3	33
56–60	5	28
61–65	5	29
66–70	4	57

From Bakay et al. In: Dunnett, Richards, eds. *Neural Transplantation from Molecular Basis to Clinical Applications.* Elsevier; 1990:603–610.

in 13 centers in North America. Although diagnostic criteria were not provided, the authors list numerous adverse behavioral effects, including changes in sleep/wake behavior, delusions, confusion, visual hallucinations, auditory hallucinations, depression, and attempted suicide (Fig. 24–3). Nearly 51 percent had one or more behavioral complications during the immediate postoperative period. By 3 months after surgery, behavioral disturbance was present in only 34 percent. At 1 year after surgery, 28 percent had persistent abnormal behavior, most commonly insomnia. The occurrence of adverse behavioral effects did not depend on type of neurosurgical technique (craniotomy vs stereotactic).

Altered Pain Perception

Two groups (Ostrosky-Solis et al, 1988; Tanner et al, 1988) noted decreased pain perception in patients undergoing adrenal medulla/caudate implant surgery. No data are provided in the Ostrosky-Solis report, but Tanner noted that average narcotic use in the implant patients was much lower than in a control group of patients who had received a cholecystectomy. This report compared narcotic use in PD patients with implantation, PD patients receiving cholecystectomy (involving a similar abdominal incision as in the implant surgery) but no implant, and nonparkinsonian patients receiving cholecystectomy. As Figure 24–4 shows, the PD implant patients required significantly less narcotic (defined as morphine sulfate equivalents) than either PD cholecystectomy or nonparkinsonian cholecystectomy patients.

Ostrosky-Solis and colleagues (1988) hypothesized that decreased pain perception after adrenal medulla/caudate implant was due to the release of metenkephalins by the graft tissue. In a report by Jankovic and associates (1989), an increased level of CSF beta-endorphin was found in one patient with increased pain threshold. The finding of increased pain threshold has been noted in animal models of adrenal medulla transplantation as well. Sagen and co-workers (1987) found that nociception was decreased in rats after transplantation of adrenal medullary cells to periaqueductal gray matter. Drucker-Colin and associates (1990) noted increased pain thresholds in transplanted rats after administration of dibutyryl cAMP, suggesting an interaction between the release of neuropeptides from the graft and endogenous AMP action.

% of Sample

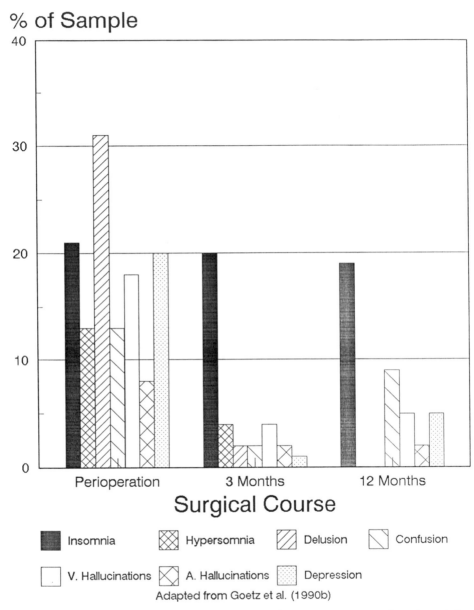

Figure 24-3. Percent of total sample from a multicenter report on adrenal medullary implant in Parkinson's disease exhibiting specific behavioral abnormalities during the perioperative period (n = 61), 3 months after surgery (n = 50), and 1 year after surgery (n = 43).

M.S.E. DOSE

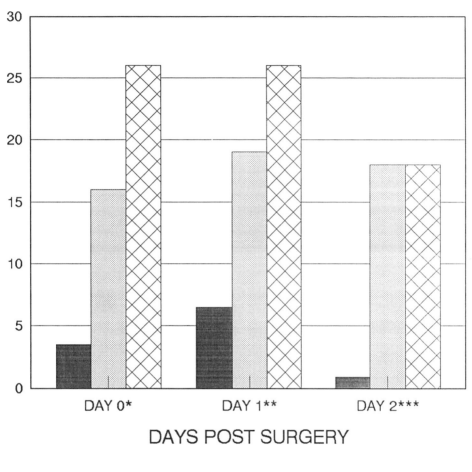

DAYS POST SURGERY

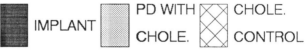

Friedman's ANOVA: *p<.001; **p<.008; ***p<.02

Figure 24–4. Use of morphine sulfate equivalents (M.S.E.) by Parkinson's disease patients receiving adrenal medullary implantation (IMPLANT), nonimplanted Parkinson's disease patients undergoing cholecystectomy (PD with CHOLE.), and nonparkinsonian patients undergoing cholecystectomy (CHOLE. CONTROL).

An alternative explanation for the increased pain threshold could be the surgical lesion itself. Kawamura and colleagues (1988) report one patient who had had a discrete lesion at the head of the left caudate and experienced denial of the resulting hemichorea. Since the implant surgery involves a small lesion of the head of the caudate, this type of denial may be present in adrenal medulla/caudate implant patients as well.

Disturbances in Sleep/Wake Cycle

Disturbances in the sleep/wake cycle after neural implant surgery have been noted by numerous authors (Penn et al, 1988; Lieberman et al, 1988; Kelly et al, 1989; Allen et al, 1989; Jankovic et al, 1989; Goetz et al, 1990a, 1990b). These changes are described either as brief periods (usually less than 7 days) of hypersomnolence or longer lasting periods of insomnia.

At Rush-Presbyterian-St. Luke's Medical Center, we specifically monitored changes in behavior in seven patients receiving adrenal implant surgery. Since most reports of behavioral changes after implant surgery do not provide detailed descriptions of the patient's condition, we supplement the review of the literature with our experiences from these seven patients.

In our sample, excessive somnolence occurred in four of the seven patients. In each case, patients could be aroused with vigorous stimulation and then would follow commands appropriately but would drift back to sleep when not stimulated. Somnolence began on the day of surgery, was most marked during the first 2 to 3 postoperative days, and abated within 7 days in every case. Neurological examination was otherwise unchanged in each case, and computer tomographic (CT) scans showed only the expected postoperative changes. In one case, treatment with intravenous naloxone and oral amphetamine was not effective in reversing somnolence. Weeks after returning to a normal level of alertness, one patient could describe in great detail events that had occurred during the somnolent state, suggesting preserved awareness. To date, no specific hypotheses as to the cause of this increased somnolence have been made, but it may be due to the release of an opiatelike substance by the graft (Penn et al, 1988; Tanner et al, 1988). In addition, disturbances in somnolence have been noted in patients receiving thalamotomy (Markham and Rand, 1963), and the currently noted changes in alertness may be related to the surgical procedure.

Patients described in the United Parkinson Foundation registry (Goetz et al, 1990a) often complained of insomnia, although the number with this problem before surgery is not known. In the perioperative period, 22 percent of the patients had insomnia, and at 3 months after implantation, 20 percent continued to have this disturbance. Insomnia persisted in 17 percent at 1 year after surgery. The mechanism of this disturbance is unknown, although disturbances in the sleep/wake cycle have been observed in thalamotomy patients. In addition, PD patients have been shown to have specific sleep disturbances, including insomnia (Nausieda et al, 1984).

Delusions and Hallucinations

Backlund and associates (1985) were the first to note delusions in PD patients after adrenal medulla implant. Since this initial report, almost all studies discussing behavioral changes in the immediate postoperative period have noted similar reactions.

In the United Parkinson Foundation registry (Goetz et al, 1990a), delusions accounted for the largest percentage of adverse behavioral changes in the immediate postoperative period. Thirty-two percent of the patients experienced delusions immediately after surgery. By 3 months after surgery, delusions fell to 1 percent of the total sample, and at 1 year, no patients were delusional.

Six of the seven patients in our series had delusions in the presence of a clear sensorium in the immediate postoperative period. The delusions began within the first few days after surgery and were absent in all cases after 8 weeks. They were typically well circumscribed and often were evident only when specifically sought. Four of the patients had paranoid delusions, such as a belief that the hospital staff was trying to harm them. One patient believed that the hospital administration was sending a salesman into patient's rooms and forcing them to buy expensive appliances. Another patient had the delusional belief that there was a farm store on the ground floor of the hospital and that he had visited this store many years ago. He also believed that his room was moved from floor to floor of the hospital every night. Other delusions included the belief that phrases overheard in conversations or read in novels had magical significance in predicting the outcome of the surgery, that the neurologist had remained at the bedside all night long, and that a patient was scheduled to give a trombone concert for the president of the medical center.

Although the report by Backlund and associates (1985) indicated that the onset of the delusion was concomitant with the administration of levodopa medications and that the paranoid reaction was due to an increase of dopaminergic effect, we and other authors have noted the occurrence of these abnormalities before the reinstitution of antiparkinsonian medications (Tanner et al, 1988; Allen et al, 1989; Goetz et al, 1990b). Delusions resembling those reported in adrenal medulla implantation have been seen in patients with right cerebral infarction (Levine and Grek, 1984; Schmidley and Messing, 1984). It is interesting to note that the damage in these patients was to the same side of the cortex as the surgical incision in the implant patients. However, the anatomical injuries in the stroke patients are much larger than the discrete lesions associated with the implant procedure.

Visual hallucinations also are common in adrenal implant patients. Eighteen percent of the patients in the United Parkinson Foundation registry (Goetz et al, 1990a) experienced these phenomena immediately after surgery. Visual hallucinations rapidly cleared, persisting in only 4 percent of the sample at the 3 month and 1 year follow-up examinations.

Among our seven patients, two had visual hallucinations in the presence of an otherwise clear sensorium. The hallucinations were phenomenologically similar to those associated with levodopa use, representing people familiar to the patients. In both cases, the hallucinations occurred immediately after surgery, when antiparkinsonian medications had not been reintroduced. In one case, hallucinations occurred episodically for 2 weeks and then resolved. The second patient developed a psychotic depression, and the content of the visual hallucinations became progressively more threatening, coincident with this affective change. Ostrosky-Solis and colleagues (1988) reported similar hallucinations in five of seven patients.

Although these phenomena were similar to those seen in levodopa use (Weiner and Lang, 1989), in all cases the hallucinations began before the reinstitution of levodopa and gradually improved over the ensuing weeks after reintroduction of antiparkinsonian medications. Before the use of levodopa, hallucinations had been reported in PD patients (Schwab et al, 1950), so the cause of this disturbance in implant patients may be associated with the disease, independent of treatment. Hallucinations have been noted also in patients after right cerebral infarction (Levine and Finklestein, 1982), but again, these patients have large areas of damage to the cerebral cortex.

Mood Changes

Both depression (Lieberman et al, 1988; Kelly et al, 1989; Tanner et al, 1988; Goetz et al, 1989) and disinhibition (Tanner et al, 1988) may follow adrenal medulla implant surgery. The depression evolves slowly over weeks after surgery (Kelly et al, 1989; Tanner et al, 1988) and resolves in most cases without treatment. However, both Tanner and colleagues (1988) and Lieberman and associates (1988) report a small number of cases with prolonged depression requiring either antidepressant medications or ECT.

The United Parkinson Foundation registry data (Goetz et al, 1990a) support these findings for depression. Depression is present in 20 percent of the series during the perioperative period but decreases to 10 percent by 3 months and 4 percent by 1 year after surgery. This report does not mention the occurrence of disinhibition or hypomanic behaviors.

In the sample of implant patients at our center, five patients experienced short-lived personality changes of a disinhibited or hypomanic nature. These inappropriate behaviors were maximal in the second through fourth weeks after surgery and resolved by the sixth month. These behaviors were distinct aberrations from the premorbid personalities of the patients. One patient, a conservative former literature professor awakened an aunt at 3 AM, demanding her credit card number so that he could purchase an item seen on a television sales show. Another patient stood in the public hallway outside the neurology office, introducing herself and shaking hands with anyone who passed by.

In one of the patients at our center, a severe psychotic depression with persecutory delusions and excessive religiosity gradually developed over the first 6 months after surgery. The depressive symptoms did not respond to antidepressant medication but did improve dramatically on two separate inpatient ECT treatments, only to recur within a few months. In the remaining six patients, mild depressive symptoms sufficient to cause a flattened affect and loss of interest but without interference with sleep, appetite, or self-care occurred at approximately the fourth month after surgery. These symptoms never required treatment and resolved in a few weeks in all patients.

Depression is thought to be a common behavioral occurrence in PD regardless of type of treatment (Mayeux et al, 1984). Whether the presence of depression in adrenal medulla implant PD patients is independent of the surgery and associated with progression of the disease is not known. To date, no theories as to the cause of depression in patients after adrenal medulla/caudate implant surgery have been postulated and no evidence of changes in serotonergic metabolism or bioavailability have been noted (Rush Research Group and Colleagues, 1990).

PUTATIVE CAUSES FOR BEHAVIORAL DISTURBANCES IN ADRENAL MEDULLA IMPLANT SURGERY

Little is known about the relationship between the occurrence of abnormal behavior and changes in neurobiology following adrenal medullary implantation. Some authors have suggested that the graft tissue produces increased levels of central dopamine that are responsible for the confusion, hallucinations, and delusions seen after transplantation (Backlund et al, 1985; Ostrosky-Solis et al, 1988). It has been suggested that release of neuropeptides by the graft is responsible for decreased pain threshold (Drucker-Colin et al, 1990) and somnolence (Ostrosky-Solis et al, 1988). However, most autopsy studies have found few if any viable adrenal medullary cells at the site of the graft to produce such substances (Cahill and Olanow, 1990; Lieberman et al, 1990; Peterson et al, 1989). In addition, many studies have failed to show elevations in dopamine or neuropeptides in the CSF of humans receiving autografted adrenal medulla tissue (Cahill and Olanow, 1990; Rush Research Group and Colleagues, 1990) or fetal mesocortical tissue (Madrazo et al, 1990).

Rather than being specific to the adrenal implant procedure, the behavioral changes reported may have been a nonspecific response to the surgical procedure. As noted, confusional episodes after stereotactic treatment of PD were reported (Cooper, 1960; Markham and Rand, 1963). In addition, postoperative somnolence in thalamotomy has been described by many authors (Fortin, 1961; Krayenbuhl et al, 1961; Riklan et al, 1966). Damage to the right cerebral hemisphere has been reported to result in delusions resembling those noted in adrenal medulla implant PD patients (Levine and Finklestein, 1982; Levine and Grek, 1984). These presentations usually are associated with extensive injuries as opposed to the small injury produced by the surgical procedure in implantation. In addition, delusions after right cerebral infarction has been associated with preexisting cortical atrophy (Levine and Grek, 1984).

Unilateral lesions of both the frontal lobe (Mesulam, 1986) and the caudate nucleus (Mendez et al, 1989; Pardal et al, 1985; Caplan et al, 1990; Kawamura et al, 1988; Pozzilli et al, 1987) can produce behavioral changes resembling those experienced by implant patients. Mendez and colleagues (1989) categorized 12 patients with nonhemorrhagic vascular lesions of the caudate nucleus into three syndrome groups; one with apathy, reduced spontaneity and initiative, accompanying dorsolateral caudate lesions; one with disinhibition, inappropriate behavior and disorganization accompanying small ventromedial caudate lesions; and one with affective disturbances, including anxiety, depression, and bipolar illness accompanying large dorsolateral caudate lesions. Although the actual size of the caudate lesion associated with adrenal medullary implant is very small and limited to the extreme medial portion of ventral caudate in most cases, the resemblance between the behavioral abnormalities seen in implant surgery and those described by Mendez and colleagues suggests that the anatomical lesion produced by the surgery may have contributed to the behavioral changes.

Finally, many of the behavioral sequelae of adrenal medulla implantation may be nonspecific exacerbations of preexisting PD symptoms. Sleep disturbances, confusion, agitation, depression, and hallucinations have all been described in PD patients regardless of treatment status (Ball, 1882; Schwab et al, 1950), and the development of hallucinations, confusion, and paranoia with the use of levodopa medication has been well documented (Weiner and Lang, 1989).

CONCLUSION

In summary, behavioral abnormalities associated with adrenal medulla/caudate implantation are common in the perisurgical period. These behavioral changes include increased pain threshold, disruption of sleep/wake cycles, hallucinations, delusions, confusion, and mood changes. Most of these abnormalities clear within a few months after surgery, although lasting insomnia and depression have been reported.

The occurrence of abnormal behaviors does not appear to be related to neurosurgical technique (stereotactic vs open craniotomy). Conflicting information is available on the effects of the age of the patient at the time of surgery. Bakay and colleagues (1990) noted a specific increase in behavioral disturbances in older patients, whereas no significant age differences were found between patients with or without behavioral disturbances in the Goetz and colleagues report (1990a). Although published reports on fetal mesocortical implantation in humans are sparse, three reports fail to note any behavioral disturbances (Hitchcock et al, 1988; Lindvall et al, 1990; Madrazo et al, 1990).

The cause of these disturbances is not known. Both neurochemical changes and response to surgical trauma have been postulated. Evidence of neurochemical changes as mediating events is not strong at this time, but the possibility of trophic factors (Gage et al, 1987) or the recovery of striatal dopaminergic fibers (Bohn et al, 1987; Fiandaca et al, 1988) may provide information in the future.

The importance of monitoring postoperative changes in behavior is highlighted by the observations of this chapter. Since the mechanisms responsible for these changes have not been identified, it is important not only to delineate the presence of abnormal behavior but also to characterize any behavioral disturbances, both before and after surgery.

REFERENCES

Allen GS, Burns RS, Tulipan NB, Parker RA. Adrenal medullary transplantation to the caudate nucleus in Parkinson's disease initial clinical results in 18 patients. *Arch Neurol.* 1989;46:487–491.

American Psychiatric Association. *Diagnostic and Statistical Manual of Mental Disorders,* 3rd ed, rev. Washington, DC: APA; 1987.

Backlund EO, Granberg PO, Hamberger B, et al. Transplantation of adrenal medullary tissue to striatum in parkinsonism. *J Neurosurg.* 1985;62:169–173.

Backlund EO, Olson L, Sieger A, Lindvall O. Toward a transplantation therapy in Parkinson's disease. Ann NY Acad Sci 1987;495:658–673.

Bakay RAE, Allen GS, Apuzzo M, et al. Preliminary report on adrenal medullary grafting from the American Association of Neurological Surgeons graft project. In: Dunnett SB, Richards SJ, eds. *Neural Transplantation from Molecular Basis to Clinical Applications.* Amsterdam: Elsevier; 1990:603–610.

Ball B. De L'insanite dans la paralysie agitante. *Encephale.* 1882;2:22–32.

Bjorklund A, Stenevi U. Intracerebral ceural grafting: a historical perspective. In: Bjorklund A, Stenevi U, eds. *Neural Grafting in the Mammalian CNS.* Amsterdam: Elsevier; 1985:3–14.

Bohn MC, Cupit L, Marciano F, Gash DM. Adrenal medulla grafts enhance recovery of striatal dopaminergic fibers. *Science.* 1987;237:913–916.

Browder J. Section of fibers of anterior limb of internal capsule in parkinsonism. *Am J Surg.* 1948;75:264–268.

Bucy PC. Cortical extirpation in treatment of involuntary movements. *Res Publ Assoc Nerv Ment Dis.* 1942;21:551–595.

Cahill DW, Olanow CW. Autologous adrenal medulla to caudate nucleus transplantation in advanced Parkinson's disease: 18 month results. In: Dunnett SB, Richards SJ, eds. *Neural Transplantation from Molecular Basis to Clinical Applications.* Amsterdam: Elsevier; 1990:637–642.

Caplan LR, Schmahmann JD, Kase CS, et al. Caudate infarcts. *Arch Neurol.* 1990;47:133–143.

Cooper IS. Results of 1,000 consecutive basal ganglia operations for parkinsonism. *Ann Intern Med.* 1960;52:483–499.

Drucker-Colin R, Garcia-Hernandez F, Mendoza-Ramirez JL, et al. Possible mechanisms of action of adrenal transplants in Parkinson's disease. In: Dunnett SB, Richards SJ, eds. *Neural Transplantation from Molecular Basis to Clinical Applications.* Amsterdam: Elsevier; 1990:509–514.

Dunnett SB, Richards SJ. *Neural Transplantation from Molecular Basis to Clinical Applications.* Amsterdam: Elsevier; 1990.

Fiandaca MS, Kordower JH, Hansen JT, et al. Adrenal medullary autografts into the basal ganglia of cebus monkeys: injury-induced regeneration. *Exp Neurol.* 1988;102:76–91.

Fortin JM. Psychological and social aspects of parkinsonians before and after surgery. *Rev Can Biol.* 1961;20:297–304.

Freed CR, Breeze RE, Rosenberg NL, et al. Therapeutic effects of human fetal dopamine cells transplanted in a patient with Parkinson's disease. In: Dunnett SB, Richards SJ, eds. *Neural Transplantation from Molecular Basis to Clinical Applications.* Amsterdam: Elsevier; 1990:509–514.

Gage FH, Wolff JA, Rosenberg MB, et al. Grafting genetically modified cells to the brain: possibilities for the future. *Neuroscience.* 1987;23:795–807.

Goetz CG, Olanow CW, Koller WC, et al. Multicenter study of autologous adrenal medullary transplantation to the corpus striatum in patients with advanced Parkinson's disease. *N Engl J Med.* 1989;320:337–341.

Goetz CG, Stebbins GT, Klawans HL, et al. United Parkinson Foundation neurotransplantation registry: multicenter US and Canadian data base, presurgical and 12 month follow-up. In: Dunnett SB, Richards SJ, eds. *Neural Transplantation from Molecular Basis to Clinical Applications.* Amsterdam: Elsevier; 1990a:611–618.

Goetz CG, Tanner CM, Penn RD, et al. Adrenal medullary transplant to the striatum of patients with advanced Parkinson's disease: 1-year motor and psychomotor data. *Neurology.* 1990b;40:273–276.

Grossman RG. Surgery for movement disorders. In: Jankovic J, Tolosa E, eds. *Parkinson's Disease and Movement Disorders.* Baltimore: Urban & Schwarzenberg; 1988:461–470.

Guiot G, Pecker J. Tractotomie mesencephalique anterieure pour tremblement Parkinsonien. *Rev Neurol.* 1949;81:387–388.

Hassler R, Riechert T. A special method of stereotactic brain operation. *Proc R Soc Med.* 1955;48:469–470.

Hitchcock ER, Clough C, Hughes R, Kenny B. Embryos and Parkinson's disease. *Lancet.* 1988;1:1274.

Hitchcock ER, Kenny CG, Clough RC, et al. Stereotactic implantation of foetal mesencephalon (STIM): the UK experience. In: Dunnett SB, Richards SJ, eds. *Neural Transplantation from Molecular Basis to Clinical Applications.* Amsterdam: Elsevier; 1990:723–728.

Hornykiewicz, O. Dopamine (3-hydroxytryptamine) and brain function. *Pharmacol Rev.* 1966;18:925–964.

Horsley V. The functions of the so-called motor area of the brain. *Br Med J.* 1909;124:5–28.

Jankovic J, Grossman R, Goodman C, et al. Clinical, biochemical and neuropathologic findings following transplantation of adrenal medulla to the caudate nucleus for treatment of Parkinson's disease. *Neurology.* 1989;39:1227–1234.

Jiao SS, Ding YJ, Zhang WC, et al. Adrenal medullary autografts in patients with Parkinson's disease. *N Engl J Med.* 1989;121:324–325.

Kawamura M, Takahashi N, Hirayama K. Hemichorea and its denial in a case of caudate infarction diagnosed by magnetic resonance imaging. *J Neurol Neurosurg Psychiatry.* 1988;51:590–591.

Kelly PJ, Ahlskog JE, vanHeerden JA, et al. Adrenal medullary autograft transplantation into the striatum of patients with Parkinson's disease. *Mayo Clin Proc.* 1989;64:282–290.

Klemme RM. Surgical treatment of dystonia, paralysis agitans, and athetosis. *Arch Neurol Psychiatry.* 1940;44:926.

Krayenbuhl H, Wyss OAM, Yasargil MG. Bilateral thalamotomy and pallidotomy as treatment for bilateral parkinsonism. *J Neurosurg.* 1961;18:429–444.

Levine DN, Finklestein S. Delayed psychosis after right temporoparietal stroke or trauma: relationship to epilepsy. *Neurology.* 1982;32:267–273.

Levine DN, Grek A. The anatomic basis of delusions after right cerebral infarction. *Neurology.* 1984;34:577–582.

Lewin R. Cloud over parkinson's therapy. *Science.* 1988;240:390–392.

Lieberman A, Ransohoff J, Berczeller P, et al. Neural and adrenal medullary transplants as a treatment for Parkinson's disease and other neurodegenerative disorders. *NeuroView.* 1988;4:1–15.

Lieberman A, Ransohoff J, Berczeller P, Goldstein M. Adrenal medullary transplants as a treatment for advanced Parkinson's disease. In: Dunnett SB, Richards SJ, eds. *Neural Transplantation from Molecular Basis to Clinical Applications.* Amsterdam: Elsevier; 1990:665–670.

Lindvall O, Backlund EO, Farde L, et al. Transplantation in Parkinson's disease: two cases of adrenal medullary grafts to the putamen. *Ann Neurol.* 1987;22:457–468.

Lindvall O, Brundin P, Widner H, et al. Grafts of fetal dopamine neurons survive and improve motor function in Parkinson's disease. *Science.* 1990;247:574–577.

Madrazo I, Drucker-Colin R, Diaz V, et al. Open microsurgical autograft of adrenal medulla to the right caudate in Parkinson's disease: a report of two cases. *N Engl J Med.* 1987a;316:831–834.

Madrazo I, Drucker-Colin R, Leon V, Torres C. Adrenal medulla transplanted to caudate nucleus for treatment of Parkinson's disease: report of 10 cases. *Surg Forum.* 1987b;38:510–511.

Madrazo I, Franco-Bourland R, Ostrosky-Solis F, et al. Neural transplantation (auto-adrenal, fetal nigral and fetal adrenal) in Parkinson's disease: the Mexican experience. In: Dunnett SB, Richards SJ, eds. *Neural Transplantation from Molecular Basis to Clinical Applications.* Amsterdam: Elsevier; 1990:593–602.

Madrazo, I, Leon, V, Torres, C, et al. Transplantation of fetal substantia nigra and adrenal medulla to the caudate nucleus in two patients with Parkinson's disease. *N Engl J Med.* 1988;318:51.

Markham CH, Rand RW. Stereotactic surgery in Parkinson's disease. *Arch Neurol.* 1963;8:621–631.

Mayeux R, Stern Y, Cote L, Williams J. Altered serotonin metabolism in depressed patients with Parkinson's disease. *Neurology.* 1984;31:645–650.

Mendez MF, Adams NL, Lewandowski KS. Neurobehavioral changes associated with caudate lesions. *Neurology.* 1989;39:349–354.

Mesulam MM. Frontal cortex and behavior. *Ann Neurol.* 1986;19:320–343.

Meyers R. Surgical experiments in the therapy of certain "extrapyramidal diseases": a current evaluation. *Acta Psychiat Neurol.* 67(suppl) 1951;1–42.

Nagaseki Y, Shibazake T, Hiral T, et al. Long-term follow-up results of selective VIM-thalamotomy. *J Neurosurg.* 1986;65:296–302.

Nausieda PA, Glantz R, Weber S, et al. Psychiatric complications of levodopa therapy in Parkinson's disease. *Adv Neurol.* 1984;40:271–277.

Nyberg P, Nordberg A, Wester P, Winbald B. Dopaminergic deficiency is more pronounced in putamen than in nucleus caudatus in Parkinson's disease. *Neurochem Pathol.* 1983;1:193–202.

Olson L. Fluorescence histochemical evidence for axonal growth and secretion from transplanted adrenal medullary tissue. *Histochemie.* 1970;22:1–7.

Ostrosky-Solis F, Quintanar L, Madrazo I, et al. Neuropsychological effects of brain autograft of adrenal medullary tissue for the treatment of Parkinson's disease. *Neurology.* 1988;38:1442–1450.

Pardal MM, Micheli F, Asconape J, Paradiso G. Neurobehavioral symptoms in caudate hemorrhage: two cases. *Neurology.* 1985;35:1806–1807.

Penn RD, Goetz CG, Tanner CM, et al. The adrenal medullary transplant operation for Parkinson's disease: clinical observations in five patients. *Neurosurgery.* 1988;22:999–1004.

Perlow MJ. Brain grafting as a treatment for Parkinson's disease. *Neurosurgery.* 1987;20:335–342.

Peterson DI, Price ML, Small CS. Autopsy findings in a patient who had an adrenal-to-brain transplant for Parkinson's disease. *Neurology.* 1989;39:235–238.

Pozzilli C, Passafiume D, Bastianello S, et al. Remote effects of caudate hemorrhage: a clinical and functional study. *Cortex.* 1987;23:341–349.

Putman TJ. Relief from unilateral paralysis agitans by section of the pyramidal tract. *Arch Neurol Psychiatry.* 1938;40:1049–1050.

Riklan M, Levita E, Cooper I. Psychological effects of bilateral subcortical surgery for Parkinson's disease. *J Nerv Mental Dis.* 1966;141:403–409.

Rush Research Group and Colleagues. The adrenal medullary transplant operation: the Chicago experience. In: Dunnett SB, Richards SJ, eds. *Neural Transplantation from Molecular Basis to Clinical Applications.* Amsterdam: Elsevier; 1990:627–635.

Sagen J, Pappas GD, Perlow MJ. Alterations in nociception following adrenal medullary transplants in the rat periaqueductal gray. *Exp Brain Res.* 1987;67:373.

Schaltenbrand G, Bailey P. *Introduction to Stereotaxis with an Atlas of the Human Brain.* New York: Grune & Stratton; 1959.

Schmidley JW, Messing RO. Agitated confusional states in patients with right hemisphere infarctions. *Stroke.* 1984;15:883–885.

Schwab RS, Fabing HD, Prichard JS. Psychiatric symptoms and syndromes in Parkinson's disease. *Am J Psychiatry.* 1950;107:901–907.

Spiegel EA, Wycis HT. *Stereoencephalotomy: Part I. Methods and Stereotaxic Atlas of Human Brain.* New York: Grune & Stratton; 1952.

Tanner CM, Goetz CG, Gilley DW, et al. Behavioral aspects of intrastriatal adrenal medulla transplant surgery in Parkinson's disease. *Neurology.* 1988;39(suppl):143.

Tasker RR. Tremor of parkinsonism and stereotactic thalamotomy. *Mayo Clin Proc.* 1987;62:736–739.

Tulipan N. Brain transplants. A new approach to the therapy of neurodegenerative disease. *Neurol Clin* 1988;6:405–420.

Weiner WJ, Lang AE. *Movement Disorders: A Comprehensive Survey.* New York: Futura; 1989.

VI
SUMMARY

25

Conclusions and Future Directions

STEVEN J. HUBER AND JEFFREY L. CUMMINGS

It is an axiomatic belief in a scientifically oriented society that human problems will eventually yield to the efforts of science. The purposes of scientific investigation in neurology are to improve the care provided to patients, to understand the cause of brain disease, to find a cure for these diseases, and to discover principles applicable to understanding and improving the human condition. Behavioral research seeks to reveal the mechanisms of intellectual impairment in neurological disorders, to alleviate cognitive dysfunction in disease states, and to understand and optimize cognition in nondiseased individuals. Neurobehavioral research in Parkinson's disease (PD) follows in this tradition and lends itself to studying dementia and depression, the two main neuropsychological manifestations of the disease. Lessons derived from these investigations may aid in treating these conditions in PD and may be applicable to understanding and managing other diseases.

The behavioral dimension of PD has had a long history, with a relatively short period of experimental investigation. In 1817, when James Parkinson first described this disease, he thought that intellectual and personality disturbances were not a part of the disorder (Chapter 1). Behavioral abnormalities were soon recognized to be common in PD, but research related to the behavioral changes did not receive serious and consistent research attention until approximately 20 years ago. Initiation of this research was coincident with an emerging interest in the physiological basis of mental activity and the development of objective neuropsychological procedures that allowed researchers to examine behavioral symptoms in a quantifiable manner.

Although progress in understanding of the neurobehavioral symptoms associated with PD during the past 20 years is undeniable, continued research advancements require systematic refinement of experimental methods and conceptual frameworks. This chapter summarizes some important research issues discussed in the preceding chapters, as well as important areas for future research. In the final section, we attempt to integrate current neurobiological information with data derived from behavioral investigations to provide insight into the mechanisms of dementia and depression in PD.

RESEARCH APPROACHES

Several areas of cognitive function commonly are impaired in patients with PD (Chapters 4–7). Much of the existing research has identified the presence and severity of particular cognitive disturbances. Recently, however, neuropsychological procedures have been designed not only to examine the presence of an impairment in a quantitative manner but also to provide information regarding the nature of the underlying cognitive processes responsible for the observed deficit. The use of such interrogative procedures is essential to advance our theoretical understanding of neurobehavioral symptoms in PD.

As discussed in Chapter 11, PD serves as an important model of subcortical dementia. This syndrome is characterized by a pattern of cognitive impairments that differ from those observed in patients with disorders involving predominantly cortical degeneration, such as Alzheimer's disease. In order to further our understanding of this distinction, it is important to examine both the pattern of behavioral differences and the nature of the underlying cognitive processes responsible for the observed behavioral changes. For example, the nature of the deficits in subcortical dementia suggests that a common disruption of a frontal–subcortical axis may underlie the abnormalities on a variety of neuropsychological tests. Specification of the nature of the observed deficits in PD may provide further insight into the role of subcortical structures in human cognition. A model of the possible subcortical mechanisms associated with cognitive impairments in PD is elaborated later in this chapter.

Another important issue concerns standardization of methodology. In certain areas of investigation, such as dementia (Part III), this is essential for research advances. Research examining the pathological, radiological, biochemical, and electrophysiological correlates of PD dementia often has lacked standardized diagnostic criteria for dementia. Research findings in these areas often are inconsistent, and this variability can be traced at least partially to the lack of standardized methodology and differing definitions of dementia. One set of objective methods to define dementia is outlined in Chapter 3. The Cummings and Benson (1983) dementia criteria are most suitable for use in PD because they can be applied in a purely objective manner and avoid subjective judgments related to occupational and social functions as required in the criteria of the *Diagnostic and Statistical Manual of Mental Disorders,* 3rd ed, Revised (DSM IIIR) (1987). Procedures to use these criteria, as well as a method to stage objectively the severity of dementia in PD, are discussed in Chapter 3. Consistent application of these or similar criteria will facilitate research into the behavioral and cognitive alterations of PD.

FUTURE DIRECTIONS

This section outlines some important areas for future research examining the neurobehavioral aspects of PD. These areas include examination of the natural history of cognitive decline, the impact of neurobehavioral symptoms on daily life, and neuropsychological and neuropsychiatric ramifications of drug therapies.

Longitudinal Studies

Although the occurrence of cognitive deficits in PD is well established, there is little known about the prevalence, range of severity, and natural history of these deficits.

Comparison of existing studies is difficult, since different methods of assessment are the rule. The use of widely different neuropsychological procedures has limited attempts to characterize the range and severity of such impairments. In addition, the vast majority of individual studies in PD are based on relatively small samples of patients that can vary in terms of several potentially important clinical variables. As discussed in Chapter 8, neuropsychological symptoms in PD may vary as a function of disease severity, age of onset, duration of disease, or type of motor symptoms. Thus, differences among patient samples also contribute to the difficulty in comparing current studies of PD.

In order to systematically evaluate these issues, serial evaluations of patients starting in the initial stage of disease are required. This will not only provide the natural history of cognitive decline in PD but also will allow an examination of the relationship between the rate of cognitive decline and clinical factors. These observations would lead to the development of useful prognostic indicators in the early stages of PD.

Longitudinal studies assessing prevalence require careful selection of the patient sample to be studied. Most studies examine patients from university settings, and such selection bias will yield prevalence estimates that may not be applicable to the general population.

Systematic evaluation of the natural history of cognitive decline in PD also requires adoption of a standard core battery of neuropsychological procedures that would facilitate large-scale multicenter studies. Suggestions for such a core battery were outlined in Chapter 3. These procedures were chosen to provide an assessment of the range and severity of impairments (e.g., memory) and to elucidate the nature of the underlying cognitive processing deficits responsible for the observed decline.

The natural history of depression in PD is essentially unknown. One study described in Chapter 3 examined whether specific features of depression change as a function of disease progression, but this study used a cross-sectional design. A longitudinal study would provide a systematic means to examine many issues related to depression. These include determining the possible existence of subgroups of patients with recurrent or ongoing depression and more systematic exploration of the neuropathological changes that distinguish depressed from nondepressed PD patients when they come to autopsy.

Ecological Validity and Impact on Daily Life

Although some degree of cognitive dysfunction occurs in the majority of PD patients, the practical significance of these changes is not well understood. There is no study that has examined systematically the impact of cognitive dysfunction on daily activities, social function, or employment.

In designing such a study, it is critical to control for the confounding effects of physical disability. This is especially important in PD since there is a trend for cognitive impairment and disease severity to progress in a generally parallel fashion. This potential confounding effect can be controlled by matching patients with and without cognitive impairment using established scales of disease severity. The common occurrence of depression in PD may represent an additional confounding variable. Changes, such as social withdrawal, decreased interest in previous activities, or inability to perform routine tasks requiring attention such as balancing a checkbook, may be influenced by mood changes. These potentially problematic issues can be controlled partially statistically using covariance procedures.

A better understanding of the relationship between cognitive and functional impairments may improve the clinical management of PD patients. There are at least four issues of interest. First, neuropsychological status could be assessed in a systematic fashion regarding work-related disability status. This may be particularly important for younger patients with PD. Second, the association of cognitive and functional disabilities may determine the value of formalized cognitive rehabilitation programs (Ben-Yishay and Diller, 1983), which have not yet been systematically explored in PD. Third, it has been demonstrated that with increasing disability, PD patients drive fewer miles but have proportionately more accidents (Dubinsky et al, 1991). The role of cognitive factors, including attention, vigilance, visuospatial disturbances, and reaction time, has yet to be examined in this context. Finally, a better understanding of the relationship between cognitive changes and daily function may help to better educate the patient and family members. As pointed out by Rao and colleagues (1991) regarding multiple sclerosis, family members tend to attribute cognitive as well as social changes to personality factors, such as obstinacy, depression, or other characteristics. This may create unnecessary stress and underscores the need to educate both the patient and the family members that cognitive impairments can be important symptoms of the disease.

Neuropsychopharmacology

Drugs used in PD have marked neuropsychological and neuropsychiatric ramifications (Chapters 21–23), and these have been underaddressed in most studies. Treatment of PD can produce adverse side effects, including visual hallucinations, delusions, and mania. Psychiatric side effects are common, occurring in 10 percent to 25 percent of PD patients. Systematic examination of these behavioral alterations may provide further insight into the neurochemical basis of neuropsychiatric symptoms.

Another side effect of PD treatment, on/off fluctuations, provides an opportunity to examine the relationship between dopamine level and behavioral alterations in the same patient. Most research related to this phenomenon has concentrated on the motoric rather than the behavioral aspects.

A recent development in the treatment of PD also deserves attention from a behavioral perspective. Levodopa is the most potent and common treatment for PD (Chapter 20). Although levodopa provides effective symptomatic treatment, it does not alter the underlying pathological process. Recent research examined a compound thought to slow the underlying pathology of PD. A multicenter study of 800 PD patients found that deprenyl slows the progression of PD in the early stages (Parkinson Study Group, 1989). This study indicated that patients receiving deprenyl had significantly slower progression of disease, defined by the need to start levodopa therapy, compared with patients receiving placebo.

Since it is well established that cognitive impairments tend to progress with advancing PD, it may be the case that deprenyl has a similar effect on cognitive symptoms. A preliminary report comparing baseline neuropsychological evaluations with a 12-month follow-up between early-stage PD patients randomized to either deprenyl or placebo has been provided by Como and associates (1990). The two groups from the study were not different on any of the neuropsychological measures at baseline. In contrast, at follow-up, the placebo group was significantly more impaired than the deprenyl group on several tests of verbal and nonverbal memory and on a test of psychomotor speed. These preliminary results suggest that deprenyl may delay cognitive decline in early-stage patients, but more research is necessary to verify these preliminary findings.

NEUROBIOLOGICAL MECHANISMS OF DEMENTIA IN PARKINSON'S DISEASE

Neuropsychological and neuropathological studies support the concept of multiple types of dementia in PD (Chapter 11) (Cummings, 1988). Mild intellectual deficits are demonstrable in a majority of patients when sought with sensitive techniques, whereas more severe cognitive alterations are evident in a minority of patients. The characteristics of the more mild and ubiquitous changes are qualitatively distinct from the Alzheimer's disease-like dementia observed in a subgroup of PD patients. At autopsy, PD patients with dementia may have neuropathological alterations limited to the classic catecholaminergic nuclei of the brainstem (substantia nigra, ventral tegmental area, locus ceruleus), combinations of changes in catecholaminergic and cholinergic nuclei (nucleus basalis), or combined PD and Alzheimer's disease-type pathology (Chapter 13).

The mental status changes evident in many PD patients are consistent with the syndrome of subcortical dementia and comprise slowing of cognitive processing, altered memory, impaired executive function, and prominent mood changes (Chapters 4, 6, 7, 11) (Cummings, 1986; Huber et al, 1989). Similar behavioral alterations occur in patients with frontal lobe dysfunction, and biochemical changes are present in both frontal and subcortical structures in PD. Thus, it may be appropriate to consider the non-Alzheimer's disease dementia of PD a frontal–subcortical systems disorder. This conceptualization is supported by recent advances in understanding the circuitry of frontal–subcortical connections (Alexander and Crutcher, 1990; Alexander et al, 1986). The dorsolateral prefrontal cortex projects to the dorsolateral region of the caudate nucleus. The caudate projects to the lateral and dorsomedial areas of the internal globus pallidus and the rostromedial substantia nigra pars reticulata. An alternate pathway projects from the caudate to the external globus pallidus, and on to the internal globus pallidus and substantia nigra reticulata. These structures in turn project to the parvicellular regions of the ventral anterior and dorsomedial nuclei of the thalamus. In the final link of the circuit, the thalamic nuclei project back onto the prefrontal cortex. Lesions in the prefrontal cortex, caudate nuclei, or medial thalamic nuclei all result in similar behavioral deficits. In PD, changes in both the caudate and the prefrontal regions may contribute to the subcortical type dementia.

Language alterations, prominent contructional abnormalities, apraxia, or agnosia is indicative of a cortical dementia and suggests the existence of superimposed Alzheimer's disease in conjunction with PD (Gaspar and Gray, 1984). Careful investigation of these cortically mediated functions may provide a premortem means of determining which PD patients also have Alzheimer's disease-type changes.

Current studies of frontal–subcortical dementia in PD suggest that dopamine may play a role in cognition as well as motor function. This conclusion is supported by the following observations: the ubiquitous presence of mild neuropsychological deficits in PD, modest improvement in mental function with dopamine replacement therapy, limited fluctuations in cognition in on/off episodes, correlation of mental status changes with akinesia, and existence of similar changes in other dopamine-deficiency diseases, such as progressive supranuclear palsy and MPTP-induced parkinsonism (Cummings, 1988). The investigations suggest that dopamine-related cognitive changes are mild in degree but consistently demonstrable. If found to be true, these observations indicate that iatrogenic mental status changes may be anticipated in patients treated with dopamine-blocking neuroleptic or gastrointestinal agents. Such implications deserve further investigation.

Other transmitters also are involved in PD (Chapter 14), and further studies in this regard may lead to mixed replacement regimens more successful than dopamine monotherapy in ameliorating the mental status changes of PD.

NEUROBIOLOGICAL MECHANISMS OF DEPRESSION IN PARKINSON'S DISEASE

A major challenge in contemporary neuropsychiatry is the translation between neuroscience observations and human subjective experience. How can observations such as low CSF 5-HIAA levels in depressed patients (Chapter 17) be meaningfully related to the pain and sadness of the depressed person?

At least three neurobiological mechanisms provide a preliminary basis for crossing the gap between laboratory observation and subjective experience. First, Febiger (1984) noted that dopamine plays a crucial role in mediating reward responses, and dopamine deficiency would interfere with this process, leading to anhedonia and loss of motivation. Second, Taylor and Saint-Cyr (1990) observed that dopamine deficiency in the prefrontal cortex in PD would create an "environmental dependency" syndrome in which the PD patient lacks initiative and is dependent on environmental influences to organize behavior. Such a dependency syndrome might result in a loss of sense of self-control, poor self-esteem, and feelings of helplessness and hopelessness. Third, dopamine has a major role in mediating physiological responses to stress (Glowinski et al, 1984). Limitation of the appropriate stress-coping responses might contribute importantly to the dysphoric characteristic of depression. Thus, most elements of the depression syndrome—poor motivation, hopelessness, worthlessness, dysphoria—can be related to the established neurobiology of PD. Variations in the severity of dopamine loss in various structures and differences in the combinations of transmitter and modulator deficiencies might determine the presence and extent of depression in different PD patients. Hereditary vulnerability, coping styles, and social–environmental supports might further influence the final mood state. These observations provide a preliminary platform for further investigations of the neurobiology of depression and relating neurobiological observations to the behavioral syndrome.

CONCLUSIONS

Parkinson's disease is a complex disorder with ramifications in the motoric, neuro-psychological, and neurobehavioral domains. It can serve as an important model for the study of brain–behavior relationships. Further investigation will help reveal the role of the basal ganglia and related structures in cognition and mood.

REFERENCES

Alexander GE, Crutcher MD. Functional architecture of basal ganglia circuits: neural substrates of parallel processing. *Trends Neurosci.* 1990;13:266–271.

Alexander GE, DeLong MR, Strick PL. Parallel organization of functionally segregated circuits linking basal ganglia and cortex. *Annu Rev Neurosci.* 1986;9:357–381.

American Psychiatric Association. *Diagnostic and Statistical Manual of Mental Disorders,* 3rd ed rev. Washington, DC: American Psychiatric Association; 1987.

Ben-Yishay Y, Diller L. Cognitive rehabilitation. In: Rosenthal M, Griffith ER, Bond MR, Miller JD, eds. *Rehabilitation of the Head Injured Adult.* Philadelphia: FA Davis; 1983:367–380.

Como PG. The Parkinson Study Group. Effect of deprenyl on neuropsychological function in early Parkinson's disease. *Ann Neurol.* 1990;28:297.

Cummings JL. Intellectual impairment in Parkinson's disease: clinical, pathologic, and bio-chemical correlates. *J Geriatr Psychiatry Neurol.* 1988;1:24–36.

Cummings JL. Subcortical dementia. Neuropsychology, neuropsychiatry, and pathophysiology. *Br J Psychiatry.* 1986;149:682–697.

Cummings JL, Benson DF. *Dementia: A Clinical Approach.* Stoneham, Mass: Butterworth Publishers Inc. 1983.

Dubinsky RM, Gray C, Husted D, et al. Driving in Parkinson's disease. *Neurology.* 1991;41:517–519.

Febiger HC. The neurobiological substrates of depression in Parkinson's disease: a hypothesis. *Can J Neurol Sci.* 1984;11:105–107.

Gaspar P, Gray F. Dementia in idiopathic Parkinson's disease. *Acta Neuropathol.* 1984;64:43–52.

Glowinski J, Tassin JP, Thierry AM. The mesocortical-prefrontal dopaminergic neurons. *Trends Neurosci.* 1984;7:415–418.

Huber SJ, Shuttleworth EC, Freidenberg DL. Neuropsychological differences between the dementias of Alzheimer's and Parkinson's disease. *Arch Neurol.* 1989;46:1287–1291.

Parkinson Study Group. Effect of deprenyl on the progression of disability in early Parkinson's disease. *N Engl J Med.* 1989;321:1364–1371.

Rao SM, Leo GJ, Ellington L, et al. Cognitive dysfunction in multiple sclerosis: II. Impact on employment and social functioning. *Neurology.* 1991;41:692–696.

Taylor AE, Saint-Cyr JA. Depression in Parkinson's disease: reconciling physiological and psychological perspectives. *J Neuropsychiatry Clin Neurosci.* 1990;2:92–98.

Index